Parenting in Global Perspective

Drawing on both sociological and anthropological perspectives, this volume explores cross-national trends and everyday experiences of parenting.

Parenting in Global Perspective examines the significance of parenting as a subject of professional expertise, and an activity in which adults are increasingly expected to be emotionally absorbed and to become personally fulfilled. By focusing on the significance of parenting as a form of relationship and as mediated by family relationships across time and space, the book explores the points of accommodation and points of tension between parenting as defined by professionals, and parenting as experienced by parents themselves. Specific themes include:

- the ways in which the moral context for parenting is negotiated and sustained
- the structural constraints of 'good' parenting (particularly in cases of immigration or reproductive technologies)
- the relationship between intimate family life and broader cultural trends, parenting culture, policy making and nationhood
- parenting and/as adult 'identity-work'.

Including contributions on parenting from a range of ethnographic locales – from Europe, Canada and the US, to non-Euro-American settings such as Turkey, Chile and Brazil – this volume presents a uniquely critical and international perspective, which positions parenting as a global ideology that intersects in a variety of ways with the political, social, cultural and economic positions of parents and families.

Charlotte Faircloth is a Leverhulme Trust Early Career Fellow, based in the Centre for Parenting Culture Studies at the University of Kent, UK.

Diane M. Hoffman is an Associate Professor of Anthropology of Education and International Comparative Education at the Curry School of Education, University of Virginia, USA.

Linda L. Layne is Hale Professor of Humanities and Social Sciences at Rensselaer Polytechnic Institute, USA.

Relationships and Resources
Series Editors: Janet Holland and Rosalind Edwards

A key contemporary political and intellectual issue is the link between the relationships that people have and the resources to which they have access. When people share a sense of identity, hold similar values, trust each other and reciprocally do things for each other, this has an impact on the social, political and economic cohesion of the society in which they live. So, are changes in contemporary society leading to deterioration in the link between relationships and resources, or new and innovative forms of linking, or merely the reproduction of enduring inequalities? Consideration of relationships and resources raises key theoretical and empirical issues around change and continuity over time as well as time use, the consequences of globalisation and individualisation for intimate and broader social relations, and location and space in terms of communities and neighbourhoods. The books in this series are concerned with elaborating these issues and will form a body of work that will contribute to academic and political debate.

Available titles include:

Marginalised Mothers
Exploring working-class experiences of parenting
Val Gillies

Sibling Identity and Relationships
Sisters and brothers
Rosalind Edwards, Lucy Hadfield, Helen Lucey and Melanie Mauthner

Teenagers' Citizenship
Experiences and education
Susie Weller

Researching Families and Communities
Social and generational change
Edited by Rosalind Edwards

Interdependency and Care over the Lifecourse
Sophia Bowlby, Linda McKie, Susan Gregory and Isobel MacPherson

Transnational Families
Ethnicities, identities and social capital
Harry Goulbourne, Tracey Reynolds, John Solomos and Elisabetta Zontini

International Perspectives on Racial and Ethnic Mixedness and Mixing
Edited by Rosalind Edwards, Suki Ali, Chamion Caballero and Miri Song

Critical Approaches to Care
Understanding caring relations, identities and cultures
Edited by Chrissie Rogers and Susie Weller

Parenting in Global Perspective
Negotiating ideologies of kinship, self and politics
Edited by Charlotte Faircloth, Diane M. Hoffman and Linda L. Layne

Forthcoming titles include:

Moving On
The changing lives of young people after parental divorce
Bren Neale and Jennifer Flowerdew

Parenting in Global Perspective

Negotiating ideologies of kinship, self and politics

Edited by Charlotte Faircloth, Diane M. Hoffman and Linda L. Layne

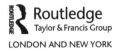

Routledge
Taylor & Francis Group

LONDON AND NEW YORK

First published 2013
by Routledge
2 Park Square, Milton Park, Abingdon, Oxon OX14 4RN

Simultaneously published in the USA and Canada
by Routledge
711 Third Avenue, New York, NY 10017

Routledge is an imprint of the Taylor & Francis Group, an informa business

British Library Cataloguing in Publication Data
A catalogue record for this book is available from the British Library

Library of Congress Cataloging in Publication Data
Parenting in global perspective : negotiating ideologies of kinship, self and politics / edited by Charlotte Faircloth, Diane Hoffman and Linda Layne.
　p. cm. – (Relationships & resources)
　1. Parenting–Cross-cultural studies. I. Faircloth, Charlotte. II. Hoffman, Diane M., 1954– III. Layne, Linda L.
　HQ755.8.P384 2013
　649'.1–dc23　　　　　　　　　　　　　　　　　　　　　2012040235

ISBN: 978-0-415-62487-9 (hbk)
ISBN: 978-0-203-10390-6 (ebk)

Typeset in Times
by Wearset Ltd, Boldon, Tyne and Wear

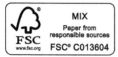

MIX
Paper from
responsible sources
FSC® C013604
www.fsc.org

Printed and bound by CPI Group (UK) Ltd, Croydon, CR0 4YY

Contents

Illustrations

Figures

Box

Contributors

Editors

Charlotte Faircloth is a Leverhulme Trust Early Career Fellow, based in the Centre for Parenting Culture Studies at the University of Kent, where her research explores parenting, gender, intimacy and equality. Based on her PhD in Social Anthropology at the University of Cambridge, her book *Militant Lactivism?* was recently published by Berghahn Books.

Diane M. Hoffman is an Associate Professor of Anthropology of Education and International Comparative Education at the Curry School of Education, University of Virginia. She received her PhD from Stanford University and her MA and BA from Brown University. Her work is situated at the intersection of anthropological understandings of childhood, parenting and education.

Linda L. Layne is Hale Professor of Humanities and Social Sciences at Rensselaer Polytechnic Institute, currently on loan to the National Science Foundation as programme officer for Science and Technology Studies. Her current research explores the management of absent presences in several alternative family forms: single mothers by choice, two-mum and two-dad families, as well as families who claim miscarried or stillborn babies as family members.

Contributors

Frank Furedi is emeritus professor of sociology at the University of Kent in Canterbury. His publications explore the problem that Western societies have in engaging with risk and uncertainty. Since the publication of *Paranoid Parenting* he has published on parenting, education and cultural life.

Rosalind Edwards is professor of sociology, University of Southampton. Her work focuses on family life, and research methods. Recent book publications include *International Perspectives on Racial and Ethnic Mixedness and Mixing* (2012) and *Key Concepts in Family Studies* (2011). She co-edits the *International Journal of Social Research Methodology*.

Val Gillies is a professor of social research and a co-director of the Families and Social Capital Research Group in the Weeks Centre for Social and Policy Research at London South Bank University. She has researched and published widely in the area of family, social class and at risk youth.

Katharine Dow is an independent researcher. She received her PhD in social anthropology from the London School of Economics in 2010, based on research into how people make ethical judgments about surrogacy and followed this with an ESRC postdoctoral fellowship at the University of Edinburgh. She chairs an interdisciplinary reading group on reproduction and is currently co-editing a collection on contemporary relationships between nature and ethics.

Tracey Jensen is a lecturer at Newcastle University, where she teaches media and cultural studies. Her research examines parenting policy, culture and advice, social citizenship and inequalities and the affective intersections of gender and class in contemporary identity and culture. Her work has been published in a number of books and international journals including *Subjectivities, Feminism and Psychology*, *Feminist Media Studies* and *Studies in the Maternal*. She is currently writing a book on parental pedagogies.

Denise Hinton is a postdoctoral research assistant working in the Maternal and Newborn Health Unit at the Liverpool School of Tropical Medicine. Her research focuses on family health and wellbeing, and young people's (im)mobilities and transitions to adulthood.

Louise Laverty is a PhD student in the Department of Sociology, Social Policy and Criminology at the University of Liverpool. The focus of her study is exploring young people's agency in negotiating dominant public health discourses.

Jude Robinson is a reader in the anthropology of health and illness, Department of Sociology, Social Policy and Criminology at the University of Liverpool, researching the health and well-being of women and their families living in poverty in the UK.

Nicole S. Berry is a medical anthropologist, who holds a position as assistant professor in the Faculty of Health Sciences at Simon Fraser University, British Columbia. Her research focuses on the study of social change through an examination of reproduction in a globalising world.

Anna Jaysane-Darr is a PhD candidate at Brandeis University. Her dissertation research with the South Sudanese former refugee community in the United States concerns reproduction, ethnicity, citizenship, personhood and subjectivity in a diaspora.

Katrien De Graeve recently completed a PhD in comparative sciences of culture at Ghent University, Belgium. Her research interests are situated at the intersection of critical kinship and family studies and the anthropology of migration and postcoloniality.

Chia Longman is lecturer in gender and diversity studies at Ghent University. Her research interests include identity politics among religious and ethnic minority women in the European context, multiculturalism, feminism, kinship and mothering. She is executive editor of the journal *Gender and Religion* and has published widely in English, Dutch, and French.

Marjorie Murray is a lecturer in anthropology, anthropology programme, Pontificia Universidad Católica de Chile. Her PhD thesis (UCL) focused on material culture and cosmology in everyday life in Madrid. Her current research project studies early mothering in different contexts Chile.

Livia Jiménez Sedano gained her PhD in 2011 and has taught social and cultural anthropology at UNED (Madrid) since 2009. She has taken part in projects about ethnicity, children, immigration and social exclusion. She is currently working on the research project on Islamophoby and gender relations in the Muslim Diaspora in Spain coordinated by Professor Ángeles Ramírez.

Maureen O'Dougherty is research associate at the University of Minnesota and adjunct anthropology faculty at Metropolitan State University. She authored *Consumption Intensified: The Politics of Middle-Class Daily Life in Brazil* (2002). Her current work concerns reproduction and parenthood in Brazil and the US.

A. Merve Göknar recently completed a PhD in social anthropology at University of Cambridge. Her research focused on new reproductive technologies and infertility. As an independent researcher she is currently exploring birth ideologies and the birth experiences of women.

Ellie Lee is reader is social policy and director of the Centre for Parenting Culture Studies at the University of Kent. She is the editor of the collections *Abortion Law and Politics Today* (Macmillan) and *Real Bodies* (Palgrave), and author of *Abortion, Motherhood and Mental Health: medicalizing reproduction in the United States and Great Britain* (Aldine Transaction). She is a co-author of the forthcoming *Parenting Culture Studies* (Palgrave).

Foreword

Frank Furedi

No one who reads this collection of essays can continue to think of parenting as a self-evident and taken for granted practice. Parenting is a cultural accomplishment – an activity that is mediated through the prevailing grammar of morality, and subject to the influence of competing groups of claim-makers. Historically the transformation of mothers and fathers into parents coexists with the rise of the tendency to reinterpret child-rearing as a skill rather than as an integral feature of an informal family relationship. Consequently the relationship of mothers and fathers with their children has become detached from the possession of parenting skills. Such skills are increasingly represented as the attributes of expertise and of science. Parents of course may acquire these skills but not through their experience as mothers and fathers. These are skills that have been constructed outside the immediate child-rearing relationships. So a good parent is someone who has willingly embraced the science and the professional advice as well as accepted the social policies through which these views are promoted.

Of course mothers and fathers are not simply passive objects of forces beyond their control. As this important collection of cross-cultural essays imply, parents are continually in the business of constructing and negotiating their identity. As I have argued in my study, *Paranoid Parenting*, the transformation of child-rearing into a constant focus of expert and political intervention tends to inflate the significance that society attaches to parenting. With so much apparently at stake, it is not surprising that mothers and fathers have tended to attach greater and greater significance to their identity as parents. What the chapters in this book indicate is that there are a variety of culturally specific strategies available for the construction of parental identity. However one important point that emerges from these studies is that the intensification of parenting is gradually becoming a truly global trend.

At the workshop where these papers were discussed it was evident that a scholarly exchange of views between anthropologists and sociologists would have to surmount the disciplinary challenges of differing methodologies, concepts and languages. Yet for me it was the very attempt at a cross-disciplinary conversation that proved most stimulating. The discussion generated by the workshop indicated that parenting culture studies provides an important intellectual terrain where discussions on child-rearing, mothering and fathering could develop a productive interaction with social and cultural theory.

It is worth recalling that from its inception in the eighteenth century, modern expertise has been interested in the relationship mothers and fathers have with their children. One of the first studies on expert authority in the English language regarded the way that children gain their opinions from their elders as potentially an important site for intervention. Nevertheless, Sir George Cornwall Lewis, the author of *An Essay on the Influence of Authority in Matters of Opinion* (1849), was hesitant about challenging what he perceived as 'the traditions of civiliza-tion' which, 'perpetuate by the implicit faith of children in their parents'.[1] Yet what was for Lewis an inviolable tradition of civilisation has become problema-tised through the process of rationalisation and modernisation of society.

During the century following Lewis's book the problem of raising children was increasingly implicated as the proximate cause of an ever-growing variety of social and political problems. By the 1930s the role of fathers and mothers was increasingly scrutinised by experts and their capacity to bring up their chil-dren was invariably found wanting. This was the era where it was precisely the 'implicit faith' that children had towards their parents that was identified as the problem. It was alleged that the family had become a site for the breeding of an authoritarian personality, which was allegedly susceptible to the influence of totalitarian movements.

In the aftermath of the Second World War intervention in family life was fre-quently presented as essential for protecting the democratic way of life from the authoritarian influence of parents. This narrative of prevention was systemati-cally advocated in a collection of essays, *Studies in Leadership: Leadership and Democratic Action*. Published in 1950 and edited by the soon-to-be famous American sociologist Alvin Gouldner, the collection contained articles by some of the most influential social commentators on the time – including Theodor Adorno, Daniel Bell, Kurt Lewin, William Whyte, Seymour Lipset and Reinhard Bendix.

In retrospect the most interesting contribution on the subject of re-educating mothers and fathers was made by the sociologist Jeremiah Wolpert. He noted that 'since personality is nourished incipiently in the family situation, and the attitudes toward authority gain their contours from this processing, a family atmosphere and structure which would generate such attitudes would seem to be an important point of attack'. He was particularly interested in influencing the middle class family because the 'middle-class is much more receptive to changes in child rearing than lower-income groups and can be persuaded to make changes in this area'. He believed that the 'lower-income groups would be much more difficult in this respect because they do not have the leeway to pay atten-tion to such problems'.[2]

In this remarkable call to subject family life to the enlightened influence of psychologists and other experts, Wolpert recognised that the middle-class mother and father would be a far easier target than their working-class counterpart. His diagnosis of a middle class that was 'receptive' to professional input and advice on child-rearing matters proved to be prescient. For a variety of reasons – some which are discussed in the chapters that follow – middle-class mothers and fathers are far more likely to become absorbed by parental identity work than their working-class counterparts. During the decade following the publication of Wolpert's essay, middle-class mothers and fathers were effortlessly recast and redefined as parents. The culture of parenting that emerged in the 1950s has crystallised into a powerful medium through which people give meaning to their experience. It is the uneasy relationship between this grammar of morality and the social construction of parental identity that constitutes the exciting theme captured in this collection of articles.

Notes

1 See Lewis, G.C. (1974) (Originally published 1849) *An Essay on the Influence of Authority in Matters of Opinion*, Arno Press: New York, p. 10.
2 See Wolpert, J. 'Towards a sociology of authority', in Gouldner, A. (ed.) (1950) *Studies in Leadership: Leadership and Democratic Action*, Harper & Brothers: New York, pp. 700–701.

Acknowledgements

This volume represents one stage in the gradual formalisation of the study of 'parenting culture'. Anthropologists by training, Faircloth, Hoffman and Layne had been working on parenting culture with research on infant feeding, education and pregnancy loss. We noted a paucity of anthropological perspectives on 'parenting' when we met at a 2008 American Anthropological Association panel 'Imagined Futures and Limited Presents: Engaging Parenting and Inequality in Contemporary North America'. This seemed surprising to us, since anthropologists have long had an interest in issues around kinship, reproduction and child-rearing.

At that meeting, Hoffman noted that the emergence of 'parenting' as a distinctive approach to child-rearing is one in which the negotiation of authority, power and social control is mediated by networks of professional expertise and shared knowledge/practice. 'Parenting' as 'public culture' is particularly apt for anthropological investigation: it is constituted by individuals (experts, parents); networks (mother-communities, parenting groups); institutions (academies, organisations); media (internet, film, TV, books, magazines) and other forms of knowledge production (research, journalism, popular and academic information and analysis). Parenting is both lived experience and an object of academic enquiry: to some extent, we have all experienced it. This curious public/private relationship means that an anthropological perspective has a particularly significant role to play, not least because we can contribute concrete ethnography to 'flesh out' more theoretical perspectives.

Since the 2008 panel, there has been a growing interest in this field, and we have been working to galvanise productive conversations. To this end the editors organised the 2010 American Anthropology Association panel 'What's New about Parenting? Kinship, Politics and Identity'. These early discussions revealed that whilst 'parenting' is a thoroughly cultured product, it nonetheless is often treated (in policy circles particularly) as transparent or value-less. Given the success of the panel, we put out an international call that was widely distributed through anthropological and sociological list-servs to gauge interest in a volume that would serve as a foundational resource, both for anthropologists and others with an interest in this topic. We selected abstracts, and were lucky enough to be awarded a Wenner–Gren Workshop Award to bring the contributors together at the University of Kent during 2012. Without the Wenner–Gren's grant, face-to-face discussion and debate amongst this group of scholars would have been impossible, and we thank them for supporting this project.

Our contributors include PhD students, independent scholars, postdoctoral fellows, lecturers and professors from a range of international and disciplinary locations. The time together allowed us to further conceptualise the study of parenting culture. How does an 'anthropology of parenting' differ from, for example, the 'sociology of parenting'? In entering into this discussion we felt lucky to be not only talking 'to ourselves' but be in real dialogue with others. Whilst one of the points that emerged in our discussions was the different ways in which we all framed parenting – some preferring lenses such as race, class, ethnicity and gender, others more seeming more comfortable with kinship, relatedness, power, identity and so on – we all agreed that one of our aims should be to foreground the experience of parents as agents, recognising the important but neglected transformations that affect them as situated within networks of kinship, material culture, ideology and beyond.

Introduction

Charlotte Faircloth, Diane M. Hoffman and
Linda L. Layne

This volume explores negotiations around 'parenting' in a variety of geographical and historical locales. By drawing on a range of disciplinary perspectives, including the sociology of the family, new kinship studies, social policy studies and medical anthropology, the contributors here think about how the new 'parenting' culture we have observed in contemporary contexts intersects with ideologies of kinship, self and politics.

Our introduction has three aims: to give a theoretical and historical context to the volume, to highlight the ways the chapters extend the existing literature on 'parenting', and to outline some of the themes that connect the contributions. We have grouped the chapters under the following headings, which we explore further below: The moral context for parenting; The structural constraints to 'good' parenting; Negotiating parenting culture; and Parenting and/as identity.

'Parenting' as a concept

The term 'parenting' is a relatively recent one; it became prominent in the 1950s in language used by psychologists, sociologists and self-help practitioners in North America, before spreading into wider usage, both in the US and elsewhere. From an anthropological perspective, which emphasises cultural variability, 'parenting' might be seen as a particular historically and socially situated form of childrearing, a product of late twentieth century ideological shifts around family, kinship, risk and social morality.

'Parenting' as we understand it problematises the traditional assumptions surrounding childrearing by forcing a re-examination of the goals, resources and relationships that constitute an emerging global set of parameters for framing personhood in contemporary times. We therefore use 'parenting' not just to refer to childrearing, or the care activities associated with traditional kinship roles, but as an activity that is increasingly taken to require a specific skill-set: a certain level of expertise about children and their care, often based on the latest research on child-development, or an affiliation to a certain 'expert-led' way of raising a child.

This inevitably ties our discussion into wider political trends, where parenting is increasingly understood as both the source of, and solution to, a whole host of social problems (a theme we develop further below). Equally importantly, however, 'parenting' also demands a discussion of reflexivity and individual 'identity work': to parent is to be discursively positioned by and actively contributing to the networks of idea, value, practice and social relations that have come to define a particular form of the politics of parent–child relations within the domain of the contemporary family. In this sense, then, how people 'parent' has implications for our conceptions of self, kinship and politics – implications that we attempt to address in this volume.

Theoretical background

Sharon Hays' *The Cultural Contradictions of Motherhood* (based on research with working mothers in the USA, 1996) and Frank Furedi's *Paranoid Parenting* (looking at US and UK parenting culture, 2002) form two of the key texts in the nascent field of 'parenting culture studies' (see also: Douglas and Michaels 2004; Lee 2007; Warner 2006).

In both Hays' and Furedi's work is the recognition that the role and meaning of parenthood has changed in recent years, so that childrearing has expanded to encompass a growing range of activities that were not previously seen as an obligatory dimension of this task. While the meaning of the word 'parenting' is often taken for granted, it is therefore more accurate to suggest that this social activity can be considered culturally and historically specific. 'Parenting' as we mean it is not just what parents do. Compared to the past, it is a time-and-emotion-expensive enterprise, that parents should find personally fulfilling, yet also one that has increasingly (and ironically) been deemed far too important and difficult to be left up to parents (Furedi 2002). In the context of debates around 'work/life balance', parents can therefore feel as if there is 'never enough time' to parent properly, even though – in the US, at least – they are spending more time than ever with their children (Gauthier *et al.* 2004).

The diagnosis these two scholars offer for the expansion of parenting is part historical and part conceptual. In *The Cultural Contradictions of Motherhood*, Hays discusses the historical construction of childhood, motherhood and fatherhood as well as their more recent permutations. She argues that 'intensive motherhood' is an emergent ideology that urges mothers to 'spend a tremendous amount of time, energy and money in raising their children' (1996: x). She suggests that this injunction remains culturally salient, despite an uneasy relationship with the logic of the work place, both because it props up the capitalist infrastructure and because mothering is perceived as 'the last best defence against what many people see as the impoverishment of social ties, communal obligations and unremunerated commitments' (1996: xiii).

She suggests that this is a dominant mode of parenting in the contemporary US and, like Furedi, she shows how this trend exercises a decisive impact on the mothering role in particular (for she recognises that 'parenting' is inherently gendered). In setting out the central features of 'intensive mothering' as the cultural norm for contemporary childrearing Hays notes that:

- 'Good motherhood' involves devoting large amounts of time, energy and material resources on the child
- 'Good motherhood' requires that the child's needs are put first: mothering must be child-centred
- 'Good mothers' pay attention to what experts say about child development. It is not enough to 'make do' and do what seems easiest.

Furedi's work in particular draws important links between these changes and the wider development of risk-consciousness. For example, he notes that the way children are constructed in this new 'parenting' culture is as being 'vulnerable' and more sensitive to risks impacting on physical and emotional development (especially in the early years of life) than was previously considered to be the case. In turn, the parent is understood as 'God like', with what parents do represented as determining each individual child's development and future. This particular construction of the parent–child dyad is summarised by Furedi with the terms 'infant determinism' and 'parent causality', themes which echo throughout the volume as a whole.

When we talk about 'parenting' we suppose that, by definition, it has 'intensive' elements (as outlined by Hays). However, we also see a continuum of intensiveness in newer versions of parenting (such as holistic parenting, attachment parenting or otherwise) that amplify (or play down) certain elements of the intensive mothering relation Hays describes. Similarly, although intensive parenting most often refers to the behaviour of mothers, both Hays and Furedi acknowledge the profound impact that parenting culture has on the constitution of both mothering *and* fathering identities as well on the relationship amongst parents (see also Dermott 2008).

The contribution of the volume: a global perspective

The trend towards 'intensive' parenting has been noted by a range of social scientists working in middle class milieu across the UK, US, Australia and Canada. (Hays 1996; Faircloth 2010; Schmeid *et al.* 2001; Wall 2001). Yet the ways in which parents' and families' experiences have been affected by this shift is not a topic that has been explored significantly in the social sciences, either within, or beyond these contexts (though see Barlow and Chapin 2010). This volume addresses this gap, by including portraits of parenting in a range of ethnographic, socio-economic and historical locales from Europe, Canada and the US, as well non-Euro-American settings (including Turkey, Chile and Brazil). In each of these settings we foreground the negotiations around the shifts towards a new 'parenting' culture – whether that is resistance, rejection, accommodation, modification or a complex combination of several forms of agency.

In short, we believe that 'parenting' deserves a discrete analytical focus in its own right, within a global perspective. While the discourses and practices of parenting may be seen as culturally and historically specific, this volume illustrates how they are currently acquiring a global significance as they diffuse and interact with local and indigenous conceptualisations of raising children. A global perspective is essential, both because parenting is at present a globalising set of ideas and practices that cannot be separated from considerations of global power inequities (as a number of contributors to this volume illustrate), and because the interactions of globally circulating discourses, and constructions of parenting with localised constructs, reveal assumptions and tensions within parenting that enhance our practical and theoretical understanding of the phenomenon. The global perspective also allows us to challenge ideas about the moral valence of particular notions of parenting, as well as revealing the many ways in which kinship, identity and cultural ideals concerning motherhood/fatherhood are challenging and resisting certain formations of intensive parenting. In a period characterised by the spread of neoliberal economic regimes around the world, parenting ideologies have a particular salience and significance, as a number of anthropologists have pointed out (e.g. Stephens 1995).

There is some evidence to suggest that parenting as a set of ideals and practices that is 'child-centred,' resource-intensive, and focused on the maximisation of individual achievement potential, are in fact associated with rising capitalist economies around the world such as China (see Hoffman and Zhao 2008) and Brazil (de Carvalho 2000). Parenting is clearly being targeted globally as an arena in which states can create new generations of workers/citizens who embody ideals integral to the success of the new capitalism: individualistic, risk-taking, entrepreneurial selves. And, as a corollary, this forces us to ask, does 'parenting', in this sense, code or represent for the parents that adopt it a set of aspirations for social mobility and – perhaps – hopes for better lives?

At the same time, it is clear that while there may be globally circulating discourses of parenting, there remain important points of resistance and confrontation, as a number of papers in this volume illustrate. The world-views of North Americans about individual needs and potentials, so powerfully enacted in schools and in parent-education seminars, for example, mesh uncomfortably with the values of nationhood and personhood that intersect among immigrant communities and in transnational contexts (De Graeve and Longman, Jiménez Sedano, Jaysane-Darr, Berry, this volume). The volume also illustrates how tensions associated with the ways parenting demand the reformulation of kinship ties, gendered identities (O'Dougherty, Layne, Göknar, Faircloth) and generational-based ideas of obligation and responsibility.

(Problem) parenting and policy

Our exploration of 'parenting' here recognises that 'the family' has, throughout modernity, been viewed with ambivalence and routinely problematised as a reliable context for childrearing (as much as it has been idealised and sanctified). While it could be argued that it is not new for there to be pronounced social anxieties about the relationships between older family members and children, the 'problem of parenting' is not simply another version of an old 'moral panic' about the private sphere, and its ability to socialise the next generation. Rather, the ascent of concern about 'parenting' indicates a preoccupation with particular sorts of relationships and bonds between individuals – parents and children. We can thus, at the same time, have a society and culture that is (relatively) more relaxed than it once was about variations in types of families, but marked by anxiety about the parenting styles and practices of individual parents – perhaps, particularly, immigrant parents (as a number of our contributors here foreground).

This expansion of the childrearing role has precipitated (and is precipitated by) the belief that 'parenting' is a problematic sphere of social life. Indeed, 'parenting' is almost always discussed as a social problem (in the UK, the prime minister talked about the summer riots of 2011 as a problem of 'broken Britain', and has recently introduced 'parenting classes' as a means of tackling this problem (*Guardian* 2012). Indeed many stakeholders (from politicians to NGOs and beyond) have sought to turn childrearing into an object of policy making, most notably in the US and the UK, but also in other OECD (Organisation for Economic Co-operation and Development[1]) countries, and beyond. This is, arguably, the new politics of 'parenting' – as an explanation for and solution to social problems. Where poverty, for example, once featured as a major policy concern in its own right, this problem is now often discussed in contrast as a 'risk factor' for the real problem, 'poor parenting'. More recently constructed social problems in the UK and the US, such as the 'obesity crisis', 'anti-social behaviour' and 'educational failure' (for boys especially) are rarely discussed by policy makers without 'parenting' featuring as a key explanatory factor. As Furedi argues (2002) the belief underpinning this development in politics is the notion that social problems are 'handed down' in cycles through generations. What was once a defining right-wing political idea has become 'common sense' across the political class and taken the form of 'evidence-based' parenting policy.

Parenting skills

The growing validation of the notion that parents need to be trained to 'parent' – and an increasing propensity to represent good parenting as a skill-set that can be both taught and learned through reference to expert, scientific evidence about 'how to' 'parent' – forms a central feature of the new parenting culture. Many of the chapters address the place of experts and advice in parenting culture, and the relationship between parenting and ideas about 'expertise'. As noted, there is clearly a contradiction here, as Furedi points out: the parent is simultaneously 'God like' (in that what the parent does is construed as determinant for the child), yet also unable to meet the demands of 'parenting' without expert guidance:

> It does not take long for parents to realise that everyone today seems to hold strong opinions about the problems of raising a child. While the politicians regularly hold forth about what they believe make a 'good' or 'responsible' parent, there is an industry of experts who bombard us with 'helpful'

insights drawn from the science of child-rearing. ... Paradoxically it seems as if the only people who feel unconfident in their opinions about what is good for children are parents themselves. The role of bumbling amateurs has been assigned them by the self-appointed experts.

(Furedi 2002: 2)

With ever more studies stressing the importance of the early (even pre-conception) environment for infant development (see Gerhardt 2004); providing children with the 'right' kind of environment turns normal activities of parenting into a series of tasks to be achieved. Touching, talking, feeding – even 'loving' – are no longer ends in themselves, but tools which parents are required to perfect to ensure proper development. Playing with a child is no longer simply an enjoyable activity for adult and child; it is also a way of ensuring positive 'long-term outcomes'. To take Rose's argument, the everyday experience of parenting becomes re-written as set of skills to be honed and perfected if one is to achieve optimum outcomes (Rose 1999). He has even argued that 'love' can be used to promote a certain type of self-understanding in children, and is duly emphasised for parents: increasing confidence, helpfulness, dependability at the same time as averting fear, cruelty or any other deviation from the desired norm (see Rose 1999: 160). The conversion of 'love' from a spontaneous sentiment manifested in warm affection into a parental function or skill is one of the key reasons parents are now routinely told to 'Enjoy their baby' (Furedi 2002: 79), with almost magical powers ascribed to 'unconditional love'.

Kinship and parenting

Ideologies of parenting are intimately tied to more traditional kinship studies in anthropology. Indeed, within anthropology, accounts of interactions between parents and children generally come under the rubric of 'kinship'. In the past, 'kinship' as politico-jural institution, was one of the mainstays of social anthropology (in the likes of Evans-Pritchard, Fortes and Radcliffe-Brown). Today, kinship is characterised by problematising that anthropological heritage (Schneider 1968) preferring to prioritise the meaning (as opposed to the structural-function) of 'relatedness' (Carsten 2000). Accounts of new reproductive technologies, mapping the slippage between 'natural' and 'cultural' groundings for this relatedness have been a major site for analysis (Strathern 1992; Rapp 2000; Ragoné 1994; Franklin and McKinnon 2001).

To the extent that these papers are concerned with 'socialisation', and ideas of nature (the child as raw ingredient) and culture (the adult as refined product), they can be said to pay homage to this tradition. But they are not a study of kinship in the sense that they look at how people consider themselves related by 'nature' or 'culture'. Rather, what we are doing here comes out of the anthropological tradition of Mead and Wolfenstein (1955) and others, as well as a wealth of sociologists and historians who question the cultural and historical contingency of parenting practices – that is, those tasks undertaken by an adult caretaker to ensure that the child is reproduced into the next generation (Ariès 1962; Badinter 1981; Hardyment 1995). As Mead states, at some fundamental level, the tasks of bearing and begetting are the same the world over (in the sense that after birth an infant requires warmth and nourishment, and protection from predators, as much as induction into about social mores). But the ways in which these tasks are carried out vary widely, despite being considered necessary and commonsensical in a given setting.

We draw on Strathern here in *Kinship, Law and the Unexpected* (2005: 4–5.) She starts with a vignette, taken from the work of Daniel Miller. He describes how in bringing up their children, middle-class mothers in North London use their knowledge of the world to shape their children's habits. They cannot do anything about the genes; they can do everything about health, hygiene and other common afflictions. Debate revolves around what food they should eat and what toys they should play with. Indeed Miller reports that mothers may regard the child's growing up as a series of defeats. The first enemy was sugar, then sweets and biscuits, then brands such as Coca Cola, and bigger temptations such as 'Barbie dolls and the ubiquitous gun': 'an unceasing struggle between what is regarded as the world of nature and the artificial world of commodity materialism' he says (1997: 75). The battles over diet and gender are regarded as efforts to resist commercialism and con-sumerism. Why the struggle in the first place, asks Strathern? She says,

> The young mother is placed in a position of responsibility by her knowledge of the effects of these substances and toys on the growing body, and on the growing mind and sets of behaviours. In other words, the child's condition depends on how the mother acts on her knowledge of the world.
>
> (2005: 4)

What the child seems to reflect and embody is the conscientiousness with which the mother has acted on her knowledge and stuck to her principles. She must carry on until the child itself is properly informed about the world. 'In the interim, both its body and its behaviour reflect the application of her own know-ledge' (ibid.). And why is this so critical for a parent? Strathern notes that a parent shares body with the child twice over.

> First is the body of genetic inheritance, a given, a matter regarded colloqui-ally as of common blood or common substance. Second is the body that is a sign of the parent's devotion – or neglect – and it is in this middle class milieu above all through the application of knowledge that the parent's efforts make this body. Miller jokes that the child grows the mother.
>
> (2005: 5)

Choice and reflexivity

Given Strathern's observations, the fact that there is a moral context for 'parent-ing' hardly needs reiterating. Where 'parenting' now encompasses a growing range of activities that were not previously seen as an obligatory dimension of this social role (Hays 1996; Douglas and Michaels 2004) they are also the subject of public, and often political, debate (Freely 2000). What parents feed their children, when they put them to bed, what they read to them, how they discipline them, how they play with them at home and how they let them play outdoors have all become contested and politicised questions. Private routines of everyday life for children and families – mealtimes, sleeping, playing, reading nursery rhymes and stories – have long been the subject of debate, but it is clear that these have become particularly intense in recent years, in their focus on the impact on future generations (Hardyment 2007; Gillies 2008; Bristow 2009).

The study of parenting therefore sits at a juncture between critiques of value, practice and ideals and critiques of power. Several papers here draw attention to the power-structures which define what constitutes 'good' parenting in the first place, and enable or inhibit its realisation, highlighting an incongruity with a typical neoliberal discourse in UK and US cultures around notions of choice, democracy and freedom. What these papers illustrate is the underlying moral tensions that surround ideas about what is 'good' for children, parents and society as a whole.

Indeed, many point to the critical nature of 'choice' in contemporary 'parenting' culture. Today, in both the US and the UK, baby and childcare can be roughly divided into styles that are 'controlling', and those that are more 'liberal'. The former, which sees children and their care as something to be structured, is characterised by scheduled feeds, formula feeding, imposed discipline and separate sleeping. Liberal models, by contrast, aim to dissolve notions of rational-efficiency in favour of more relaxed styles of care, often characterised by long-term, on-cue breastfeeding, a family bed and 'positive' discipline (Buskens 2001: 75).

Of course, the distinction between the models may be more heuristic than descriptive, as many parents will attest, since one can adopt characteristic elements of one style (breastfeeding) and deploy them as part of the other (on schedule, as part of separate sleeping, for example). Similarly, there may be a gap between intention and outcome (formula feeding not always being a deliberate, reflexive choice, but a necessary intervention if breastfeeding is not possible). But because the plurality exists, at a heuristic level at least, mothers are accountable for the choice they make both within and between these 'competing normalities'. In Foucault's language, in contemporary liberalism the responsible moral actor is not one who conforms blindly to expert or even popular recommendations; 'Rather, she is expected to subject such recommendations to evaluation and questioning, operating as an informed consumer' (Murphy 2003: 457). Those who are not reflexive, informed consumers are deemed irresponsible or in need of education.

Identity work

Parenting, as these chapters show, is therefore closely tied up with our ideas about ourselves. Our theoretical interest in this volume – an engagement with mothering and fathering as 'identity work' – is partly a product of historical circumstance: only recently has mothering or fathering been an 'identity' which women can 'work at' (Arendell 2000; Avishai 2007, 2010; Lee and Bristow 2009).

The concept of 'identity' has a long trajectory in the social sciences (see for example Giddens 1991; Jenkins 1996; Mead 1934; Strathern 1992; Stryker 1968), a term typically used to denote an individual's comprehension of selfhood. In particular, there has been a focus in these accounts on the ways in which individuals (and indeed groups) constitute their identity in negotiation with wider society. For Stryker (1968), for example, the purpose of 'identity negotiation' (between the individual and society) is to develop a consistent set of behaviours that reinforce the identity of the person within the wider social context.

Many of the discussions around 'identity' have been aimed at destabilising the notion that it is a natural, fixed or objective criteria; asserting instead that 'identity' itself is a political project in which individuals and groups engage in accordance with social and historical contingencies (Giddens 1991). In their critique of 'identity' as a concept, Brubaker and Cooper (2000) note that there remains a tendency in scholarly writing to confuse identity as a category of practice, and as a category of analysis, leaving it as something of an ill-defined term, floating between the poles of reification and ambiguity.

It is for this reason that the focus here is on 'identity work' and notions of 'selfhood' rather than on 'identity' per se. This is intended to highlight the active processes by which identity is constructed, and the inherently social nature of this enterprise (as opposed to being simply a means of self-expression). Thus whilst 'identity' itself may be an abstract entity, its manifestations and the ways it is exercised are often open to view: in language, dress, behaviour, use of space and so forth. During social encounters individuals assert elements of their identity through these mechanisms, and it is in this sense that 'identity work' is used to refer to the range of *activities* in which individuals engage to create, present and sustain personal identities, with particular reference to the constitution of relatedness (Goffman 1959).

The chapters

The volume considers how recent historical transformations illuminate classic anthropological and sociological questions about the construction of personhood and selves, kinship and political economy. In particular, we ask what kinds of 'mothers', 'fathers', and 'children' are being produced in this new culture of 'parenting'? How are parents produced through discourses of what they are not, of what they (seem to) fail to do? What moral obligations are entailed in these categories and what are their consequences for the daily enactment of kinship? How might reproductive technologies intersect with these debates about parenting and identity? What kinds of cultural assumptions and authoritative claims are made by 'parenting experts' and how do parents negotiate and experience these expectations in their daily lives? What kinds of political economic relations are being reproduced through 'parenting' and how do these affect the construction of gender, race and social class? How does the relationship of 'parenting experts', government policy targeting 'parenting' and the daily concerns of families as they engage in 'parenting' ultimately shape the 'nation' (cf. Carsten 2000; Wade 2007)?

We have divided the chapters into the following themes:

I The moral context for parenting

Edwards and Gillies provide an historical context against which to view the emergence of a new parenting culture, with a focus on the UK. They critique contemporary political rhetoric about a past 'golden age' of responsible and committed parenting norms and practices, and concommitant ideas that neglectful mothering and fathering is to blame for contemporary social ills. In particular, they consider prevalent ideas about constant parental (usually maternal) presence and attention; knowing where your children are. They explore accounts of everyday parenting in the 1960s to show the way that even young children were often left to their own devices without judgement about immoral parents and neglectful parenting. Their analysis highlights a distinct change in understandings of children's needs and expectations of intensive parental engagement. Ideas about the investment of constant child-centred physical and emotional attention as 'good parenting' are distinctly contemporary conceptions.

Dow's chapter, which looks at people's ideas around parenting in rural Scotland, foregrounds negotiations around 'good parenting' through a focus on preparation: that is, what does it take to create a 'stable environment' into which to bring a child? In particular, she explores how notions of appropriate parenting are tied to wider cultural trends around ecologism, which is itself used as a basis for moral decisions (a theme picked up by Faircloth's contribution, which follows below). Dow observes that part of the preparation people do, which is itself gendered, is reorienting themselves towards a more altruistic, rather than individualistic, ethic; both in how they expect to parent and in their lives more generally (around issues such as consumption decisions or caring for the environment, and so on).

Jensen's chapter, which also takes the UK as a focus, highlights the negotiations that go on around expertise-led parenting culture. She looks in particular at how groups of parents respond to television programmes that are intended both as educational and entertaining. Jensen's chapter foregrounds this contradiction through a rich analysis of the narratives of parents themselves, pointing to the more pervasive contradiction of this expert-led culture.

II The structural constraints to 'good' parenting

A key axis running through all of the chapters is the relationship between pedagogy and reflexivity, exploring this negotiation on the part of parents themselves. Hinton, Laverty and Robinson bring these debates to life in their rich portrayal of parenting in north-west England, to highlight the divergent ways in which 'good' parenting is interpreted, discussed and challenged in relation to health 'risks'. Drawing on a number of case-studies, they argue that simplistic public health messages around alcohol and tobacco ignore complex family dynamics, including the barriers mothers *and* fathers may encounter when attempting to emulate 'healthy' lifestyle behaviours, and children's reactions to dominant narratives of 'good' parenting and health. In particular, this chapter emphasises the way in which parents manage their accountability for a child when they are unable to fulfil a moral obligation to 'protect' their child's health and satisfy their own and others' 'intensive' parenting ideals. Moreover, it demonstrates that children may also actively seek to 'regulate' their parents (un)healthy behaviours in line with these ideals. In doing so, they challenge two key assumptions about 'intensive parenting': first that parents have full control of risk management and health within the home; second that children are passive agents in this process.

Berry and Jaysane-Darr's chapters look at these issues in a cross-cultural perspective, by examining the experiences of undocumented Hispanic migrant families and Sudanese refugees in the United States respectively. In looking at how these two groups negotiate their own parenting with that of their host nation, they elucidate the ways in which 'parenting' is tied to questions of politics and nationhood. Berry points to the importance of reflecting on the power dynamics inherent in labelling 'good' parenting. She analyses kin obligations that guide parenting among undocumented immigrants and experts to demonstrate how expert-led parenting strategies are presented as technical skills rather than dominant cultural ideologies concerning who should do what for whom.

While Berry emphasises how kinship impacts parenting within the family, Jaysane-Darr explores how kinship mediates relations between nation and family. Her chapter examines South Sudanese experiences of and responses to intensive parenting discourses in the United States, and particularly the 'culture of expertise' that defines contemporary American parenting. It shows how a local nonprofit's parenting workshops try to structure South Sudanese parent–child relationships in a way that replicates a middle-class American way of understanding infancy, childhood and the individual person, even as they ignore the socio-economic and racial realities that structure South Sudanese diasporic life. Through analyses of conversations and interactions with volunteers from a local nonprofit, as well as childrearing practices in the home, this chapter shows how South Sudanese seek to glean knowledge about how to raise their children in American society at the same time as they strive to reshape the parenting sessions according to South Sudanese ideals of sociocentricity, hospitality and respect. Likewise, South Sudanese parents work to fashion their children's behaviour, comportment and speech to embody ethnic and national identity.

III Negotiating parenting culture

These themes bring us nicely to our third section, which explores negotiations around parenting in a local/global framework. Faircloth, De Graeve, Longman and Murray all look at the relationship between global trends in parenting and the ethics of intimate relationships. Looking at how an 'intensive motherhood' ideology is (or rather, is not) being adopted in France, Faircloth highlights the wider cultural differences which allow or prevent new ideologies from 'sticking' and becoming salient. In this case, the very different history of feminism in France (when compared with the UK or the US) and the place of nature in the history of the Enlightenment proves to be a block on the adoption of 'natural' ('attachment') parenting.

De Graeve and Longman have as their case-study Ethiopian children who are adopted by Belgian parents, looking in particular at how non-biological parenting works across racial and ethnic boundaries in the new parenting culture. They point to the contradiction here, in that narratives around intensive motherhood are invoked to justify the transfer of poor Ethiopian children to affluent families in Belgium at the same time that these narratives problematise their non-biological relationship. Their chapter shows how these parents magnify the injunction to parent 'intensively' as a means of mediating this contradiction. By describing the ambiguity and complex contradictions of the parenting practices, they show the ability of the parenting work to both endure and re-imagine essentialist conceptions of identity, relatedness and belonging.

Murray's chapter looks at how a group of mothers in Santiago de Chile take on the new 'intensive' mothering edict by inserting it into their own existent and transforming ideas around appropriate care (see also Göknar). She argues that several intensive mothering mandates encouraged by the state and by private practice (particularly attachment mothering) reinforce and reframe an already existing sense of being good mothers involving long-term rationales of motherhood, religion and kinship in Chile. These women's routines of 'intensive mothering' and 'child-centredness' question the newness of new intensive parenting understood as a recent ideological movement taking place in contexts such as the UK and USA. Murray suggests that these women's priorities regarding mothering should also be considered along their social mobility aims in neoliberal Chile; aspirations that somehow match, but are also in contradiction with various values of mothering. This chapter reminds us of the need to focus on the interplay of ideologies and political economy rather than on the wholesale export of Western ideologies and replacement of peripheral ideologies.

IV Parenting and/as identity

Sedano's chapter acts as a bridge between these third and fourth sections in exploring the experiences of Dominican mothers in Madrid. Like Jensen's chapter, it shows how these mothers do not accept or take on intensive mothering in a wholehearted way. Instead, she foregrounds the negotiations they undertake in defining 'good' parenting (seeing their own methods as providing better care), and the ways in which this is internalised in the course of their 'identity work'.

In her research with Brazilian women, O'Dougherty found that for many, becoming mothers entailed a struggle for a selfhood separate from motherhood, and for some, a crisis which they came to identify as postpartum depression. O'Dougherty employs narrative analysis to trace the women's emergent theories of what caused or precipitated postpartum depression and what resolved it. The women who became mothers through depression experienced emotions completely at odds with the enduring idealisation of motherhood as women's ultimate fulfilment. Some of what the women describe – the weight of their responsibility to be perfect mothers, a sense of inadequacy with mothering skills, suggests that perinatal distress might be seen in part as a response to the contemporary model of intensive motherhood. The resolution to their crises developed by resuming professional work and by critical reflection on motherhood. O'Dougherty points out that the Brazilian context is one where the globally defined postpartum depression is of restricted circulation in the national media and where there is little social acceptance of the medicalised concept. She asserts that rather than constraining of their agency, in this context, the diagnostic label, mainly self-assigned, seemed to provide a means for the women to claim their negative experiences of motherhood.

O'Dougherty suggests broadening the definition of intensive mothering to include the 'identity work' entailed in this life crisis event. She argues that the women's distress registers that the transition to motherhood entails a powerful process of gender regulation. The 'failure' among these Brazilian middle-class women to emotionally perform according to the idealised model for mothers might be said to constitute unvoiced objection or resistance partially to intensive mothering and more broadly and directly to the imperative of motherhood. She concludes from the women's narratives that the 'new' model of intensive mothering reinvigorates the older imperative of the self-sacrificing woman dedicating herself to motherhood.

This resonates with the contribution from Layne, which is a case-study of a 'single mother by choice' in the US. She shows how motherhood is not only a key source for identity work, but explores the ways in which a couple relationship can be perceived as a threat to the 'intensive' mother–child relationship. In light of this, she asks whether single mothers might actually be able to better fulfil the demands of 'intensive' mothering, posing interesting questions around the logical conclusion of the 'dyadic' approach to parenting we observe here, and its implications for 'identity work'.

Göknar's chapter has a dual lens: she looks at how an 'intensive' parenting ideology slots into traditional Turkish ideas around sacrificial motherhood in the context of IVF treatment. At the same time, she explores her own experiences as a pregnant Turkish woman, living in Los Angeles, who is adopting the 'intensive' mothering ideology.

The final chapter, from Hoffman, considers parenting through an exploration of a central cultural trope among privileged mothers in the United States: the so-called parent–child 'power struggle'. Her analysis highlights the ways in which white, upper-middle-class mothers, while vehemently describing themselves as 'non-mainstream', still accept a set of assumptions about the need for emotional management strategies and choice that are very much a part of 'mainstream' parenting discourse as represented in US parenting advice literature. In part, mothers attempt to differentiate themselves from other parents through what they consider to be their more 'child-centred' approaches, yet Hoffman shows that the actual strategies used to support their child-centredness paradoxically undermine children's genuine emotionality and power. Ultimately, Hoffman suggests that the power struggle is not just between mothers and their children, but among mothers themselves, and even in the culture at large, in its unresolved tensions over the place of emotions and power in the self and in human relationships. She thus weaves together concerns over self, power and identity that are central to our explorations of parenting in contemporary societies.

Concluding thoughts

Taken collectively, the chapters in this volume broaden, extend, deepen and challenge the ideas and practices that we have come to know as 'parenting'. In sum, they do so in a number of important ways. First, they show how parenting maps onto different societal and cultural contexts, sometimes generating resistances and sometimes building on pre-existing indigenous notions of mothering (such as sacrificial mothering) to create hybrid ideologies. In this sense, some chapters challenge the idea that 'intensiveness' is solely the province of Western, privileged parenting. Others also challenge the individualistic mother–child model of intensive parenting by showing how parenting is locally constituted at the nexus of kinship relations extending far beyond the mother–child dyad. Still others show how parenting ought more properly be viewed along a temporal continuum, extending even to pre-conception period, as mothers attempt to perform 'ideal motherhood' and in fact achieve 'mother' status through pre-conception efforts.

Other chapters show how institutionalised assumptions about best parenting practice intersect with locally constituted, minority and ethnic understandings of appropriate roles for parents. Parents in these contexts may adopt and adapt superficially to the messages of institutional and state agents, but at the same time remake these messages and transform them into ideas that are more culturally comfortable.

Second, chapters present a diverse and deepened view of pedagogy in relation to parenting. They raise the question, collectively, of who is teaching whom? Is it about the state or media teaching parents to perform properly? Or parents teaching children the 'essential' lessons of socialisation? Or about children – acting as agents – teaching parents just what it means to care and to parent? Chapters in this volume suggest that the agency of children in the parenting process is an important and yet neglected arena for investigation into parenting culture. They also suggest that parents are important critics of state- and media-delivered parent pedagogy, simultaneously consuming yet critiquing representations of themselves, and other parents.

Third, the chapters deepen our understanding of how parenting – even when ostensibly child-centred – is also just as importantly about parental identities.

These identities are sometimes constituted through social class differentiation, through assertions of personal uniqueness, through 'choices' made to ascribe to particular parenting ideologies or styles, through the acceptance or rejection of diagnostic labels, or through the maintenance or establishment of ethnic borders or boundaries. They also suggest that parental identity should be viewed not in isolation as an individual project, but constituted through relations with children, kin and diverse others who constitute the social 'field' in which parenting is played out.

Finally, the chapters highlight the politics of parenting in transnational spaces. As parents remake themselves and their families through processes of crossing borders through adoption and/or immigration, they variously grapple with the hegemony of national and state visions of best parenting that often position them as 'other' and simultaneously as deficient. They – or their children – risk being defined as pathological, somehow at risk of 'not succeeding', whether that be in school or in life.

These are narratives about parenting that privilege developing skills of social interaction, cognitive development, getting one's needs fulfilled, emotional control, individual achievement, etc. but that hide deep assumptions about the kinds of selves that are socially and culturally desirable. The chapters suggest that the latter need to be highlighted and revealed as political, because ultimately they are connected to the power of some to determine what is good and best for others and, by implication, what is to be deemed in need of repair or remediation. In drawing attention to the multiple meanings of parenting in complex societies, then, this volume has articulated the need for a closer and more refined inquiry into a set of cultural practices and ideologies central to the emergence and maintenance of communities, societies and nations.

Note

1 An organisation based in France, with 30 member countries including France, Germany, Italy, Japan, New Zealand, Australia, the UK and the United States, committed to democracy and the market economy.

References

Arendell, T. 2000. Conceiving and Investigating Motherhood: The Decade's Scholarship. *Journal of Marriage and Family.* 62(4): 1192–1207.

Ariès, P. 1962. *Centuries of Childhood; A Social History of Family Life.* New York: Vintage Books.

Avishai, O. 2007. Managing the Lactating Body: The Breast-Feeding Project and Privileged Motherhood. *Qualitative Sociology.* 30(2): 135–152.

Avishai, O. 2010. Managing the Lactating Body: 'The Breastfeeding Project in the Age of Anxiety', in P. Liamputtong (ed.) *Infant Feeding Practices: A Cross-Cultural Perspective.* London: Springer, pp. 23–39.

Badinter, E. 1981. *The Myth of Motherhood: A Historical View of the Maternal Instinct,* trans. Roger De Garis. London: Souvenir Press.

Barlow, K. and Chapin, B. 2012. *Ethos* Special Issue: Mothering as Everyday Practice 38(4).

Bristow, J. 2009. *Standing Up to Supernanny*. London: Imprint Academic.

Brubaker, R. and Cooper, F. 2000. Beyond 'Identity'. *Theory and Society.* 29(1): 1–47.

Buskens, P. 2001. The Impossibility of 'Natural Parenting' for Modern Mothers: On Social Structure and the Formation of Habit. *Association for Research on Mothering Journal.* 3(1): 75–86.

Carsten, J. (ed.) 2000. *Cultures of Relatedness: New Approaches to the Study of Kinship.* Cambridge: Cambridge University Press.

De Carvalho, M.E.P. 2000. *Rethinking Family–School Relations: A Critique of Parental Involvement in Schooling*. London: Routledge.

Dermott, E. 2008. *Intimate Fatherhood, A Sociological Analysis*. London: Routledge.

Douglas, S. and Michaels, M. 2004. *The Mommy Myth: The Idealization of Motherhood and How it has Undermined All Women*. New York: Free Press.

Faircloth, C. 2010. What Science Says is Best: Parenting Practices, Scientific Authority and Maternal Identity. *Sociological Research Online* Special Section on 'Changing Parenting Culture'. 15(4)4, online, available at: www.socresonline.org.uk/15/4/4.html.

Franklin, S. and McKinnon, S. (eds) 2001. *Relative Values: Reconfiguring Kinship Studies.* London: Duke University Press.

Freely, M. 2000. *The Parent Trap: Children, Families And the New Morality*. London: Virago.

Furedi, F. 2002. *Paranoid Parenting: Why Ignoring the Experts May be Best for Your Child*. Chicago: Chicago Review Press.

Gauthier, A., Smeeding, T.M. and Furstenberg Jr., F.F. 2004. Are Parents Investing Less Time in Children? Trends in Selected Industrialized Countries. *Population and Development Review* 30(4): 647–671.

Gerhardt, S. 2004. *Why Love Matters: How Affection Shapes a Baby's Brain.* London: Routledge.

Giddens, A. 1991. *Modernity and Self-Identity: Self and Society in the Late Modern Age.* Cambridge: Polity.

Gillies, V. 2008. Childrearing, class and the new politics of parenting. *Sociology Compass* 2(3): 1079–1095.

Goffman, E. 1959. *The Presentation of Self in Everyday Life*. New York: Doubleday.

Guardian. 2012. *Do we need Parenting Classes?* Online, available at: www.guardian.co.uk/lifeandstyle/2012/mar/31/do-we-need-parenting-classes.

Hardyment, C. 1995. *Perfect Parents: Baby-care Advice Past and Present*. Oxford, Oxford University Press.

Hardyment, C. 2007. *Dream Babies: Childcare Advice from John Locke to Gina Ford.* London: Francis Lincoln.

Hays, S. 1996. *The Cultural Contradictions of Motherhood.* New Haven/London: Yale University Press.

Hoffman, D.M. and Zhao, G. 2008. Global Convergence and Divergence in Childhood Ideologies and the Marginalization of Children. In J. Zajda, K. Biraimah and W. Gaudelli (eds) *Education and Social Inequality in the Global Culture*. Dordrecht: Springer, pp. 1–16.

Jenkins, R. 1996. *Social Identity.* London: Routledge.

Lee, E. 2007. Health, Morality, and Infant Feeding: British Mothers' Experiences of Formula Milk Use in the Early Weeks. *Sociology of Health and Illness.* 29(7): 1075–1090.

Lee, E. and Bristow, J. 2009. Rules for Feeding Babies. In S. Day Sclater, F. Ebtehaj, E. Jackson and M. Richards (eds.) *Regulating Autonomy: Sex Reproduction and Family.* Oxford: Hart, pp. 73–91.

Mead, G.H. 1934. *Mind, Self, and Society.* Chicago: University of Chicago Press.

Mead, M. and Wolfenstein, M. (eds.) 1955. *Childhood in Contemporary Cultures.* Phoenix Books Vol. 124, Chicago: University of Chicago Press.

Miller, D. 1997. How Infants Grow Mothers in North London. *Theory, Culture and Society.* 14(4): 67–88.

Murphy, E. 2003. Expertise and Forms of Knowledge in the Government of Families. *The Sociological Review.* 51(4): 433–462.

Ragoné, H. 1994. *Surrogate Motherhood, Conception in the Heart.* Oxford: Westview Press.

Rapp, R. 2000. *Testing Women, Testing the Fetus: The Social Impact of Amniocentesis in America.* London/New York: Routledge.

Rose, N. 1999. *Governing the Soul: The Shaping of the Private Self,* 2nd edition. London: Routledge.

Schmeid, V., Sheehan, A. and Barclay, L. 2001. Contemporary Breast-feeding Policy and Practice: Implications for Midwives. *Midwifery.* 17(1): 44–54.

Schneider, D. 1968. *American Kinship: A Cultural Account.* Chicago: University of Chicago Press.

Strathern, M. 1992. *After Nature: Kinship in the Late Twentieth Century.* Cambridge: Cambridge University Press.

Strathern, M. 2005. *Kinship, Law and the Unexpected: Relatives are Always a Surprise.* Cambridge: Cambridge University Press.

Stephens, S. 1995. Children and the Politics of Culture in 'Late Capitalism'. In S. Stephens (ed.) *Children and the Politics of Culture.* Princeton: Princeton University Press.

Stryker, S. 1968. Identity salience and role performance: The importance of symbolic interaction theory for family research. *Journal of Marriage and Family.* 30(4) 558–564.

Wade, P. 2007. *Race, Ethnicity and Nation: Perspectives from Kinship and Genetics.* Oxford/New York: Berghahn Books.

Wall, G. 2001. Moral Constructions of Motherhood in Breastfeeding Discourse. *Gender and Society.* 15(4): 592–610.

Warner, J. 2006. *Perfect Madness, Motherhood in the Age of Anxiety.* London: Vermilion.

Part I

The moral context for parenting

1 'Where are the parents?'

Changing parenting responsibilities
between the 1960s and the 2010s

Rosalind Edwards and Val Gillies

Introduction

In 1947, in the immediate aftermath of the Second World War, British Pathé Pictorial produced a short film, a mass-distribution filler shown in cinemas, entitled 'East and West'. It was built around the symbolic and long-standing confluence of space and class in London, with its affluent middle- and upper-class 'West End' and poor working class and immigrant 'East End'. The film contrasted life for the pampered children and dogs of the West End, constantly cared for and watched over, and isolated, with the carefree children and dogs of the East End, allowed to roam and part of a (romanticized) strong community. Over clips of a gang of rather grimy and scruffy young boys playing cricket on rubble-strewn waste ground 'down' in the East End of London, without an adult in sight, followed by shots of individual or pairs of clean, well-dressed children accompanied by nanny, feeding ducks or driving small replica boats on a lake in a park 'up' in the West End, the commentator enunciates:

> [The East End kids'] playground is all too often the place where the bomb dropped. He learns to take his pleasure where he can. What have [the West End children] got that the other fellow hasn't? Probably a nanny keeping an eye on them, a nanny who never lets them out of her sight, these children of the west who must dress up even to play in the park.[1]

Later, he muses about both children and dogs: 'Perhaps there is such a thing as too much kindness, too much care'.

It truly is difficult to envisage a film with such sentiments being made today and treated as uncontentious. Not only would the equation of children and dogs be unacceptable, the contemporary wisdom would have the film turned on its head. Rather than constructed as admirably carefree, the East End 'kids' would be posed both as being in danger and a danger to others. They would be regarded as potentially at risk from neglectful parents who allow them unsupervised play in hazardous conditions, and a risk to others with their anti-social behaviour. In turn the West End 'children' would be seen as well-cared for, supervised and safe, brought up to be the well-behaved neo-liberal citizens of the future as a result of contemporary intensive parenting practices (Hays 1996) that are the focus of this edited collection. Contemporary wisdom also seems to have rewritten Pathé's perhaps overblown contrast of the time, posing the immediate post-war period as an undifferentiated model of parenting along the West End lines.

In this chapter, it is not our intention to endorse a particular view of the best conditions for children. We are not going to argue that the East End past was a golden age for both children and parents akin to ideas about 'free range' parenting (e.g. Skenazy 2009; see also Jiménez Sedano this volume) that ostensibly challenge overprotective intensity, or champion techniques of contemporary parental responsibilization, for example. Rather, our concern here is the way that the immediate post-war past has become mobilized in dominant ideas about the state of parenting and children's upbringing in contemporary Britain. In particular, we are concerned with a critique of the particular claim that the last fifty years or so have seen a deterioration in the transmission of parenting skills, no longer passed down from generation to generation because of the fracturing of traditional support systems with dire consequences for society. It is this claim that helps to undergird parental pedagogy television programmes such as 'Supernanny', discussed by Tracey Jensen in her chapter in this collection – which, returning to British Pathé Pictorial's conflation of children and dogs, have been likened to dog training programmes (Hendrick 2012).[2]

We outline and assess those claims through an exploratory analysis of parents bringing up children, drawing on in-depth data from community research studies carried out in the 1960s; the 'classics' of British sociology (Thompson and Corti 2004). In particular, we focus on a comparison of prevalent ideas about parents' responsibilities in relation to knowing where their children are.

Contemporary ideas about parenting deficit

The construction of family as a problem is a long-standing, remarkably consistent feature of British public, political and academic debates (Rodger 1996; Welshman 2007). Part of this construction is the notion that the strength of the family and thus its ability to fulfil its true function lies in the past (see also Coontz, 2000, as well as contributions to this volume from Faircloth, Dow and Jiménez Sedano respectively, for discussions of nostalgia for the past of family life and parenting in different national contexts). Quite what the problem of family is has shifted over the years, according to the ideal that is being harked back to. Nonetheless, the story remains structured broadly around the calamitous moral consequences of social and economic transformations for family life. Most recently, concern has focused on childrearing. Contemporary family life is said to be characterized by a decline in values of duty and responsibility, undermining good parenting, placing great strain on the institution of the family, drastically undermining supports for good parenting and thereby damaging social cohesion more generally (Gillies 2005).

This theme has been ramped up and powerfully articulated as part of the 'Broken Britain' thesis of the Conservative-led coalition government (a coalition between the Conservative and Liberal Democrat parties). Under this thesis, poor parenting is held to account for a range of social ills, including poverty, crime, irresponsibility and selfishness. This blame reached a height in the aftermath of the English riots in the summer of 2011, with social commentators and politicians attributing youth disorder to a crisis in parenting skills and commitment. For example, the Conservative prime minister, David Cameron, commented that the rioters were the product of 'neglect and immorality', with parents not caring where their children are, let along what they are doing. In a speech given in the aftermath of the riots, he said:

> The question people asked over and over again last week was 'where are the parents? Why aren't they keeping the rioting kids indoors?' Tragically that's been followed in some cases by judges rightly lamenting: 'why don't the parents even turn up when their children are in court?' Well, join the dots and you have a clear idea about why some of these young people were behaving so terribly. Either there was no one at home, they didn't much care or they'd lost control ... So if we want to have any hope of mending our broken society, family and parenting is where we've got to start.
>
> (15 August 2011[3])

This narrative of deterioration in parenting has a cross-party consensus, from the left as well as right of politics. It has featured prominently in policy reports, with an emphasis on early intervention as a cost-effective measure for tackling social problems. For example, in a report for the government on child poverty, the Labour Member of Parliament (MP) leading the review – Frank Field – recommended that, 'a modern definition of poverty must take into account those children whose parents remain disengaged from their responsibilities' (2010: 15). This focus on parenting is a 'modern' definition because in Field's view, disengaged parenting was not the issue in the past that it is now:

> Since 1969 I have witnessed a growing indifference from some parents to meeting the most basic needs of children, and particularly younger children, those who are least able to fend for themselves. I have also observed how the home lives of a minority but, worryingly, a growing minority of children, fails to express an unconditional commitment to the successful nurturing of children.
>
> (2010: 18)

Field's mention of 1969 is interesting. In Britain, it is the year of student protests forcing the closure of the London School of Economics, violent political and sectarian rioting in Northern Ireland, and sentencing of the notorious 'East End' gangland Kray twins for murder. This is hardly a picture of a wholly stable, ordered and respectful society. 1969 is also the year in which Frank Field became Director of the Child Poverty Action Group (serving for a decade), a voluntary organization set up in 1965 to raise awareness of family poverty and campaign for action to alleviate it.

Field's report resonates with long-standing interpretations by those on the political right, particularly in its invocation of a 'golden age' of parenting and family in the 1950s and 1960s. As we consider in this chapter, however, such claims have little basis in evidence of everyday parenting practices of the time. Furthermore, crucially, they fail to engage with the dramatic change in understandings of children's capacities and needs over the last half century. We will be discussing some insights from a research project, working with data from archived classic British community studies of the 1960s, that we undertook with the intention of exploring social change and continuity in family relationships and parenting support systems.

Assessing social change in parenting through working with archived data

In the main, theorists derive evidence of social change in family lives from large scale, longitudinal quantitative social surveys such as the UK Millennium Cohort and Understanding Society studies (Gillies and Edwards 2005; Savage 2007). This emphasis on macro, demographic change rarely is accompanied by a detailed exploration of those lives as they actually were lived in the past. Without such detail, however, it is difficult to assess the nature and extent of social shifts in community, family life and parenting (Charles *et al.* 2008; Crow 2008). Family forms may change but their content may well stay the same, or vice versa. What is deemed acceptable or unacceptable may shift but the distribution of liberal and conservative views may remain much the same. For example, Simon Duncan (2011) shows that the majority of people in both 1950 and the present day held/hold 'pragmatic' views about extra-marital sex and divorce, within the context of the debates prevalent at each time point. Further, cyclical patterns might be mistaken for linear change, as Liz Stanley (1992) notes in relation to family structures. And enduring concerns may be reframed in new language and understood as different, which Harry Goulbourne (2006) reveals in exploring the way that African-Caribbean families' marginalization from mainstream society has been explained through assertions of, variously, their lack of 'culture' in the 1970s and their lack of integrative 'social capital' in the 2000s. These sorts of issues highlight the need for careful revisiting of past family relationships to better understand current experiences.

Given these pitfalls, we have been working with material from archived British classic community studies from the 1960s in an attempt to provide insights into the nature and extent of social change in parenting practices. Interestingly, in the light of contemporary assertions about social change, social research carried out in the 1960s also was often preoccupied with what were regarded as major shifts occurring in society. The current sense of seismic social and material transformations in family life and parenting that provided the context for our work, then, is a continuous political theme across the post-war period.

In what follows, we will be bringing insights from our analysis of some of these 1960s research studies into dialogue with the prevalent contemporary policy picture of a decline in parenting commitment. We will be drawing in particular on illustrative data from two of the archived collection of classic studies carried out by Dennis Marsden, which offer valuable insights into a range of experiences of family life and parenting at the time.[4] The 'Salford Slum and Re-housing' study was carried out between 1962 and 1963[5] and focused on the consequences of the rehousing programme for traditional working class communities. The extensive archive of fieldnotes and accounts of interviews contain material on family and community life, and employment. The 'Mothers Alone' study was carried out between 1965 and 1966[6] and examined the lives of lone mothers drawing the National Assistance welfare support benefit. There are 116 accounts of in-depth interviews with the mothers, addressing living standards, poverty and support networks, notably relationships with fathers and wider family and friends.

It is important to note that the 1960s research materials bear little resemblance to the standard audio-recorded and verbatim transcribed data familiar to today's researchers. The material from Dennis Marsden's studies consist of a hand- and type-written mix of remembered quotes recorded after the event alongside descriptions, reflections and conjecture. Figure 1.1 provides an example. As Mike Savage (2010) points out, the 1960s was a period in which the qualitative social research interview about everyday life was emergent practice. Researchers did not distinguish between the narratives that they elicited from interviewees and their own observations, value judgments and moral evaluations as appropriate data. In order to analyse the material from his studies then, it was necessary to treat Dennis as a respondent in his own right rather than simply as a researcher (Gillies and Edwards 2012).

This issue is to the fore especially where investigators' lives were deeply intertwined with those they were researching. For example, in the Salford study, Dennis Marsden, his then wife, Pat, and their two young children spent a year and a half living on a public housing estate alongside his research subjects. Dennis and Pat each kept diaries containing detailed descriptions of everyday life and the families they lived amongst, providing a powerful and vivid insight into their experiences and practices.

Their accounts of lives on the estate were inevitably founded on their assumptions, values and expectations, which are in themselves revelatory. Dennis and Pat clearly felt empathy for these disadvantaged families and had a strong commitment to social change. But, as with all researchers, their narrations often reflect their class trajectories and standards, and most likely the preoccupations of the day. For example, Pat keeps track of how many sweets the estate children are given to eat and how often they are sent to Mr Chippy (the van that came round the estate in the early evening selling chips) for their tea, while Dennis documents drinking habits, swearing in the presence of children and any hint of sexual impropriety among women.

From a current perspective, accounts of the research subjects in the original collections are often shockingly frank, consisting of unfiltered and highly personal descriptions of their appearance and perceived intelligence. Sexist and

can manage, I'm alright. I had so much debt when my husband left me, and it
took me so much worry and trouble, sorting it all out that I said to myself, 'If
I got turned round, I'd never go into doubt again'. And I haven't done, I've
never had any clubs since then because it's not worth it, the worry it causes.
I've no time going looking what other people have, either. I think that you
find, when you're in my position that the children take all your time. I might
say to myself, 'Well, I think next week, I'll buy so-and-so'. But then, the
children come home from school, and they want 3/6d. for this, or they've torn
their coat on a piece of railing, or something like that, and there it goes. And
I'm not much at a hand for sewing, but I've tried my best. Look at this." Proudly,
she produced a Brownie's uniform. "I asked them how much it would cost to buy
a dress like this, and they said 15/-. So I thought, I can do as well as that,
and I bought a piece of material for 5/-, and I ran it up myself. Same with
this." She produced another, a romper suit for the baby. "Round here, with
them all working in the mill, they can all get bits of cloth, and they sell it
to me cheap, or give it me." She can do this for the two little ones, but she
can't do it for the older boy, Michael, who is very particular about what he
wears.

Family

        Her father has had cancer for eight years, and this strictly limits what
her mother can do for her. Also, her mother lives at three-quarters of an hour
away, over on the other side of the town. Last night when I called, to try and
get an interview, the mother, and an aunt, had just come over for the first time
in 18 months to allow Mrs. Campbell to go out to a Church meeting, which she
was particularly anxious to attend. "They'll never come to eat my things. They
always say, 'What you've got is for you, and for your own, and we're not going
to start living off you'. Whenever they come they bring a bottle of milk, and
they always bring their own tea. They always bring enough food to cover what
they eat, and a bit over. And when I was out last night, the children were
supposed to have had their supper but when I came back, they had fish and chips,
and cream slices. They got spoilt last night." My aunty's just like a second
mother to us, because she got married, and she never had any children, so when
we were little, she always used to bring us up. And she's very good." Her
mother was a widow, and had to bring the children up by herself. Then she got
married again, a man with two children of her own, much younger. And these two
children, "They are really better than my own. My step brother and sister are
more used to me." The step sister works, or used to work, up at the mill nearby,
Joseph Hoyles. Before she started courting, Mrs. Campbell saw her every day,
and quite often she'd collect the little girl and take her down to her Grandma's.
As it is, Michael goes down to his Grandma's every Tuesday and Friday, and has
his tea. "And she always gives him a couple or oranges and a bag of spice."
(Spice = sweets) And there are always small sums of money which Mrs. Campbell
can't really compute, or affects not to be able to, which amounts to 1/6d. to
2/- a week for each child. The brother and sister are always handing out six-
pences and shillings and the children get a great deal of pocket money in this
way.

Figure 1.1 Extract from Marsden's interview notes for Mrs Campbell, March 1966
(Interview No. 014), SN: 5072.

racist assumptions pervade the accounts, offending both present day moral sensibilities and conventions around research ethics (Gillies and Edwards 2012). For example, mothers are often rated on their physical attractiveness (or lack of it), described as (amongst other things) greasy, spotty, fat, simple, spineless and lacking sex appeal. While these comments can make for uncomfortable reading, they provide useful insights into the sensitivities and insensitivities of the time. They also highlight the relative sterility of today's research field notes, which are routinely self-censored. The comments and evaluations made by the original researchers would now be considered unacceptable, but at least they are owned, clearly stated and can be factored into any analysis. Indeed, they have been an important purchase for us in generating insights about acceptable practice in bringing up children in the early 1960s – a time of unconditional commitment to parental nurturing in Frank Field's chronology of poor parenting.

Ideas about parental responsibility: knowing where your children are

Given the judgemental tone characterizing much of the original research material from the 1960s, a lack of moral commentary could be even more telling, highlighting how parenting practices considered dubious today were taken for granted at that time. More specifically, children often were left to their own devices in a way that would be considered positively neglectful today, even within notions of free-range parenting, where the idea is that parents consciously enable their children's freedom to roam while maintaining accountability for ensuring this is achieved safely (e.g. Skenazy 2009).

In contrast, parents in the 1960s did not appear to be reflexive free-range practitioners. For example, in July 1963 Dennis Marsden wrote the following description of an accident that happened to the six-year-old boy, Sam, who lived in the flat above him and his family on the Salford housing estate:

> Sam had an accident that nearly killed him. A builder's ladder had been left and some boys of around 10 and 11 were manhandling it when it fell over (or was pushed) and fractured Sam's skull. It happened at 10.05 at night and he had to be rushed into hospital for a brain operation. ... From the newspaper accounts it appears that no blame can be pinned on anyone (although the original story was that the ladder had been pushed over deliberately perhaps).

From a contemporary perspective most striking about this account is the absence of discussion around parental responsibility. Where Dennis Marsden makes moral judgments in other circumstances, he does not question whether a six-year-old boy should have been left without adult supervision, outdoors and late in the evening. A similar incident today would likely lead to a child protection investigation and potentially even court proceedings against the parents. Indeed, recent UK research on 'risky behaviour' focuses on children age ten to fifteen who have stayed out 'late' – defined as past 9 PM, without their parents knowing their whereabouts (found to be well under 5 per cent of the sample as a frequent occurrence) (Iacovou 2012). Six-year-olds out at 10 PM are beyond contemporary (data collection) conception it seems. In contrast, in 1963 speculation about blame appears to have centred on the intentions (or otherwise) of the older boys rather than parents and the time of night.

Another striking example of this very different context for understanding parental care and children's capabilities can be found in the 'Mothers Alone' study, with Dennis Marsden reflecting on the actions of seven-year-old June's mother:

> With the little girl June she seems rather over protective … she takes June all the way to school which is quite a long way, possible half an hour's trip, just so that she can see her across the road

While these excerpts point to a distinct change in understandings of children and their welfare needs, also highlighted is the contingent and present-centred nature of the topic framing our work with classic archived studies – parenting – which does not transfer easily to the 1960s. During this time 'parenting' was not a commonly recognized term. Rather, the word 'parent' – or more often mother or father – related to an ascribed relationship rather than as the practice or 'job' it tends to be described as now (Ramaekers and Suissa 2011). Families in the classic studies were also considerably larger; significant numbers had upwards of seven children, with siblings or grown-up children commonly providing considerable domestic and childcare support. The average number of children born per woman estimated for 1961 is 2.6 children as against 1.7 in 2005 (Diamond 2007).

As we have outlined, policy debates about contemporary parenting deficits are notably ahistorical in that they fail to acknowledge or engage with these changing understandings and expectations. Influential claims from Frank Field MP that 'Britain is witnessing a rupturing in its once strong parenting tradition' (2010: 18) conjure up an era of taken for granted standards and values in relation to good parenting. Yet our analysis of the classic studies reveals widely accepted practices and values from the 1960s that would today be viewed at best in terms of benign neglect and at worst as child abuse. Young children were regularly left home alone; babies and toddlers were often cared for by very young siblings. For example in the 'Mothers Alone' study, one mother describes how she managed to work without her husband's knowledge. Mrs H was living with her husband and had three children at the time, the eldest being Jack who would have been around eight years old. Dennis Marsden records her telling him:

> I'll tell you the sort of thing when I was living with me husband. He didn't want me to work. He didn't mind me going out and helping an old lady that had heart trouble at night time, but he didn't like me to work anywhere where there was any men. So, when he was out in the morning, and I had

our Cynthia I used to put her to bed at 9 o'clock for her morning sleep. I used to kid myself that she was ready for a sleep at that time and I used to go off down the pub and clean them for two hours, and then I'd rush off home. She'd always be asleep. And that's how I used to do. The only trouble was, I used to have to go Sundays as well. So Sunday mornings, what I did, I used to get all the kids ready, put them in the pram, and go down past the pub and I'd nip in and do the cleaning for a bit, and Jack would take the pram down to Greenhead Park, and push it around and I'd join him there. That's how me husband never found out.

Again it is significant that Dennis Marsden makes no comment on what would be experienced today by researchers as an extremely worrying disclosure. In fact, later on in the interview he describes her as 'very soft hearted and basically a simple soul'. While it would now be considered morally unthinkable for a baby to be left home alone, it would also be viewed as inflicting permanent damage in relation to the child's brain development. Policy literature extolling the importance of early intervention stresses the crucial function of parental 'attunement' to a child's needs in the early years. For example, the independent review of early intervention conducted for the UK government by Labour MP Graham Allen sets out what he describes as the 'dire lifelong consequences of a parents' failure to respond sensitively':

Although poor parenting practices can cause damage to children of all ages, the worst and deepest damage is done to children when their brains are being formed during their earliest months and years. The most serious damage takes place before birth and during the first 18 months of life when formation of the part of the brain governing emotional development has been identified to be taking place. ... If a child does not experience attunement, their development is retarded, and they may lack empathy altogether.

(2010: 17)

This expectation of intensive, science-led and attentive parenting was nowhere to be found in accounts from the 1960s. Children generally roamed free without adult supervision and serious accidents, like the one that befell Sam, were common. In the mid-1960s around 70 per 100,000 child pedestrians aged nine or under were killed or seriously injured, in contrast to about 1 per 100,000 aged under nine in the early 2000s (Ministry of Transport 1967; Department for Transport 2010).[7] Road traffic has increased but children playing out on the street has decreased.

In the Salford study, parents were depicted as drinking heavily and arguing loudly. Children were often filthy and sometimes smelly, they had bad teeth, irregular bedtimes and often missed school. For example, Dennis Marsden wrote the following description of six-year-old John and his younger sister, Mary, and baby brother, William:

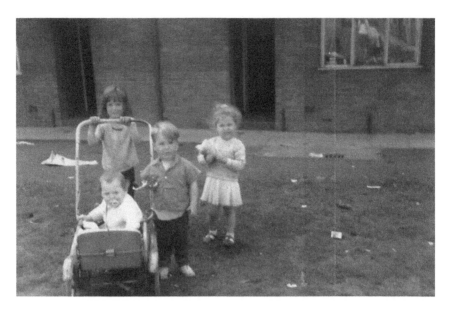

Figure 1.2 Children playing outside on the estate in the Salford rehousing study (source: photo taken by Pat Marsden and reproduced with her permission).

They're left to their own devices most of the day. Their mother sets them off in clean clothes in the morning, pushing the baby in the pram or walking him, and when it's fine they're out nearly all the time. William has a sleep 'on the couch' in the afternoon. William who's two and very, very fat goes off by himself. I've seen him being wheeled and led off by other children (a neighbour's child seems to take him for a walk) riding with a group of boys on a lorry cart. But usually there's John or Mary to look after him. John sometimes has to stop in to mind William while his mother goes to the shops and both can be seen at the window standing on the couch.

Further, as we now discuss, while we can make observations about the kinds of help that parents accessed then as opposed to now, any comparison is senseless without a detailed understanding of the historically located meanings attached to childrearing.

Taking care of the children

Another significant difference between then and now concerns the extent to which 1960s lone mothers spoke about relying on the local authority social services care system to tide them over challenging times. While having a child taken into care today carries considerable stigma, it appears to have been a more commonplace, acceptable practice in the 1960s.[8] Many of those participating in the

'Mothers Alone' study had children admitted to care homes, while others struggled to get what was referred to as the 'welfare office' to accept them. For the lone mothers, care homes seem to have been viewed as a necessary and valuable support, and efforts were commonly focused around persuading the authorities to keep children for longer. For example, Mrs W from the 'Mothers Alone' study had been hospitalized with meningitis and had complained that her children were sent back to her even though she was still very ill: 'I went down there and I cried, I begged and prayed for them to take them but they say "they're your children, and you've got to bide by that."' Mrs H, again from the 'Mothers Alone' study, was more concerned to avoid her children being taken in to care when the National Society for the Prevention of Cruelty to Children – a long-established voluntary agency whose inspectors maintain the legal power to intervene and take children into care – became involved as a result of her husband's cruelty, but even she emphasized how well provided for they would have been:

> Oh, to think of children in one of them homes. Although they are very nice, I'm always meeting someone and she said, 'Don't be sorry for them, they've got seven pairs of different sorts of shoes, and they have two holidays a year, and at Christmas-time they are going for this trip, and that trip. They have a lot more than what ours have'.

Notably, there was little consideration of children's emotional well-being detectable in the studies in contrast to the much greater concern over their physical appearance (whether or not they were wearing clean clothes and looked healthy). This emphasizes again how current concerns over intensive parenting warmth, attunement and attachment lack continuity with 1960s. Similarly, expectations that parents should actively cultivate cognitive and emotional skills in their children reflect uniquely contemporary preoccupations.

Yet the claim that parenting standards have dropped is presented as a key explanation for a perceived increase in social problems. As the MPs Graham Allen and Iain Duncan Smith contended in a collaborative report that brought together members of the Labour and Conservative parties, entitled *Early Intervention: Good Parents, Great Kids, Better Citizens*:

> Britain's dysfunctional base is expanding. ... The transmission of parenting skills from generation to generation has changed considerably, and while the middle classes can read the guide books, those with lower educational and social skills are finding parenting skills squeezed out as extended families reduce and more one parent households have smaller knowledge bases on which to draw. ... As a society, we seem to have reduced the standards of responsibility which we expect parents and households to meet when children are born. This has produced tacit acceptance (particularly from those who do not have to face the consequences) of many of the dysfunctional conditions least favourable to successful childrearing
>
> (Allen and Duncan Smith 2008: 30)

While contradicting this claim, our research also finds little evidence to support the alleged root cause of this perceived parenting deficit – that parenting skills are no longer passed down from generation to generation because of the fracturing of traditional support systems.

The types and extent of support received from wider family in the 1960s, whatever parents' backgrounds, appears to have been no more widespread or intensive than it is nowadays, and followed a remarkably similar pattern (Edwards and Gillies 2004). As is still the case, parents in the 1960s classic studies could receive little or no help from their families because of bereavement or illness, the geographical distance they lived from each other, or estrangement, while others relied heavily on their mothers and/or sisters for everyday support.

Unlike the present day, however, there appeared to be little expectation that family should exist as an unconditional support system. Contemporary parents often express a strong ideal of family as providing unqualified support, which rarely matches the reality (Edwards and Gillies 2004). Mothers in particular tend to portray other, 'normal' families as providing the kind of unreserved support that few parents actually receive. Back in the 1960s though, lack of support from family members was not dwelt upon or particularly problematized by parents or the researchers. For example, there is little comment on the fact that impoverished Mrs H from the 'Mothers Alone' study had very little contact other than a Christmas card exchange with her local and relatively well-off brother and sisters. Rather, there seems to have been more value attached to notions of privacy and independence.

Working class mothers in the classic studies described dense networks of highly reciprocal supportive relationships, as do contemporary working class mothers (Edwards and Gillies 2005; Gillies and Edwards 2011). However, contemporary mothers were much more likely to talk about these relationships in terms of emotional bonds than those from the 1960s, who were distinctly less sentimental about friendships. There was no real conception in those days of emotional support as a distinct need. Nevertheless, mothers and especially fathers appear to have had a more active social life fifty years ago. It appears to have been common for both parents to go out to the local pub of an evening, popping back occasionally to check on the children who had been left alone.

Conclusion

In this chapter we have discussed some of the insights that have emerged from an in-depth investigation of bringing up children five decades ago, in a context where claims about the model state of parenting at the time have been mobilized to position contemporary parenting uniquely as culpable in social disorder and breakdown. While our study is a small and exploratory endeavour, we contend that these insights seriously undermine any claim that the 1960s represent a golden age of engaged parenting. By today's standards the parenting norms and practices that are revealed in the data from some of the classic, well-regarded community studies of the 1960s would likely be condemned as irresponsible, personally damaging and, in some cases, criminal. Particularly noticeable is the absence of moralized discussions of parental liability that are so central to contemporary social commentary.

In highlighting these differences our research findings reflect the political step-change that has occurred in the way family and parenting is envisaged and targeted, with public understandings and expectations having undergone substantial revision to better fit neo-liberal ideals of individualized choice and therefore of individualized accountability. Emphasis has been placed on the interpersonal realm of family as the formative site through which competent personhood is cultivated, with intensively parented children better able to navigate and capitalize on new post-industrial economic landscapes. A key feature of this new public politics of family is the way in which attention has moved away from concerns with structure and economic function, towards an emphasis on personal knowledge and proficiency. As a result 1960s preoccupations with 'family values' and strengthening the traditional nuclear family have largely been replaced by a new culture of parenting focusing on the 'well-being' of children, in a context where the rearing of children is linked to the economic and moral destiny of the nation. As part of this shift mothers and fathers are depicted, and held accountable, as the architects of family, while children occupy a new visibility and significance as its core subject. A crucial feature of this change is a reframing and centring of childrearing as a job requiring particular know how and expertise. Policy makers have sought to establish parenting as a complex skill which must be learnt, with 'knowledge' about childrearing portrayed as a necessary resource that mothers and fathers must have access to in order to fulfil their moral duty as good parents.

This politicization of parenting over recent years renders evaluative analysis across the two timeframes impossible. As we have demonstrated, direct comparisons cannot be made between everyday practices then and now, to say that one is worse or better than the other, because conceptions of children's needs and capacities, and what is involved in taking care of children, have shifted so radically across the past fifty-odd years. Such comparisons require the past to be explained through reference to the present, an endeavour that could be described as looking at history through the wrong end of the telescope (Casey 1989). Nevertheless, our study illustrates the potential value of revisiting of past family relationships and resources to better understand current experiences. Indeed, overall there are important messages here about the ahistorical assumptions embedded in the policy debates and wider concerns about contemporary parenting deficits and fractured support systems that provide a context for the new parenting culture.

Notes

1 Available at: www.britishpathe.com/record.php?id=47622 [accessed 6 November 2011].
2 For another recent counterposing of children and dogs, see Smith (2011) on ethical reasoning about parenting.

3 Available at: www.conservatives.com/News/Speeches/2011/08/David_Cameron_We_are_all_in_this_together.aspx [accessed 6 January 2012].
4 The Marsden Collection is held at ESDS Qualidata, UK Data Archive, and the Alfred Sloman Library at the University of Essex.
5 Marsden, D. Salford Slum and Rehousing Study, 1962–1963 [unprocessed study]. Colchester, Essex: UK Data Archive [distributor], SN: 6225.
6 Marsden, D. Mothers Alone: Poverty and the Fatherless Family, 1965–1966 [computer file]. Colchester, Essex: UK Data Archive [distributor], February 2005, SN: 5072.
7 Thanks to Anita Plumb, Information Assistant at the Royal Society for the Prevention of Accidents, for help with accessing statistics for the 1960s.
8 Limited information was collected on number of children in care in the 1960s, particularly with regards to those who were looked after by the state for temporary periods. This does not detract from the key point that the care system appears to have been viewed by 1960s lone mothers at least, as a commonplace support in a way that would not be recognized today.

References

Allen, G. (2010) *Early Intervention: The Next Steps. An Independent Report to Her Majesty's Government*, London: Cabinet Office.
Allen, G. and Duncan Smith, I. (2008) *Early Intervention: Good Parents, Great Kids, Better Citizens*, London: Centre for Social Justice.
Casey, J. (1989) *The History of the Family*, Oxford: Blackwell.
Charles, N., Aull Davies, C. and Harris, C. (2008) *Families in Transition: Social Change, Family Formation and Kin Relationships*, Bristol: Policy Press.
Coontz, S. (2000) *The Way We Never Were: American Families and the Nostalgia Trap*, 2nd edition, New York, NY: Basic Books.
Crow, G. (2008) 'Thinking about families and communities over time', in R. Edwards (ed.) *Researching Families and Communities: Social and Generational Change*, Abingdon: Routledge.
Department for Transport (2010) *Road Accidents and Safety Annual Report 2010*, online, available at: http://webarchive.nationalarchives.gov.uk/20120926002851/ www.dft.gov.uk/statistics/releases/road-accidents-and-safety-annual-report-2010/ [accessed 18 November 2012].
Diamond, I. (2007) 'Total fertility rate, England and Wales, 1841–2005', GSS Conference Paper, Economic and Social Research Council, online, available at: www.powershow.com/view/6ef54-NThiM/GSS_Conference_Ian_Diamond_ESRC_25_June_2007_powerpoint_ppt_presentation.
Duncan, S. (2011) 'The world we have made? Individualisation and personal life in the 1950s', *The Sociological Review*, 59(2): 242–265.
Edwards, R. and Gillies, V. (2004) 'Support in parenting: values and consensus concerning who to turn to', *Journal of Social Policy*, 33(4): 623–643.
Edwards, R. and Gillies, V. (2005) *Resources in Parenting: Access to Capitals Project Report*, Families & Social Capital ESRC Research Group Working Paper No. 14, London: London South Bank University.
Field, F. (2010) *The Foundation Years: Preventing Poor Children Becoming Poor Adults. The Report of the Independent Review on Poverty and Life Chances*, London: Cabinet Office.
Gillies, V. (2005) 'Meeting parents' needs? Discourses of 'support' and 'inclusion' in family policy', *Critical Social Policy*, 25(1): 70–90.

Gillies, V. and Edwards, R. (2005) Secondary analysis in exploring family and social change: addressing the issue of context (30 paragraphs), *Forum Qualitative Sozialforschung: Qualitative Social Research Forum* (on-line journal), 6: 1, Art. 44 – available at: www.qualitative-research.net/fqs-texte/1-05/05-1-44-e.htm.

Gillies, V. and Edwards, R. (2011) *An Historical Comparative Analysis of Family and Parenting: A Feasibility Study Across Sources and Timeframes*, Families & Social Capital Research Group Working Paper No. 29, London: London South Bank University.

Gillies, V. and Edwards, R. (2012) 'Working with archived classic family and community studies: illuminating past and present conventions around acceptable research practice', Special Issue: Perspectives on Working With Archived Textual and Visual Material in Social Research, *International Journal of Social Research Methodology*, 15(4): 321–330.

Goulbourne, H. (2006) 'Families, communities and social capital: past and continuing false prophecies in social studies', *Community, Work and Family*, 9(3): 235–250.

Hays, S. (1996) *The Cultural Contradictions of Motherhood*, New Haven: Yale University Press.

Hendrick, H. (2012) '"It's me or the dog": me, myself and child training in an uncertain world', paper presented in the Social Policy seminar series, University of Edinburgh, 27 April.

Iacovou, M. (2012) 'Does your mother know? Staying out late and risky behaviours among 10–15 year olds', in S.L. McFall (ed.) *Understanding Society: Findings 2012*, Colchester: Institute for Social and Economic Research, University of Essex.

Ministry of Transport (1967) *Road Accidents 1967*, London: Her Majesty's Stationery Office.

Ramaekers, S. and Suissa, J. (2011) *The Claims of Parenting: Reasons, Responsibility and Society*, Heidelberg: Springer.

Rodger, J. (1996) *Family Life and Social Control: A Sociological Perspective*, Basingstoke: Macmillan.

Savage, M. (2007) 'Changing social class identities in post-war Britain: perspectives from Mass Observation', *Sociological Research Online*, 12(3)6. Published online at: www.socresonline.org.uk/12/3/6.html.

Savage, M. (2010) *Identities and Social Change in Britain Since 1940: The Politics of Method*, Oxford: Oxford University Press.

Skenazy, K. (2009) *Free Range Kids: Giving Our Children the Freedom We Had Without Going Nuts With Worry*, San Francisco: Jossey-Bass.

Smith, R. (2011) 'On dogs and children: judgements in the realm of meaning', *Ethics and Education*, 6(2): 171–180.

Stanley, L. (1992) *The Auto/biographical I: The Theory and Practice of Feminist Auto/biography*, Manchester: Manchester University Press.

Thompson, P. and Corti, L. (2004) Special Issue: 'Celebrating Class Sociology: Pioneers of Contemporary British Qualitative Research', *International Journal of Social Research Methodology*, 7(1).

Welshman, J. (2007) *From Transmitted Deprivation to Social Exclusion: Policy, Poverty and Parenting*, Bristol: Policy Press.

2 Building a stable environment in Scotland

Planning parenthood in a time of ecological crisis

Katharine Dow

Sitting in a pub in a small town in north-eastern Scotland, Erin told me about her experience of becoming a mother five years previously. In the course of our interview, I had asked her whether she felt that becoming a mother had affected the way she thought about herself. She responded at some length:

ERIN: Absolutely, beyond a doubt. In a good and a bad way. Good way – you feel very proud, you know, somebody that's related to you, that you love, that you've created, so immensely proud and it's immensely positive because you are given a chance for another identity if you like.

In a bad way, I'd lie if I didn't say that there are sacrifices, there are compromises, that come with being a parent and they sometimes can be really, really difficult and costly.… It's not life and death, but sometimes you feel that, whether it's the old you that you don't recognise so much any more, you know, as you change and as you evolve and become a parent, there are times when you sort of get glimpses of, if I wasn't a parent, I might be doing this, or, I might take this opportunity or that opportunity.

…the most responsibility I think is … not just the basic to be warm and fed, watered, you know sort of healthy and in a stable environment, some of it comes from, I think there's a notion of, with each generation, you want to, as good as things my parents gave me, I'd like to extend that further. That's part of my – I feel – my personal responsibility.

Amongst those I spoke to in researching this chapter, Erin was not alone in feeling that an important part of becoming a parent was to create a 'stable environment'. All agreed that the first steps in becoming a parent should be to plan and get everything ready. This stable environment, to borrow Erin's phrase, is an ethical concept that condenses gendered and classed ideals of good parenting. In this chapter, I will explore how concerns about caring for children reflect not only dominant ideologies of parenting, but, in this case, also relate to our responsibilities to care for the environment and lead good lives.

This chapter is based on ethnographic research that I undertook between 2006 and 2007. I was investigating how people think, and make ethical judgements about, surrogacy. In contrast to many ethnographies that have examined people's experiences of undergoing assisted conception treatment, my research responds to the fact that surrogacy is also a subject of intense moral interest even for those not involved. I was based in a small coastal village in north-eastern Scotland, which is home to a wildlife centre run by an international conservation charity. Most of the people I came into contact with there are connected to the centre through paid or voluntary work and they therefore share an interest in environmentalism and leading 'good' lives. They are all white, broadly speaking middle class and university educated and almost all of the centre's volunteers work in the public sector or 'caring' professions. Most are migrants to the area, largely from England but also from other parts of Scotland and Western Europe.[1]

I collected data through participant observation and interviews. As a participant observer, I was involved to a varying extent in the lives of around sixty people and I carried out interviews with thirty women and men of various ages whom I met through my initial network at the wildlife centre. I used this mixed methodology to formulate a contextualised analysis of how people make ethical judgements, relating my observations of their everyday practice to the claims they made about surrogacy in interviews, tracing the connections between their moral values and ethical decisions in claims and in practice. In the course of my discussions with these people, we did talk about much more than surrogacy and a subject that frequently came up was respondents' own experiences of, or plans for, parenthood. In this chapter I will narrow my focus upon responses from women in their twenties and early thirties who did not have children at the time of interview. These women were all at a stage in their life where they were focused on building careers that offer opportunities to fulfil their interests, to 'make a difference' and be economically self-sufficient. Their deliberations about becoming a parent demonstrate the assumption that parenthood can, and should, be planned – that planning parenthood is a sign that one intends to be a *good* parent. If something has been planned, these people assume, that means it is less likely to be risky, more likely to be stable and that the individuals involved have been responsible. In looking at these women's plans, I will show that judging when and how to become a parent is not necessarily straightforward, but usually entails a precise negotiation of ideals and realities.

Writing in the 1990s, Sharon Hays argued that intensive parenting, which is 'child-centred', expert-guided, emotionally absorbing, labour-intensive and financially expensive, was the dominant ideology of socially appropriate childrearing in the US (1996: 8–9, *passim*; see Introduction, this volume). As she noted, while this is ostensibly an ideology of parenting, *women* are expected to be the primary caregivers of children and so this ideology is primarily relevant to mothers. Crucially, Hays identified two 'contradictions' of motherhood within this milieu: that its intensification is coterminous with women's increased participation in the paid labour-force and that the valorisation of selfless nurturing exemplified by the 'good mother' has come about in a late capitalist context in which it is assumed that human behaviour is led by rational choices and profit maximisation. As this and other chapters in this volume will show, the culture of intensive parenting is not confined to the United States, nor is it in abeyance now we have settled into the twenty-first century. It has, if anything, been amplified.

In many OECD countries, there is a sense that children exist in risky, or even toxic, environments (see Furedi 2002; Lee *et al.* 2010; Lyerly *et al.* 2009; Hoffman 2010; Shirani *et al.* 2012; Faircloth 2010; Lupton 2011). In this ideology, good parenting is a means of mitigating myriad environmental risks and doing too little to protect one's child from external risks is 'bad' or 'neglectful' parenting. In this context, which is also one of greater visibility of (in)fertility, access to family planning, assisted reproductive technologies (ART) and 'alternative' family forms (see Göknar, this volume), parenting has become contested and politicised. The unprecedented level of public articulation of parenting is a characteristic aspect of the culture of intensive parenting. Although, the ability to label, and thereby rationalise, how one cares for one's child as a particular style of parenting – whether that be 'attachment parenting', 'free range parenting' or being a 'tiger mum' – is not equally available to all (see Berry; Jaysane-Darr; Murray; Jiménez Sedano this volume).

Implicit in the vision of a parent protecting her child from its risky environment is the assumption that children are naturally passive and innocent (see also Miller 2004; Zelizer 1985) and that ageing is a battle against the corrupting and tainting influences of the outside world. It often indexes nostalgia (Edwards and Gillies, this volume), along with an assumption that future stability can be achieved through good choices. This sense of loss, and the idea that forward planning and taking certain actions in the present can create a better environment, also resonates with environmentalist ethics, as we shall see.

With intensification, parenting has become highly moralised. As a number of scholars have pointed out, there are significant congruities between the norms and aspirations of intensive parenting culture and those of the white middle-classes of OECD countries (see Hoffman 2010; Lee *et al.* 2010). The ideology of parental responsibility, which underlies intensive parenting, is highly gendered (Shirani *et al.* 2012) and classed (Hays 1996); it also rests on a vision of empowerment through consumption. Intensive parenting is enabled by having a certain amount of money – whether that be to afford extracurricular ballet lessons, to access the services of experts such as child psychologists or the ability to survive on a single income while one parent stays at home to parent intensively.

As parenting has intensified in its expectations and its moral weight, it has also extended its reach backwards in time to before the child is even born. An emerging literature on this has examined examples including foetal alcohol syndrome (Lowe *et al.* 2010), food choices during pregnancy (Lee 2007; Miller 2004), pregnant women's exposure to environmental risks (Kukla 2010), women's reasons for taking the contraceptive pill (Boydell 2010) and the 'better safe than sorry' approach of contemporary obstetrical care (Lyerly *et al.* 2009; see also Davis-Floyd 1992). This shows the deep penetration of intensive parenting, as well as the importance of the surveillance of oneself and others that this ideology provokes (Hinton *et al.*; Jensen, this volume). Unlike the others in this volume, this chapter is centred on people's ideas about parenting, rather than their practices. Yet, in reflecting upon what becoming a parent means for these people, I hope to show that, in a cultural context in which good parenting is intensive parenting, parental – and particularly, maternal – responsibility increasingly begins long before conception, in ideals, expectations and plans.

The everyday life of the people I met during fieldwork is inflected by a sense that they, and any future children they might have, live in an increasingly unstable environment. They believe that the world is facing future crisis because of the cumulative effects of anthropogenic activity on the natural environment. Through their work in the wildlife centre and the way they use resources in their everyday lives, from 'ethical shopping' to recycling waste and minimising fossil fuel consumption, they are making efforts to conserve natural habitats and prevent climate change. For them, the stability that parents should offer their future children relates to sustainability, security, planning and the proper management of resources – not just in the child's domestic set-up, but also in the wider world. These women's plans for parenthood reflect not only the ideology of intensive parenting that dominates their wider cultural milieu, but also the particular values of the environmentalist movement. Indeed, one of my aims here is to show that many of the overarching principles of environmentalism and intensive parenting overlap, and that running through both ethics is a sense that 'nature' and 'the natural' can provide ethical guidance. In terms of practice, or everyday ethics, the key point of contact between these two sets of principles is the basic assumption that goodness comes from being oriented towards others' needs. Taking the decision to embody the values of the environmental movement and to be a good parent both entail a reorientation of the self towards altruism and away from individualism or 'selfishness', which goes along with a temporal reorientation towards the future rather than the present.

A few years before Hays' work on intensive parenting was published, Marilyn Strathern identified the expectation that parents should provide their children with the right environment in which to develop as an 'axiom' of Euro-American kinship (1992: 24). In *After Nature*, she says that the late twentieth century was characterised by a sense that there was less nature in the world (1992: 37) as it, like everything else, had become inextricably linked with choice and visible only as personal style (1992: 177). Strathern's crucial claim about nature in this time is that its 'grounding function' had been lost, so that it 'no longer provide[d] a model or analogy for the very idea of context' (1992: 195). By examining people's plans for parenthood in a context of intensive parenting and environmentalist ethics, I will show that nature has not, in fact, been flattened as Strathern predicted, but continues to have a grounding function. This is not to imply a return to earlier ideas of nature, but it does suggest that ideas about nature have subtly shifted in the two decades since the publication of *After Nature*. With environmentalism and ethical living, nature has become invested with a particular kind of moral authority, but also acts as the ultimate source of goodness and hope in an increasingly risky environment.

A stable environment

At the time I interviewed her, Sophie was in her late twenties and in a hetero-sexual relationship. After some years working on conservation projects around the world, she had moved to Scotland to work in the wildlife centre. I asked her whether she perceived a relationship between contemporary lifestyles and low birth rates in Western societies. She said:

SOPHIE: I think if you start saying that it's the way people live their lives it makes it sound a bit like, 'you're doing something evil', it sounds like that … when I was at university we had a couple of classes which talked about fertility and we were talking about farm animals, the lecturer was then just bringing into play that actually humans are pretty crap at being fertile if you compare them to the farm animals and the fact that we breed those over the successive generations to be really fertile. And because there are maybe some things that don't naturally select out because people who can have some help to allow fertility – maybe there is an element of that, that they're all going a bit down the scientific route. So I'd be a bit averse to say, to go down the line that says, 'oh well, we've almost asked for it', but I do think that there are some things that we can't get away from, that probably we are going to find it harder and harder. Then again, I suppose the other part would be from the ecologist's point of view, I might say, well, there's quite a lot of humans and maybe this is just the way it goes, maybe this is the way the cycle goes.

In this response, Sophie not only brings together ecology, agriculture and demography, drawing on her undergraduate education, but, in her opening comment, demonstrates her awareness of the ethical implications of judging other people's reproductive choices. This quote eloquently expresses her complex apprehension of nature (cf. Edwards and Salazar 2009): nature can be managed highly successfully and fruitfully, as agricultural breeding demon-strates, yet people should be careful about venturing too far 'down the scientific route'. Sophie's concerns about the environment and runaway technological development were shared by her friends, yet they all also felt great sympathy for the desire to have children 'of one's own', which they saw as natural and time-less. I will return to these concerns after outlining Sophie and her friends' own plans for parenthood.

The participants in my research are generally left of centre in their politics and do not believe there is one ideal template for parenting, although there are some general expectations about what makes an appropriate environment.

Perhaps most obviously, parents should have some regular income that will cover the expenses of having a child as well as a suitable home in which to bring it up. They also assume that parents should feel ready. For those who were not already in stable relationships, having a partner and father for the child – even if the relationship turned out not to be forever – was crucial. This reflects an assumption that the father would support the family financially and the mother would be the primary caregiver, though mothers could return to work later if that was right for them.

The importance of choice, timing and money were readily apparent when I asked Sophie's colleague, Lauren, about her plans for parenthood:

KD: Do you plan or expect to become a mother at some point?

LAUREN: Financially? Clearly, no! I mean, I live at the bottom of my overdraft. I mean, I think, although I don't actively plan to have kids, I now have a number of friends who are married and having children, and it does start to occur to you how many years it would take, you know, to have a child. Like, best – well, shortest – scenario, you decide today that you want to have a child, you find out you're pregnant in months, if you're lucky, and then, so, basically best scenario would be a year until you get, until you have your child, and for most people that's not the case, particularly with the amount of birth control that we've all had, sort of – 'forced down our throats' is a little bit violent – but there's been so many, there have been all the reasons why you may not conceive as quickly as you might, and if you're starting at a later age,... so if I'm ready in two years and then it takes me three years to get pregnant, it's suddenly five years away, which occurs to me now, but not in a way like, 'I want a child at age thirty-one, therefore I should start'. I haven't reached that particular stage in my life.... And if I can't have a dog, then I certainly can't have a baby! That's the way I feel about it: I'm not stable enough to have a puppy – no baby either.

Despite not being at the right 'stage' to actively plan for parenthood, Lauren had clearly given it careful consideration. She was aware that one cannot completely control the process of getting pregnant, but only try to provide the right conditions for it to occur. Her ambivalence about this is evident in her vivid suggestion, though she immediately dismisses it, that women have had contraceptives 'forced down our throats'. Lauren co-habits with her partner, Jack, who was much less concerned about planning parenthood, despite the fact that he was, at the time, unemployed. He explained to me that his older sister had recently given birth after an unplanned pregnancy and that it had worked out, so he knew that people do cope with such events.[2]

I asked Sophie if she felt it would be appropriate for the Scottish government to try to actively increase fertility levels in the country. She felt that the best thing for public bodies to do would be to provide as much information as possible about risks to fertility so that women could make informed choices about when to get pregnant (see also Friese *et al.* 2006). She explained:

SOPHIE: I suppose the variety of reasons why people might decide to delay having kids are so vast and it may be something that's absolutely critical for them to feel like they could support a kid in the future. And in that case, they're really trying to do something good and I always try and think about the child's future as well. I don't know what kind of, well I suppose then we're talking about money, but it's not just that, is it? It might be other things that they're trying to gain experience of.

Sophie told me that when she was younger she had assumed she would not have children, but as she had got older she had changed her mind.

SOPHIE: I think my reasoning at the time would have been quite selfish and I would have said, [having children] just gets in the way of my life, actually, and also I don't need kids to be happy. And it was a bit of rebelling from that which seems to be the norm. And I still feel that I don't need them to be happy, but I just feel like I've changed on the view of whether I could see it in the future and I can now, rather than just me thinking … I can hardly look after myself, I'm not sure I can look after any kids. … But I think I feel a bit more, now, that what is most important is being able to care for them and that's something I feel a bit more able to do.

Amy, who was single and in her early thirties, spent many years travelling and working in conservation projects around the world before starting her current job in the wildlife centre. While she enjoyed this exciting phase of her life, she felt that her decision to have this lifestyle meant she might have missed out on some of the positive aspects of settling down:

AMY: I think people need to do what they need to do. But then again, I feel it's a bit of a shame as well, 'cos it's like, I've enjoyed travelling and I think it's taken me a while to get the job I want, but then, kind of, I do think it might have been nicer if I'd settled down maybe a couple of years ago…

Yeah, I think when I do have children, I think I'll be ready for them, 'cos I have done what I've wanted to do beforehand, instead of kind of, 'oh, I'll have children' then 'oh my god, but I still haven't done stuff'. 'Cos I have got one friend of mine who, I guess theirs was an unplanned pregnancy and I think, they're not regretting having the child, but I think they're regretting giving up a bit of their freedom.

In the quote at the beginning of this piece, Erin talked about how motherhood was a positive new phase in her life, in which her needs became secondary to her daughter's. She talked about motherhood as a reinvention of identity, but she did not simply mean that her status as a woman or her relationship to her husband had changed. Motherhood brought not just a change in lifestyle, but a whole new personal and interpersonal ethic. Crucially, Amy, Lauren and Sophie's comments indicate that they anticipate and accept such fundamental change as part of their futures as mothers. That they feel they must build stable environments for their future children reflects a specific assumption about what parenthood does to parents' lives. Embedded in this expectation is a split between life as a childless adult – which includes fulfilling experiences, meaningful work and self-development – and life as a parent, in which everyday life, and personal fulfilment, is characterised by responding to the needs of a dependent child.

As successful career women in a competitive, if not lucrative, field, Amy, Lauren and Sophie typify the group that might be expected to have internalised and benefited most from feminism and the increased participation of women in the paid workforce over the last century. They nonetheless expect to be the primary caregivers of their children. They assume that they will display self-abnegatory levels of maternal responsibility in caring intensively for their children, while their children's fathers' primary responsibility remains as providing economic security. In highlighting the sacrifices of being a good mother, then, they are both noting the losses to the self that this change of identity brings about, but also valorising the choice to take on that loss.

Time and the stable environment

Willow was in her mid-twenties, single and working in the wildlife centre at the time I interviewed her. She said:

WILLOW: I think our generation is quite lucky in some ways, 'cos we have got all these opportunities. I know that my mum said that when she was at uni., she had a choice of either doing nursing or teaching, and now we've got a lot more choice. So we've ... suddenly been opened up to all these possibilities, but at the same time, we're hemmed in by biology [she laughs ironically], so it's really hard. We go and get educated and we think, well, hey, we want to do something with that now, but at the same time, you know, you have to start having kids at some point. But I can totally understand why people are having kids later. By the time my parents were my age they were married. I think they would be a bit shocked if I turned round and said I was getting married, you know, they'd [say], 'oh, you're far too young!'

This tension between choice and expectation that Willow identifies in her own reproductive options was also apparent when we discussed the example of older women using assisted conception when they could no longer conceive 'naturally'. Comparing these people's ideas about older mothers with their own plans for parenthood demonstrates the significance of maternal age in good parenting. In their view, Willow and younger women like her at the beginning of their careers are naturally ready to parent yet they are not ready to offer their children the right conditions in which to be *good* parents. Meanwhile, older women who need to use assisted conception to help them conceive may have the right material conditions but their natural capacity to parent (intensively) will be impaired because of their age.

On the subject of post-menopausal women using assisted conception, Sophie remarked:

SOPHIE: Personally, although it goes right against some of my right-on views, I think that [not being able to have children past menopause] *is* nature, and – unless this is some medical condition which has meant that menopause has come in way earlier in life, if it's natural – no, I don't think there should be any intervention then, especially when there are kids who need homes and all those things.

[Original emphasis]

As these comments demonstrate, timing parenthood is a delicate balancing act because nature should not always be left to run its course, but in fact needs to be managed. Sophie told me subsequently about her discomfort with the 'conservatism', as she put it, of her views on this issue, as did Amy when I interviewed her. They both experienced a conflict between what they feel is right according to their political self-positioning and what is right according to their conceptions of naturalness. When nature and morality do not neatly map onto each other, this creates ethical and political dilemmas. These dilemmas would not arise were nature not seen as a source of moral guidance.

Lauren's keen sense of the importance of age was evident in the earlier quote in which she reckoned out how she might time her own future pregnancy. She was also concerned about older women using assisted conception:

LAUREN: I don't really like that medical science is pushing us beyond sort of natural human boundaries as far as it is ... there have to be some lines that you let nature take its course, and, you know, as hard as it is for the woman who doesn't want, choose to have a child 'til she's fifty, there are some natural limits there and there are kind of reasons why your body doesn't want you to have a child when you're fifty, and that partially is because you'll be sixty-five when your child's fifteen and, you know, you are pushing those situations. The sticky point – that men can still conceive at that point in time, so why ... can you say that a man can do it but a woman can't? But that, that's the way, I mean, I hate to say it but that's the way it is, is how I think I feel and I think that I quite like that there are some things, I s'pose, that are just, 'that's the way it is'.

The scenario of post-menopausal women using assisted conception represents a risk, because a child's mother may not be able to fully give her time, care and attention to her child as there is a greater likelihood that she may have to depend on others' help herself. So, in this scenario, personal choice and natural expectation are unbalanced. As Lauren's idea of 'natural human boundaries' suggests, it is best to time parenthood while nature can still 'take its course'. Choosing to have a child past an age when you would ordinarily be able to naturally seems to these women to be a prioritising of one's own desires over the future child's needs.

These quotes show that, in the complex and sometimes 'sticky' world of reproductive decision-making, nature acts as a common reference point, yet sometimes this creates dilemmas. In discussing ethical judgements in contemporary capitalist cultures, Michael Lambek says, 'Practice emerges through evaluation, the sizing up and fitting of action to circumstance. Yet judgment selects among alternatives not by means of a binary logic of exclusive acceptance or rejection but by balancing among qualities' (2008: 137). The examples here expose this process of weighing up and balancing ideal principles against the constraints of our everyday commitments, the contingency that inheres in building a good life and planning parenthood. There is always a gap between ideals and realities, and everyday ethics is about managing this gap by achieving a stable balance. In reproduction, the stakes are so high because the ideals being balanced are the 'natural' drive to reproduce (becoming a parent) and individual aspirations for parenthood and childhood (being a good parent).

An unstable environment?

Participants shared the assumption that having children 'of one's own' is an understandable, if 'selfish', choice, in a context in which there are, as Sophie put it, 'kids who need homes' and increasing pressure on natural resources. This concern was eloquently expressed by Andrew, who was volunteering full-time in the wildlife centre at the time of our interview. He was in his mid-twenties, in a long-term relationship and childless. In talking about assisted conception, Andrew expressed a conflict between sympathy for infertile couples' 'natural' desire to have a child and his concern that in achieving this, science might take over from nature:

ANDREW: I think, in our society, or the human race as a whole, we've evolved beyond evolution. The fact that now, people who naturally can't conceive can now conceive with science. There's huge pressure on this planet in terms of resources for a number of people and so one part of me says, 'if you can't do it naturally, you shouldn't do it at all'. On the other hand, I can totally, entirely understand on an individual level that if you want a kid then you're gonna do everything that you can possibly do to have that child.

These comments and the concerns about older women using assisted conception I have just outlined point to a shared sense that, while nature can be managed and assisted, people should be careful about taking this too far (see also Hirsch 1993).

We have seen the importance of time in achieving a stable environment for parenthood. This is also evident in these people's concerns about the wider environment, as Andrew indicates in his stark comment that we have 'evolved beyond evolution'. In Sophie's earlier comments about farm animals she juxtaposed different temporalities, drawing on the linear, progressive temporality of science and animal husbandry but also referred to a cyclical ecological time in her suggestion that humans will eventually make themselves extinct by relying excessively on science to reproduce (see also Macnaghten and Urry 1998: 143 on glacial time and its links to environmentalism and globalisation).

Andrew's comments return us to these people's sense of impending ecological crisis. These women's sense of the costs of motherhood reflects the intensive parenting culture in which they live, but also resonates with the demands of living a good, environmentally friendly, life. Although they might think of themselves as being in a 'selfish' period of their lives, these women are not in fact living self-indulgent and hedonistic lives. They have moved across the country (or even the world) to work in conservation and are enacting and embodying particular ethical principles, by making choices that do least harm to their social and natural environment. Most importantly, this is an orientation of the individual towards others' needs. The ideal of building stable environments permeates their lives now, before they have children; it also structures their plans for parenthood.

These women want their future children to live in secure families, cooperative communities and healthy environments and they expect to effect this through careful planning that will allow them to balance their material conditions with their emotional maturity and natural drives. I have noted that there is, necessarily, a gap between ideals and reality in this; Lauren's comment about having contraception forced down our throats is just one example of this uneasy tension. Building an environment that is structured by a stable balance of nature and choice is an act of maternal responsibility that demonstrates the capacity and intention to be a good parent. It also indexes the fact that parents, and their future children, live in a risky world which can be stabilised through making responsible choices. In this model motherhood marks the transition from being a selfish adult towards becoming a caring and altruistic parent.

Conclusion

Environmentalist ideas posit a time of imminent climactic chaos and ecological crisis, but the fact that these women are nonetheless planning for parenthood suggests that they think of the future as a time of stability, in their personal lives if not the wider environment. Despite their concerns about impending environmental catastrophe, they are not at sea in a meaningless world, as nature provides ethical guidance. By working with, rather than against, it, they can implement good lives and envisage a good future.

These women see parenthood as something that should be carefully planned because they anticipate taking on the primary responsibility for childcare, despite the fact that they expect to be treated as equal to men in their careers and other relationships. This inequality was rationalised with reference to nature and biology. Similarly, in explaining their concerns about certain uses of ART, they also referred to nature to ground their claims. They turn to nature for ethical and moral guidance, even though nature does not mean exactly the same thing to each of them. This slipperiness of nature is demonstrated by the tension they perceive between the natural desire to procreate and the fact that this need may be threatened by excessive human activity through technological intervention or inappropriate personal choices. Yet, despite their different ideas of what nature is and what the consequences of 'interfering' with it might be, they all refer to it as if it were a self-regulating whole with discernable limits, boundaries and order, suggesting it is fundamentally timeless and transcendent. It is this that gives it its purchase. Nature is for these people a real, tangible thing that exists 'out there' in the trees, mountains and seas and which requires conservation and care, but also a transcendent force, at once benign and dangerous. It is for this reason that it needs to be managed through careful planning.

While these people invest nature with a great deal of moral authority and often elide naturalness with goodness, they do not think of nature as straightforwardly benign. Similarly, while they are critical of excessive consumerism and the unsustainable use of natural resources, for them both individual choice and money can be put towards ethical ends. Responsibility and choice are inextricably linked – individuals have the capacity to choose to do the right thing, by being responsible consumers and living their lives in ways that have minimal negative impact on others. While creating a stable environment for future generations represents a heavy burden of responsibility and a foreclosing of certain pleasurable experiences, it also indexes an expectation that individuals *can* control their environments. Intensive parenting is an ideology that makes most sense within a middle-class milieu; the same can be said for environmentalism. While these women have in a sense chosen to live on the margins by relocating to a rural, sparsely populated area of the country, they are also educated, professionally employed and socially and politically engaged. Their sense that they *can* plan the future is premised on the agency that comes with having access to a certain amount of cultural and financial capital.

Strathern argued that, in the late twentieth century, moral choices were no longer tied to stable reference points such as nature and that as a result, 'the norms and canons of behaviour ... no longer need lie in institutions outside the individual' (1992: 162). In the late twentieth century, she said, the individual looked beyond herself for moral guidance but, because nature had become destabilised by human activity and so could no longer act as a stable reference point, she could not find anything better than her self in which to locate her desires and choices. The people I have described here do not turn inwards in making moral decisions and find sufficient grounds to support their claims or structure their lives, but look out into their environment and see nature. Using nature in order to ground particular claims entails referring to a realm beyond humanity and it is by managing the elastic gap in between themselves and nature that they can make 'good' choices and judgements.

Having a good life is about living up to ethical principles and enacting moral choices, but also about finding fulfilment and having meaningful experiences. Similarly, in intensive parenting culture, mothers talk about the 'reward' of mothering as receiving unconditional love, experiencing emotional fulfilment and the satisfaction of producing a happy, stable child. There are clear congruities between the image of the good mother posited by intensive parenting culture and the principles of environmentalist ethical living practised by the people I have discussed here. The common ground between intensive parenting and environmental ethics goes deep, because they share a sense that nature is a source of goodness.

In this intensive parenting culture (and see Miller 2004), the child is assumed to be naturally pure and innocent. Good parenting is child-centred because children are closer to nature than their parents, who have been exposed to the risky external world for their whole lives. Both environmentalism and intensive parenting valorise nature and, implicitly, critique the outside world as being greedy, selfish and corrupting. In this way, they reinforce long-standing associations between nature and love, purity, compassion and fulfilment. As Hays (1996: 154) argues, the 'contradiction' of parenting intensifying in a context of late capitalism is no paradox. Intensive motherhood is, in fact, indexical of profound ambivalence about the universal penetration of market values. Valuing natural, pure children and the parenting methods that make them is not only a positive move, but also an implicit critique of dominant cultural mores.

We have seen that these pre-parturient women feel that they can only be ready for motherhood once they have learnt to be independent, responsible adults. Having the opportunity to be 'selfish' by living their own lives before becoming parents seems to be a pre-emptive response to the knowledge that their lives will be changed irrevocably by parenthood, but also suggests they believe that becoming less selfish is a general good. Building a good life is a project that looks towards a relational future in which the self is oriented towards others' needs.

We are all familiar with the idea that children symbolise the future, and this may be one reason why they represent a glimmer of hope through their parents' very real sense of crisis. However, I would suggest that it is not only the children themselves that provide hope in an unstable world, but the responsible choices their parents have made in building stable environments for them. For the women we have met here, good parents produce good children who know the importance of thinking of others and caring for their environment and the others they share it with. So, if having children is an inevitable, natural event in people's lives and futures, the least that parents can do is to face up to their responsibilities to plan, care for and stabilise the environments into which they are born, and to pass that on to future generations.

Notes

1 This region of Scotland experiences quite high turnover in its population. While migrants to the area are certainly a minority, the percentage of English-born migrants in Moray as a county is twice that as for Scotland as a whole: 16 per cent compared to 8 per cent (GROS 2009).

2 Lauren is unusual amongst these women in that she had moved to the area with her partner. The single women perceive there to be a dearth of potential partners in this area and there is a tacit acceptance amongst them that, while this area might offer the best kind of life for a young family, if they stay there forever they run the risk of never finding a father for those future children.

Bibliography

Boydell, Victoria. 2010. 'The social life of the pill: an ethnography of the oral contraceptive pill', unpublished PhD thesis, London School of Economics.

Davis-Floyd, Robbie. 1992. *Birth as an American Rite of Passage*. Oxford: University of California Press.

Edwards, Jeanette and Carles Salazar (eds). 2009. *European Kinship in the Age of Biotechnology*. Oxford: Berghahn Books.

Faircloth, Charlotte. 2010. 'If they want to risk the health and well-being of their child, that's up to them': long-term breastfeeding, risk and maternal identity.' *Heath, Risk and Society* Special Issue: 'Child-rearing in an Age of Risk.' 12(4): 357–367.

Franklin, Sarah. 1997. *Embodied Progress: A Cultural Account of Assisted Conception*. London: Routledge.

Friese, Carrie, Gay Becker and Robert D. Nachtigall. 2006. Rethinking the biological clock: eleventh hour moms, miracle moms, and meanings of age-related infertility. *Social Science and Medicine* 63(6): 1550–1560.

Furedi, Frank. 2002. *Paranoid Parenting: Why Ignoring the Experts May be Best for Your Child*. Chicago: Chicago Review Press.

GROS (General Register Office for Scotland). 2009. *Grampian Migration Report*, Edinburgh: General Register Office for Scotland, online, available at: http://s3.amazonaws. com/zanran_storage/www.gro-scotland.gov.uk/ContentPages/ 20112457.pdf.

Hays, Sharon. 1996. *The Cultural Contradictions of Motherhood*. London: Yale University Press.

Hirsch, Eric. 1993. Negotiated limits: interviews in south-east England. In Jeanette Edwards, Sarah Franklin, Eric Hirsch, Frances Price and Marilyn Strathern (eds) *Technologies of Procreation: Kinship in the Age of Assisted Conception*. Manchester: Manchester University Press.

Hoffman, Diane M. 2010. Risky investments: parenting and the production of the 'resilient child'. *Health, Risk and Society* 12(4): 385–394.

Kukla, Rebecca. 2010. The ethics and cultural politics of reproductive risk warnings: a case study of California's Proposition 65. *Health, Risk and Society* 12(4): 323–334.

Lambek, Michael. 2008. Value and virtue. *Anthropological Theory* 8(2): 133–157.

Lee, Ellie. 2007. Infant feeding in risk society. *Health, Risk and Society* 9(3): 295–309.

Lee, Ellie, Jan Macvarish and Jennie Bristow. 2010. Risk, health and parenting culture. *Health, Risk and Society* 12(4): 293–300.

Lowe, Pam, Ellie Lee and Liz Yardley. 2010. Under the influence? The construction of foetal alcohol syndrome in UK newspapers. *Sociological Research Online* 15(4)2, online, available at: www.socresonline.org.uk/15/4/2.html.

Lyerly, Anne D., Lisa M. Mitchell, Elizabeth Mitchell Armstrong, Lisa H. Harris, Rebecca Kukla, Miriam Kupperman and Margaret Olivia Little. 2009. Risk and the pregnant body. *Hastings Center Report* 39(6): 34–42.

Lupton, Deborah A. 2011. 'The best thing for the baby': mothers' concepts and experiences related to promoting their infants' health and development. *Health, Risk and Society* 13(7/8): 637–651.

Macnaghten, Phil and John Urry. 1998. *Contested Natures*. London: Sage.

Miller, Daniel. 2004. How infants grow mothers in North London. In Janelle S. Taylor, Linda L. Layne and Danielle F. Wozniak (eds) *Consuming Motherhood*. London: Rutgers University Press.

Shirani, Fiona, Karen Henwood and Carrie Coltart. 2012. Meeting the challenges of intensive parenting culture: gender, risk management and the moral parent. *Sociology* 46(1): 25–40.

Strathern, Marilyn. 1992. *After Nature: English Kinship in the Late Twentieth Century.* Cambridge: Cambridge University Press.

Zelizer, Viviana A. Rotman. 1985. *Pricing the Priceless Child: The Changing Social Value of Children.* Chichester: Princeton University Press.

3   Creating distinction

Middle-class viewers of *Supernanny* in the UK

Tracey Jensen

In a wide range of government policy and public fora, training people to become 'good parents' is now envisaged as a central means through which the economic costs of delivering social welfare might be radically reduced, through a transfer of responsibility from the state to 'parent-citizens'. These 'parental pedagogies' are imagined as a means to address the problems of stagnant social mobility and in the past decade there has been an explosion of these pedagogies across public, private and voluntary sectors. The widely accepted public and policy narrative is that these parental pedagogies are so popular because contemporary parents are helpless and hungry for professional advice.

This chapter draws on research to argue that the relationship between parents and parental pedagogy is in fact far more complex. I examine how parental pedagogy is adopted, transformed, reconfigured, shaped and made meaningful by parents themselves, and explore how these meanings are central to their identities as parents. Drawing on innovative audience research data collected with parents as they consume parent pedagogies delivered through popular representational genres, this chapter examines the sociocultural meanings that circulate around parent training.

Whilst the parents in this research seem to have absorbed the broader logic of intensive parenting (Hays, 1996), their sociocultural relationships with parenting experts and parent pedagogy were far from clear-cut. Indeed, this research finds that it is *through* negotiations with different experts and philosophies – resisting, refusing, disclaiming – that parents produce versions of themselves as 'choosing to become' specific kinds of parents and attach themselves to particular forms of moral value. This essay examines how parental pedagogies and professional expertise provide (some) parents with an opportunity for social distinction, a space to reproduce/reconfigure moral assumptions about parenting and a potent framework for late-modern discourses of 'choice'.

Parent pedagogy: entertainment and education

Parental pedagogies have been with us for many generations: from 'mothercraft' manuals of the eighteenth and nineteenth centuries, through multiple knowledge paradigms around the 'science of babycare' incorporating advances in hygiene and nutrition, to new vocabularies around the self such as those offered in psychotherapy (Hulbert, 2003; Apple, 2006; Grant, 1998). What distinguishes contemporary parental pedagogy as 'new' is its hypervisibility and its extension into popular representational forms such as television, thus fusing education with entertainment and promising to train and teach its participating on-screen families how to 'parent better' even as it amuses and delights its viewers and voyeurs. This new intimate inflection of parent pedagogy complicates older models of pedagogical consumption and invites parents into new processes of morality-making and voyeurship (Dovey, 2000; Skeggs and Wood, 2012). The larger research project from which the discussion in this chapter is drawn was concerned with one specific example of parent pedagogy, the television programme *Supernanny* (2004–2011, Channel 4, UK).

As well as being phenomenally successful in terms of both audience share in the UK and overseas franchises, *Supernanny* is enormously significant in terms of parenting culture because has been politically seized upon as evidence of a new kind of hunger and demand from parents for state interventions into their intimate lives. One 2006 survey, conducted on behalf of the National Family and Parenting Institute (NFPI),[1] found that 55 per cent of all adults (72 per cent of all parents) had watched at least one parenting programme, with *Supernanny* 'emerging as a clear winner' having been watched by 42 per cent of all adults. *Supernanny* has come to serve as political shorthand for the explosion of parent pedagogy, on television and in other popular forms and for a new appetite for being taught how to parent 'better'. In a keynote speech to the Institute for Public Policy in 2006, Children's Minister Beverley Hughes stated that 'government too must extend the opportunities for parents to develop their expertise; the popularity of *Supernanny* exemplifies the hunger for information and for effective parenting programmes that parents often express to me' (Hughes, 2006). In a *Guardian* interview that same year, Louise Casey, leader of the Respect Task Force, drew parallels between *Supernanny* and examples of advocacy television, stating that

> Jamie Oliver rightly landed on school meals and said 'we are feeding children such bad food that they cannot sit down in the classroom' and I think the millions watching TV about parenting are saying the same thing to government
>
> (Wintour, 2006)

Shortly after this interview, Casey's department announced that a central part of their anti-social behaviour and social mobility strategy would be implemented by funding an 'army of Supernannies' across the UK. In the foreword to *Every Parent Matters* (2007), Education Secretary Alan Johnson stated that 'parents are demonstrating a growing appetite for discussion, information and advice, as we see from the increasingly vibrant market in television programmes, magazines and websites' (DfES, 2007: 1). There are many more examples of this desire to cast the watching of *Supernanny* as politically meaningful – as if watching can be interpreted as making the statement 'I need help with my parenting' – and to treat the successful ratings of a highly voyeuristic (and some might argue exploitative) reality programme as evidence, *in and of itself*, of the need to intervene and regulate intimate life.

As researchers we should rightly ask, why are people watching popular parent pedagogy such as *Supernanny* in such numbers? But we also need to ask who these parents are, how they are watching the programme and what the relationship is between who they are and how they watch. What tools can we use to get behind audience ratings and begin to understand the meaning of parental pedagogy in contemporary parenting culture? Both the NFPI survey and the politicians who enthusiastically drew on its findings presume that the relationship between parents and parent pedagogy is rational, elective and purposive: that parents consume parent pedagogy because they choose it and they want it. This replicates all kinds of problematic notions about a particular ideal respondent who has clear viewer preferences that can be isolated from the rich and complex moments of viewing. It assumes that *Supernanny* holds the same meanings at a textual level for each member of its audience, and that being a *Supernanny* viewer at a contextual level means the same thing for each member of that audience. These notions have been usefully troubled by innovative audience research which demonstrates the emotional messiness and complexity of media and cultural consumption (Hermes, 1995; Devine and Savage, 2005; Hill, 2005; Seiter, 1999). This research examines both the preferences that viewers might *report* to a survey or poll, and the actual encounter they have during viewing itself, in order to explore how parent pedagogy serves as a constitutive spaces through which parental identities are formed. Such encounters are frequently fraught, complex and troubling, and *how* one views *Supernanny* viewers is part of a complex affective process within the wider field of parenting pedagogy, which operates as a site of division and distinction.

Methods: watching *Supernanny*

The research uses multiple methods to get behind audience ratings and explore how parent pedagogy is consumed and made meaningful. This chapter draws on research with fifteen parents, who were interviewed, either alone or within peer groups that they had assembled, about their experiences of and relationship with contemporary parenting advice. These interviews were semi-structured, often moving into organic and tangential discussions, around the topics of self-definitions, parenting philosophy, good and bad parenting, parenting television viewing, and finally some direct questions about *Supernanny*. I then offered the participant(s) a choice of three episodes of *Supernanny*[2] and captured the viewing session – both the audio track of the episode and the corresponding talk of participants – with a digital recorder: an innovative audience method, 'text-in-action', developed by Helen Wood (2009). Interviews were followed immediately by viewing sessions, and viewing sessions were followed by post-interview group discussions. My analysis draws on transcripts of the interviews and viewing sessions, as well as reflective fieldnotes that were written immediately after data-gathering. My intention was to map in more complex ways how parental pedagogy occasion and prompt parental subjects forth.

Participating parents were mostly white, middle-class women, recruited through contacts at a community-run mothers' support group, pre-school art club and my daughter's primary school; securing a more representative sample proved difficult despite sustained efforts. These sampling problems may be bound up with the ways in which both the genre of 'talk' and the formats of reality television are gendered (Skeggs *et al.*, 2008; Gray, 1992) and in which the topic of 'parenting' itself euphemises what is really 'mothering' (Lawler, 2000; Hays, 1996; Sunderland, 2006). For these reasons, perhaps, it proved very difficult to interest fathers in the research; the only two that participated were the spouses of women who had already agreed to participate. All participants described themselves as 'white', except one who defined herself as 'mixed-race', which reflects my difficulties in recruiting more representatively. On reflection, I have come to see the whiteness of my respondents (and more specifically, my initial failure to interrogate it) as an illustration of how whiteness is able to remain assumed, silent and unmarked in parenting culture. While this chapter demonstrates how parenting culture positions subjects (and enables them to position themselves) in *classed* registers, it also positions them in racialised formations (see for example Byrne, 2006), which I acknowledge but do not discuss here.

In terms of social class, the sample became increasingly narrow: some parents who at first agreed to participate gradually slipped out of contact, stopped replying to phonecalls and emails and on one occasion simply going out on the scheduled day. There are many possible reasons for these absenting strategies, but it is important to note the classed patterns of the participants who dropped out (mainly working-class). Where other researchers working in the field of classed subjectivities have faced similar recruitment problems, they have suggested that research is read differently by working-class subjects, as unwanted surveillance, a situation exacerbated by the intensifying of governmental scrutiny in the lives of those defined as 'socially excluded' or 'marginalised' (Skeggs *et al.*, 2008).

Whilst all participants self-defined as 'middle-class', I noted that these classifications were shaky and hesitant. According to most 'objective' systems for qualifying social class, it could be argued that these parents were securely middle-class; homeowners living in gentrified suburbs; holding a range of 'professional' employment positions, as furniture designers, teachers, advertising project managers, photographers; university educated; some employing cleaners or gardeners. These classificatory systems though are riven with complexities gestured to in hesitant accounts of occupations, childhoods, background, 'roots' and cultural values, and sometimes wealth, pointing to the elasticity of the meaning of 'wealth', the complexity of mobility and the relationality of social class. Class cannot be easily isolated and placed within a stratification table, but rather it is given meaning through its position to other classes (Lawler, 2000; Devine and Savage, 2005; Biressi and Nunn, 2008; Gillies, 2007) and the respondents in this research made remarks which point to disjunctures between material wealth and classed feelings. These complexities indicate both evasive embarrassment around social class (Sayer, 2002) but also to the paucity of vocabulary around social class in the UK at this historical moment; a moment in which social class distinctions have become 'increasingly codified, displaced and individualised' (Gillies, 2005: 835).

Informed as this research is by the work of Pierre Bourdieu, these narrations of middle-class identity might better be seen as reflecting a classed 'becoming' rather than a classed 'being'. Bourdieu (1998) theorises social class as neither a matter of essential attributes nor voluntary choices, but as divisions that must be constantly reproduced; 'classes exist in some sense as a state of virtuality, not as something given but as something to be done' (1998: 12, cited in Lawler, 2004). I asked participants to 'give' me their social class in the interviews, but I also excavate how they 'did' social class in the subsequent viewing encounter with *Supernanny*. Social class is not simply a set of categories of which one is a member, but is a set of complex, ambivalent and emotional processes of distinction and judgement. These respondents 'made' themselves as classed subjects by drawing distinctions between themselves and the families they watched on *Supernanny*, and between themselves and other viewers (the 'real' audience) of the programme. These distinctions were transcribed into subtle codes of value, rarely explicitly naming social class; had I not asked participants to identify their social class (amongst their definitions of other vectors of difference) it may have gone unmentioned. But it was social class, and its intersections, spoken through other categories of worth and value, which saturated the encounters.

Watching/not watching and the 'real' *Supernanny* audience

Of the participants, only two of the fifteen parents had never seen the programme before (Vanina and Fiona). The remainder were evasive about identifying as loyal viewers, and consciously accounted for having ever watched at all:

> We only watch it when it's on [...] it's a *real* fascination for me. After a long day, and we're having teas-on-knees sort of thing. We've never done that purposively, just sort of stumbled across it.
>
> (Helen, interview)

> I don't make a *point* of watching it. Just if it's on and I happen to catch it.
>
> (Louisa, interview)

> I haven't watched it *religiously*. I've seen, heard of quite a few [parenting programmes], but that [*Supernanny*] is the only one I know – I don't actually know any of the others. But just when it's on and I catch it.
>
> (Clara, interview)

These disclaimers were important themes, where the relationship to television is accidental not deliberative. In these accounts, *Supernanny* has not commanded any loyalty and viewing is casual. This was a way of perhaps retreating from the programme's disturbing or upsetting content, but it was also a strategic way of holding the format at a distance and of dismissing its significance for oneself. This is significantly complicated by the subsequent viewing sessions, where most of the parents seemed in fact to be highly engaged with the programme and deeply familiar with the narrative, offering predictions in moments of drama and providing often ironic commentary alongside the Supernanny Jo Frost's diagnosis and to-camera monologues.

At the same time, consuming other parent pedagogy *was* narrated as purposive and in making these accounts participants constructed a version of themselves as discerning subjects. Patrizia, for example, draws on a common hierarchy of value between different pedagogical forms – in this case, between parenting books and parenting television – in order to generate certain kinds of value in terms of her parental pedagogies:

> I don't watch much television. I do have two *Supernanny* books at home, but I only read one, I didn't have time to read the other one. If you're doing other things with your child, you don't watch much. And there aren't many parenting shows on in the evening.
>
> (Patrizia, interview)

We might interpret this at face-value – an issue of scheduling and time – but Patrizia's dismissal of parental television (and employment of parental books) also invokes other more complex cultural meanings about the relative worth of different media forms. While books are attached to cultural worth, implying knowledge, literacy and so on, television often is seen as worthless. Television ethnographies have demonstrated the ambivalence of feelings towards television in everyday life (Silverstone, 1994) and these ambivalences are powerfully classed, with middle-class subjects in particular articulating critical concern towards television as a 'bad object' (Skeggs *et al.*, 2008). In the UK there is a 'commonsense' assumption that middle-class parents read parenting books and working-class parents watch parenting television and this assumption is formative in some of the remarks I explore here. Patrizia dismisses television throughout the interview, stating her preference for learning about parenting from books. Through this narration of oneself as a critical consumer and negotiating viewer, these parents used a variety of strategies to dismiss the significance of the programme for their own lives.

In order to create cultural value from these dismissals, comparative evaluations were made of the programme's meanings for other parents, parents who were not imagined to be as critical or thoughtful. Although I did not initiate (or anticipate) any discussions of why respondents thought *Supernanny* was popular, *all* the interviews moved onto this topic and the broader *Supernanny* audience. This presumed, broader audience emerged in these discussions as a significant counterpoint to the respondents' own viewing; who this broader audience is (and how they are presumed to watch) provided important (imagined) contrasts to how these respondents accounted for their viewing. The popularity of *Super-nanny* was interpreted apocalyptically, as heralding the ways in which 'people' (that is, 'other people') are taken in by voyeuristic and damaging reality television:

> And then you think, there are some people who actually have to *learn* this. I mean, who *are* these people?
>
> (Louisa, during viewing)

> People would rather watch car crash television.
>
> (Amy, during viewing)

> The only reason people watch it is for the drama really … parents who haven't got a clue really.
>
> (Phillip, interview)

There is a palpable sense here of the 'real' *Supernanny* audience: those that this parental pedagogy form is created for and aimed at, and who *are* (or at least presumed to be) – fanatic, purposive viewers. While *these* viewing groups did not *really* have to learn lessons from *Supernanny*, the 'real audience' does; while the 'real audience' prefers high-drama, 'car-crash television', these groups have more elevated preferences and watch critically and cautiously. A few minutes into the viewing session, the Supernanny Jo Frost enters, striding along the street and Phillip calls out triumphantly 'ah here comes the theatre!' His marking of this moment as 'theatre' sets him apart from the parents who he presumes 'haven't got a clue'. It is a key moment in his production of himself as a critical viewer.

Displaying one's critical abilities and knowingness around the machinations of reality television is one of the multiple pleasures of watching reality television. Performing as a 'savvy viewer/voyeur' creates the critical distance that is necessary in order to participate in reality television without succumbing to its illusions (Andrejevic, 2004; Couldry, 2011). Samuel jokes about how the camera crew elicited the correct dramatic 'bad behaviour' from children, suggesting that 'they're giving them sugar, right?' In doing so, he both demonstrates his knowledge of filming techniques and signals his caution around taking the screen as evidence of 'real life'. In a different session, Amy draws attention to the narrative conventions of the obligatory happy ending, enquiring with mock-innocence if anyone else has noticed that the sun always shines at the end. Both Samuel and Amy have worked in television professionally (as a camera technician and researcher, respectively), and so I was not surprised by their evaluative display. However, most of the other participants *also* demonstrated their critical abilities in similar ways, demonstrating that they too could 'see the strings' of artifice in reality television. Fiona, who had never even seen *Supernanny* before, was familiar with the use of a camera close-up at dramatic points to produce an emotional climax – 'the money shot' of reality television (Grindstaff, 2002) and this familiarity enabled her to joke about the on-screen tears she was expecting:

See I think maybe I lack empathy. I'm just like, come on, give us the tears, give us the tears, it's not a proper programme without the tears.

(Fiona, during viewing)

Through making and taking opportunities to exercise a kind of mastery over the programme, respondents can claim not to be duped by reality television. Louisa states/confesses her pleasure in crying at *Supernanny*, then makes a series of distancing moves from the programme: she can enjoy it and cry 'at an epiphanic moment, because I'm able to suspend that I'm being wrapped around a television producer's finger.' In other words, she is able to suspend *her usual mastery* of the programme and *allow herself* to succumb to tears. These accounts of critical mastery are echoed throughout audience research (Hermes 1995; Gray, 1992; Skeggs *et al.*, 2008) which find that middle-class cultural consumption must be authorised and legitimated through reflexive performance and critical evaluation. Through critical reflexivity, these respondents distinguish themselves from the 'real audience'.

Amy was one of the most consistently critical of the participants. In the first dramatic montage of bad behaviour during the viewing session, she excitedly articulated her misgivings;

See! There! That's *exactly* what I mean! They've clearly just selected the edited highlights ... the way telly works ... set him up as an absolute monster. [...] They've done everything they can, in the same way as documentaries do [...] this is a kind of extreme version, whether that's done through nice editing or if it's real, an extreme version of toddler behaviour. So red-top. You know, tabloid.

(Amy, during viewing)

Amy explicitly draws on an 'effects' model of media consumption and links here between the visual logic of the programme, which repeats footage of the same tantrum two and sometimes three times across the course of a single episode, with the ways in which tantrums are read and interpreted in the wider world. The 'real' *Supernanny* viewer, Amy insists, leaves the programme changed; ready to judge other stranger-children as monsters. Her use of the word 'tabloid' situates the visual logics of the programme at the bottom of a cultural hierarchy of value.

The cultural hierarchy of parental pedagogy

Both in interview and during viewing then, a cultural hierarchy of parent pedagogy was constructed within which *Supernanny* was ambivalently cast. These respondents differentiated themselves from others in several ways, through expressing their preferences for parenting books over parenting television, and by drawing distinctions between their critical, cautious viewing practices and the presumed viewing practices of the 'real' *Supernanny* audience. But they also created cultural value through drawing comparisons between *Supernanny* and other parenting experts, and in doing so they productively staked their support and conferred legitimacy on their preferred experts. This evaluation is part of the work of 'intensive parenting' (Hays, 1996) in which parents must sift through, weigh up and assess which advice and parenting orthodoxy they will follow. The techniques proposed by *Supernanny* were critically appraised in every viewing session and other experts were frequently referenced: in particular the parenting expert and writer Gina Ford, whose *Contented Baby Book* several participants had read. Others referred to pedagogical programming, in particular programmes made by either developmental psychologist Professor Robert Winston or clinical psychologist Dr Tanya Byron. Phillip and Amy, in different viewing groups, made these comments about Winston's programme:

> We've watched some of the Professor Winston one. Er, was it *Child Of Our Time*? He's less sort of ... prescriptive. And dictatorial.
>
> (Phillip, interview)

> There's some reality television that I love. Like Jamie's dinner thing. I just feel that there's some integrity about them. I'm sure *Child of Our Time* doesn't have such a big audience. They're not being made just for entertainment. It's done with so much more integrity, it just has a much more positive view of children and their parents.
>
> (Amy, interview)

We might read these comments as simply statements of viewer preferences, but they also represent opportunities for social distinction: what kinds of programmes you watch, what kinds you enjoy and what those choices say about the kind of person, and parent, you are. Although many participants produced an ambivalent or hesitant account of whether and how often they watched *Supernanny*, often littered with provisos, they found it easier to profess their love and loyalty of other parenting programmes, which were described in comparatively glowing terms. Not all reality television or parenting television was deemed problematic. Amy's example of the programmes made by UK celebrity chef Jamie Oliver as having 'more integrity' than *Supernanny* is something we might take issue with, not least because of Oliver's infamous fiery on-screen confrontations and off-screen outbursts. Oliver's presentational style aside, the campaigning purpose of his programmes as a front for his nutrition missions resonates with Amy's sense of integrity. The 'smaller audience' commanded by Winston's highbrow programme, as opposed to the mass appeal of *Supernanny*, reassures Amy about her cultural choices. Susan too spoke of other parenting programmes 'resonating' with her:

> I related quite a lot to Tanya Byron, and *Little Angels* and all that. I just thought, whatever she was saying, just sort of resonated with me, I thought, yes that sounds right, and I took that on board [...] anything with Tanya Byron.
>
> (Susan, interview)

I want to expand here on the significance of the *Supernanny/Little Angels* comparison as it cropped up in every session. Dr Tanya Byron, the parenting expert behind more 'highbrow' pedagogy television (*House of Tiny Tearaways*, 2005–2007: *Little Angels*, 2004) served as a counterpoint to *Supernanny* Jo Frost in terms of qualifications, professional experience and the claims to 'expert' status. It is this dyad of expertise that had clearest resonance in the research sessions and this is profoundly important in terms of the argument I am making about parent pedagogy being a key site of social distinction. Byron herself withdrew from parenting television in 2007, making several public statements which commented on how parent pedagogy television had become too 'well-marketed', begun to 'go too far' and referring to other parenting 'experts' in suspicious quotemarks. The actual pedagogy offered in Frost and Byron's programmes shares broad similarities and the premise of their programmes overlap in many ways: yet they are constructed in press reviews (and in these research sessions) as in opposition.

This opposition demonstrates the often obscured ways in which classed contempt continues to pervade culture and parenting culture in particular. In some ways, these two parenting experts have had similar public career trajectories. Both have hosted reality television programmes, became celebrity experts, write newspaper columns and have published a number of parenting advice books. Whilst the respective programmes are styled, packaged and promoted differently, both use therapeutic and confessional narratives to organise episodes, centre on almost identical behavioural strategies (although the basis upon which the expertise is validated is different) and are similarly paced in terms of editing. The same issues of voyeurism, children's consent, vulnerability and the problematic transforming of 'dysfunction' into 'entertainment' might be equally levelled at the popular pedagogy of each. Yet in television reviews and interviews, Frost's experience as a nanny for fifteen years is often derided whilst Byron's status as a professional psychologist is acclaimed (see for example Carey, 2007). A pair of interviews, conducted with each a year apart by the same journalist, demonstrate this pattern: Frost is described as 'an unqualified nanny ... who has never trained formally' and at odds with childrearing advice (Aitkenhead, 2006) while Byron's expertise and experience as a clinician is 'calmly authoritative', 'compelling', 'thoughtful', with 'professional integrity', 'brilliant in her field, but with the polymath's gift for making complicated ideas accessible' (Aitkenhead, 2007). Byron, whom Aitkenhead tellingly describes as 'the respectable face of parenting television' reflects a classed vision of education, professional success and domestic respectability:

> At 38, her CV is a paean to alpha-female achievement, with a doctorate in clinical psychology and her first child at 27. She has been with her actor husband Bruce, DC Terry Perkins in The Bill, since she was 21, and they live with their two kids in a rambling north London house, which she shows me round with an unaffected charm.
>
> (Aitkenhead, 2007)

The work of Jo Frost, meanwhile, is described by Aitkenhead as an irresponsible and sensationalist departure from 'scientific motherhood', which Aitkenhead presents as harmonious and conflict-free (although many historical accounts demonstrate the antagonism of this 'science', see for example Hulbert, 2003). Aitkenhead describes Frost as uneducated – 'she has never read – or even heard of – any of the leading theorists I mention' – and inexpressive, mispronouncing words that the journalist painstakingly documents with obvious delight:

> 'I don't just want to know on the surface why. I need to know and find out exactly where the root of that lies. So in retrospective [*sic*] of that I do that mandatorially [*sic*] within the families' [...]. 'Nothing is ever set up or derived [*sic*]'. I think she means contrived.
> (Aitkenhead, quoting Frost and adding '*sic*' annotations, 2006)

While the purpose of this chapter is not to rescue or defend *Supernanny*, I do want to highlight this classed contempt that is reserved for Frost and point to where it resonates in other (classed) navigations of the programme. These two newspaper interviews draw on discourses of good and bad science, scientific and natural mothering, entertainment and 'real' expertise. As such, they demonstrate the wider cultural politics of parent pedagogy and cultural value which was readily reproduced by parents in our viewing sessions. Many of the parents referred to Jo Frost's verbal errors, in tones ranging from delight to irritation: but they also reproduced the special valuing of professional status. Susan for example makes an implied connection between Frost and Byron, stating that her 'problem' with the Supernanny is her questionable qualifications. When challenged by another mother in the group, Susan retorts with 'yeah, but she's not a child psychologist'.

Refusing *Supernanny*

There were several moments in the research sessions which suggested an embryonic kernel of criticism leveled at parenting culture more widely. The act of refusing *Supernanny* – refusing to be 'taken in' by it, drawing attention to its artifice – was linked, at points explicitly, to dissatisfactions with everyday experiences of parenting, in particular of feeling hypervisible and surveilled. Rather than offering any final answers to these dissatisfactions, watching *Supernanny* – even if only to refuse its pedagogy – seemed to simply heighten the sense of inescapability of parenting culture, despite the reservations expressed about the ethics or artifice of the programme and in spite of the critical distance produced. Evaluating parent pedagogy might create some cultural value and even social distinction, but it is also labour-intensive, time-demanding and emotionally exhausting and is another place where mothers (in particular) become 'manacled to sensitivity' (Walkerdine and Lucey, 1989; Hays, 1996). The exhaustion created by parent pedagogy is illustrated in the following statements:

I suppose throughout the years people have always looked on and disapproved or whatever, but you knew you were just going to be left to get on with it, but *now* it's like, ooh you should be doing this and you're doing that, and complete strangers have got an opinion.

(Jane, in interview)

We are getting obsessed, and *Supernanny* is fuelling this obsession … that, as parents, we're absolutely obsessed with kids being well-behaved, and good, and behaving in a social situation as, you know, we'd like them to. As opposed to letting them be kids, and talking to them and being creative with them. It's all about curtailing them, and stopping them. It's all about discipline and nothing about being creative with them and exploring … who they are.

(Louisa, post-viewing discussion)

I find advice quite nauseating. I got a book from [mutual friend] no less! I nearly bloody threw it back at her. I said, it's all very well reading the book but [son]'s not read it. So the book tells me what to do and then he doesn't perform to type! I mean!

(Helen, interview)

Supernanny is a programme which, compared to other parent pedagogies, offers an alternative to intensive parenting and insists upon discipline and authority, rather than negotiation. Whilst there were certainly moments when some of the participants revelled in the newly discovered authority of the parents on the screen, related with humour their own parental 'failings', and joked about their possible need for the *Supernanny*, overall the refusals of *Supernanny* did not translate easily into refusals of parenting culture per se. Refusing, critiquing and assessing *Supernanny* rather, was one incoherent and contradictory part of producing oneself as a particular kind of parent (too informed/educated/sensitive to take *Supernanny* seriously) and a particular kind of viewer (one who is critically attuned to the artifice of reality television).

Furthermore, I would also suggest that the evasiveness around watching *Supernanny* (and not being part of the 'real' audience) is tied in complex ways to the shameful emotions evoked through watching other parents on the screen fail. In interview, the programme was dismissed as rarely and casually watched and as diversion: yet the subsequent text-in-action viewing sessions revealed a much more emotional and intensive encounter. Attempting to hold the programme at a critical distance, and speaking of it as a 'guilty pleasure', may then also be about attempting to hold the shameful emotions it generates at a distance from oneself (see Jensen, 2011 for a lengthier discussion).

Supernanny cannot be treated in isolation of the parenting culture from which it has emerged. The account of oneself as a savvy, reflexive viewer who remains untouched by the material on-screen is an unstable one. Silences in the viewing sessions at particularly emotional points indicate, I would argue, both an embarrassment at the on-screen melodrama *and* an excess of affectivity that cannot always be verbalised. In one session (as the on-screen mother reads out a moving note from her daughter), Louisa whispered to me, 'I think I'm going to cry': this was *both* an ironic comment on the cloying sentimentality of the scene *and* an attempt to master the desire to cry by drawing attention to it (I had tears in my eyes when Louisa said this). The affectivity of the material on the screen and the emotionality it provoked could not always be contained within this fantasy of critical mastery.

Parent pedagogy and parent research: feeling like the Supernanny

Finally, I want to turn to how the research encounter itself adds another complex layer of distinction-making opportunity. Although as researchers we could be seduced by the everydayness of the research setting – in participants' homes, watching television, surrounded by peers – and although having *Supernanny* as a focus allowed me to retreat somewhat (Skeggs *et al.*, 2008; Walkerdine, 1986; Gray, 1992), it is important to attend to how my very presence impacted upon what was speakable and unspeakable. The artifice of the interview/viewing situation (however discrete the voice recorder, however domestic the research setting) itself called forth a particular critical discourse. Although I endeavoured to stay as silent as possible during these viewing sessions, this was not straightforward and I loom large in the textual encounters as a self-conscious and performative subject. These parents often sought my opinion and my reaction, either addressing me directly or asking questions about the episode. I was an integral part of the encounter, sometimes being asked to verify details of the programme, offer my opinion of it, or corroborate suspicions about the host, Jo Frost;

Do *you* use Supernanny?

(Clara, during viewing)

Do *you* watch them? I know you do for this [research], but do you still watch, just for yourself?

(Helen, during interview)

Who is this woman? Do you know what her qualifications are?

(Louisa, during viewing)

Asking me to position myself in relation to the programme might have served as a kind of benchmark for participants; was it acceptable to watch this programme? Was it acceptable to *use* this programme? My responses to these questions and suspicions served as legitimations for subsequent opinions. I had a complex status, as a researcher and as an 'expert' on the programme. This status was certainly not guaranteed though, with some participants wanting to contribute, or challenge, the research design itself, making suggestions or asking questions about their role as a participant and my intentions as a researcher:

> So ... are you trying to find out if there's sufficient advice available for parents, is *that* what this is about?
>
> (Elizabeth, during viewing)

> Is that all you need from us?
>
> (Clara, during viewing)

> What do you want us to do? Just watch it?
>
> (Susan, during viewing)

> So much of it is about the bloody naughty bench. I mean, I don't know, have you *counted* how many times the word naughty bench is used?
>
> (Amy, during viewing)

These comments reveal the anxieties, excitement and engagement of being a research participant, but some, particularly those delivered in a dismissive or disbelieving tone, created a good deal of anxiety for me. Did I really just want participants to watch *Supernanny? Should* I count how many times the naughty step was referenced by the narrator in the programme? Amy, perhaps the most critical of the respondents, suggests this alternative method, implying that quantitative data might be more convincing. Illustrating the actively critical discourse that this research setting seemed to invite, Amy stated her interest in the subsequent analysis of the data that the sessions would yield, even offering to proofread my thesis and contacting me some months later requesting any publications. Agreeing to take part in research on parenting culture carries its own opportunities for distinction and for producing value which we should attend to.

Research methods have historically been used to produce 'scientific' accounts of gender and class, with the middle-class researcher at the centre remaining an untouched pillar of objectivity (Skeggs, 1997; Thornham, 2001). Through interrogating rather than erasing our presence as researchers of parenting culture, as stranger/other parents/authority figures, we might trouble these presumptions and to take account of the complex emotions, fantasies and projections in a research encounter means, including our own (Walkerdine, 1986: Reay, 1997). As in much emerging research into parenting culture, I was constantly unnerved by fantasies, confusions and misreadings of me by respondents, caught in the 'double-bind' (Reay, 1997) of a shaky class location and complicated by the fault-line of mother/researcher within me. The pull of researcher and of mother coalesced in difficult ways, creating something of a 'borderland identity' (Behar, 1993) which complicated the research sessions. Two sessions involved children. In one, I brought my daughter and she played with the daughters of the participants in the neighbouring house: a texture of parental camaraderie settled in our session. After the interview and viewing session, we shared a meal and the conversation, inevitably turning to *Supernanny*, went some way to neutralise the 'difficult' behaviour of our increasingly tired children. Without romanticising, it *is* important to gesture to the fact that I was a researcher *and* a mother for this session, and to acknowledge the difference this made for participants.

In the other, I was the parent in the room *without* her child, and this too made a difference to the texture of the session. The parents involved had brought their children: we all presumed that they would play together while we talked in peace (of course they did not!) That these parental demands happened *while* a researcher asked questions *about* their parenting – and requested they watch a television programme designed to provoke anxiety around parenting – may have contributed to the frequency with which they must have felt compelled to respond to their children. During what was ostensibly our 'viewing' session, one of the mothers 'viewed' very little of the programme. Instead, she busied herself with fetching snacks, playing games and ferrying children back to the living room (where we had installed them in front of a children's television pro-gramme): in my fieldnotes I recorded my irritation at her 'sabotage', but of course my presence is central to her behaviour. Just as my presence undoubtedly impacted upon her attentiveness, so too did her attentiveness prompt feelings of guilt in me: indeed, in order to attend this particular viewing session, I had to make arrangements for my daughter to be picked up from school.

Parenting, and particularly, *mothering* always involves comparisons, judge-ments and self-accounting in reference to other parents. As an outsider in these sessions, I may have been a source of anxiety, a potential scrutiniser, but I also felt scrutinised as a possible source of evaluative knowledge about advice itself: as I waited on the doorsteps of an impending viewing sessions, I felt like a visit-ing Supernanny myself.

Conclusions

Why are parents watching *Supernanny*? The answers are not simple and cannot be fully evidenced and excavated by poll, survey or even interview; these methods too rehearse a reflexive, coherent subject. By employing the interview *and* text-in-action methods in tandem, I suggest that we are able to complicate our tidy conclusions about why people are watching, and to think through more fully *how* we watch and what watching *does* for the watchers. Choosing which parenting advice to use, and then negotiating with that advice – as in these encounters – is not simply evaluating 'the best way' to raise children, but rather involves a whole range of investments, judgements and evaluations that enabled these parents to do identity work. Contemporary parenting culture is less the 'science' of perfect parenting and more the promotion of a certain kind of parent, a certain kind of parental subjectivity, a certain orientation towards one's parent-ing. This chapter has attended to the 'classed' and 'classing' processes through which parent pedagogy is consumed and evaluated.

These viewing sessions, while full of camaraderie and humour, were con-stantly haunted by the toxicity of parent pedagogy, the individualising weight of judgement and the maternal figurations (see Tyler, 2011) against which the parental self is defined. I have discussed the importance of approaching parent pedagogy in its popular representational forms as part of a broader parenting culture which is often treated as a supermarket of advice (Hulbert, 2003; Murkoff, 2000). This culture is threaded through with an injunction to 'choose' a parenting approach autonomously, as a path to becoming empowered and emboldened by advice, but not cowed by it; of choosing to 'buy-the-book' rather than going 'by-the-book'. This compunction emerges here in terms of approaching *Supernanny* as a critical viewer, drawing distinctions between one's own viewing and the imagined viewing of others. As I have demonstrated here, whilst parent pedagogy offers a key site for pursuit of social distinction, there is much material which does not fit into the fantasy of the critical viewer and what could not be contained within the critical discourse that the research setting appeared to invite. Although the popular directions that parent pedagogy has taken – including but not limited to *Supernanny* – have been interpreted as hunger/demand for advice, this kind of ethnographically intentioned audience research demonstrates that parent pedagogy takes hold in ways we are not entirely conscious of and in ways we cannot entirely master. Moreover, it operates as a site where social divisions and antagonisms are reproduced and circulated.

Notes

1 For a full report of the 'Happy Families?' poll, conducted on behalf of the National Family and Parenting Institute see www.ipsos-mori.com/researchpublications/ researcharchive/348/Happy-Families.aspx; 'The power of parenting TV programmes – help or hazard for today's families?' National Family and Parenting Institute, archived at: http://familyandparenting.web-platform.net/item/document/8.
2 For convenience I used the episode synopsis offered through the Channel 4 'on demand' online watching facility, see www.channel4.com/programmes/supernanny/4od.

References

Aitkenhead, Decca (2006) 'You've been very, very naughty' *Guardian* 22 July.
Aitkenhead, Decca (2007) 'Playtime's over' *Guardian* 8 September.
Andrejevic, Marc (2004) *Reality TV: The Work of Being Watched* Lanham, MD: Rowman and Littlefield Publishers.
Apple, Rima D. (2006) *Perfect Motherhood: Science and Childrearing in America* New Brunswick, NJ/London: Rutgers University Press.
Behar, Ruth (1993) *The Vulnerable Observer: Anthropology that Breaks your Heart* Boston, MA: Beacon Press.
Biressi, Anita and Nunn, Heather (2008) 'The bad citizen: class politics in lifestyle television' in G. Palmer (ed.) *Exposing Lifestyle Television: The Big Reveal* Aldershot: Ashgate, pp. 15–24.
Bourdieu, Pierre (1979) *Distinction: A Social Critique on the Judgement of Taste* Cambridge, MA: Harvard University Press.

Byrne, Bridget (2006) *White Lives: The Interplay of 'Race', Class and Gender in Everyday Life* London: Routledge.

Carey, Fiona (2007) 'Arrogant. Utterly unrealistic. It's the TV parenting guru who should be sent to the naughty step' *Daily Mail* 27 September.

Couldry, Nick (2011) 'Class and contemporary forms of reality production' in H. Wood and B. Skeggs (eds) *Reality Television and Class* London: Palgrave Macmillan/British Film Institute.

Devine, Fiona and Savage, Mike (2005) 'The cultural turn, sociology and class analysis' in F. Devine, M. Savage, J. Scott and R. Crompton (eds) *Rethinking Class: Culture, Identities and Lifestyle* Basingstoke/New York: Palgrave Macmillan.

DfES (Department for Education and Skills) (2007) *Every Parent Matters* London: DfES.

Dovey, J (2000) *Freakshow: First Person Media and Factual Television* London: Pluto Press.

Gillies, Val (2005) 'Raising the "meritocracy": parenting and the individualization of social class' *Sociology* 39(5): 825–853.

Gillies, Val (2007) *Marginalised Mothers: Exploring Working-class Experiences of Parenting* Abingdon: Routledge.

Grant, Julia (1998) *Raising Baby by the Book: The Education of American Mothers* New Haven, CT/London: Yale University Press.

Gray, Ann (1992) *Video Playtime: The Gendering of a Leisure Technology* London: Routledge.

Grindstaff, Laura (2002) *The Money Shot: Trash, Class and the Making of TV Talk Shows* Chicago, IL: University of Chicago Press.

Hays, Sharon (1996) *The Cultural Contradictions of Motherhood* New Haven, CT/London: Yale University Press.

Hermes, Joke (1995) *Reading Women's Magazines: An Analysis of Everyday Media Use* Cambridge: Polity Press.

Hill, Annette (2005) *Reality TV – Audiences and Popular Factual Television* Abingdon/New York: Routledge.

Hulbert, Anne (2003) *Raising America: Experts, Parents, and a Century of Advice About Children*, London: Vintage.

Hughes, Beverley (2006) 'The best years? Children, young people and family policy', keynote speech to Institute for Public Policy delivered on Wednesday 19 July.

Jensen, Tracey (2011) '"Watching with my hands over my eyes": Shame and irritation in ambivalent encounters with "Bad Mothers"' *Radical Psychology* 9(2), online, available at: www.radicalpsychology.org/vol9-2/jensen.html.

Lawler, Steph (2000) *Mothering the Self: Mothers, Daughters, Subjects* London: Routledge.

Murkoff, Heidi (2000) 'The real parenting expert is … you' *Newsweek* 5 June.

Reay, Diane (1997) 'The double-bind of the working class feminist academic: the success of failure or the failure of success?' in P. Mahoney and C. Zmroczek (eds) *Class Matters: 'Working Class' Women's Perspectives on Social Class* London: Routledge.

Sayer, Andrew (2002) 'What are you worth? Why class is an embarrassing subject' *Sociological Research Online* 7(3) online, available at: www.socresonline.org.uk/7/3/sayer.html.

Seiter, Ellen (1999) *Television and New Media Audiences* New York: Clarendon Press.

Silverstone, Roger (1994) *Television and Everyday Life* London: Routledge.

Skeggs, Beverly (1997) *Formations of Class and Gender: Becoming Respectable* London: Sage.

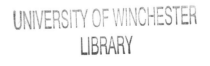

Skeggs, Beverly and Wood, Helen (2012) *Reacting to Reality Television: Performance, Audience and Value* Abingdon: Routledge.

Skeggs, Beverly, Wood, Helen and Thumim, Nancy (2008) 'Oh goodness, I *am* watching reality TV': how methods make class in audience research' *European Journal of Cultural Studies* 2(1): 5–24.

Skeggs, Beverly, Wood, Helen and Thumim, Nancy (2009) ' "It's just sad": Affect, judgement and emotional labour in "reality" television viewing' in Stacy Gillis and Joanne Hollows (eds) *Feminism, Domesticity and Popular Culture* New York/Abingdon: Routledge.

Sunderland, Jane (2006) ' "Parenting" or "mothering"? The case of modern childcare magazines' *Discourse and Society* 17(4): 503–527.

Thornham, Sue (2001) *Feminist Theory and Cultural Studies: Stories of Unsettled Relations* London: Arnold.

Tyler, Imogen (2011) 'Pramfaced Girls: the Class Politics of "Maternal TV" ' in Beverly Skeggs and Helen Wood (eds) *Real Class: Ordinary People and Reality Television Across National Spaces* London: BFI.

Walkerdine, Valerie (1986) 'Video replay: families, films and fantasy' in V. Burgin, J. Donald and C. Kaplan (eds) *Formations of Fantasy* New York: Methuen.

Walkerdine, Valerie and Lucey, Helen (1989) *Democracy in the Kitchen: Regulating Mothers and Socialising Daughters* London: Virago Press.

Wintour, Patrick (2006) 'No more misbehaving' *Guardian* 26 July.

Wood, Helen (2009) *Talking with Television: Women, Talk Shows, and Modern Self-Reflexivity* Urbana/Chicago, IL: University of Illinois Press.

Part II

The structural constraints to 'good' parenting

4 Negotiating (un)healthy lifestyles in an era of 'intensive' parenting

Ethnographic case studies from north-west England, UK

Denise Hinton, Louise Laverty and Jude Robinson

Sonia

Sonia lives with her partner Tom and their two young children Sam and Daniel in north-west England. Her youngest son, Daniel, has respiratory and ear problems and attends regular appointments at the nearest children's hospital for monitoring and treatment. Sonia has been told by healthcare staff that exposure to second-hand smoke may cause and exacerbate Daniel's condition and that she must keep Daniel away from cigarette smoke. Sonia has never smoked but her partner and other family members do. She has asked her partner, her mother and her mother-in-law not to smoke around Daniel to help protect his health. Although Sonia's partner, Tom, has said he will stop at some point he hasn't set a quit date and has repeatedly told Sonia 'not to nag at him' about quitting. Similarly, her mother-in-law has 'brushed off' her concerns and continues to smoke in front of Daniel when he visits her. Only her mother has responded to her request and does not smoke in front of the children anymore.

This case study portrays a compelling but nonetheless complex and contradictory picture of parenting that, we will argue, helps develops a more nuanced understanding of how normative discourses of intensive parenting (Hays, 1996) and health 'risks' (Lupton, 1999) are transmitted, discussed, managed and enacted in the 'doing' of family and relatedness (Carsten, 2004; Mead, 1962). While Sonia articulates a strong desire to protect her child from a health risk, she is unable to enact this responsibility because her partner and other family members interpret this risk differently. Informed by societal expectations of how mothers 'should' behave, Sonia repeatedly states 'I should put my children first and not be bothered about other people's feelings' believing she ought to challenge her partner's and mother-in-law's behaviours while being unsure how to go about this. In doing so, Sonia positions herself as both fundamentally responsible for nurturing and protecting her child's health (irrespective of the detrimental actions of others) and ultimately failing in her goal to be a 'good' mother.

Through a detailed examination of families' (un)healthy lifestyles, this chapter outlines the moral obligations that underpin parents' and children's interpretations of 'intensive' parenting discourse and their multiple responses to current health messages in the United Kingdom. In doing so it provides an interesting insight into the way in which parents manage their accountability for a child's health while identifying the barriers which prevent mothers and fathers fulfilling a moral obligation to 'protect' their child and thus satisfy their own and others 'intensive' parenting ideals. Moreover, it demonstrates that children may also actively seek to 'regulate' their parents (un)healthy behaviours in line with these ideals.

Risk-averse parenting

Modern day parents are beset by 'expert' guidance on the best way to raise children and perform model parenthood (Hays, 1996; Hoffman, 2003). What was once considered a largely private and unremarkable affair (See Edwards and Gillies this volume), parenting in the United Kingdom and the United States has now become an increasingly publicised, politicised and contested issue that is both time and resource intensive (Bristow, 2009; Hattery, 2001; Furedi, 2008; Warner, 2006; Miller, 2005; Douglas and Meredith, 2004). As Lee *et al.* (2010) and Lupton (2011) note, risk has emerged as a central tenet in the intensification of parenthood where the actions of parents, especially the behaviours of mothers, are deemed crucial to the survival of 'vulnerable' offspring.

Yet, conversely, children are also increasingly considered to be at risk from their parents due to 'poor parenting' (see Jaysane-Darr and also Berry this volume), thereby justifying outsider intervention in the family. For example, due to growing concerns about the long-term health implications of modern lifestyles, parents are under increasing pressure to practise and promote a 'healthy' lifestyle that protects children from preventable health risks such as exposure to cigarette smoke, obesity and alcohol misuse (Bell *et al.*, 2009; Department of Health, 2010; Royal College of Physicians, 2010). This has led to a plethora of health promotion campaigns and interventions designed to encourage parents to modify their lifestyle, such as stopping smoking, that will improve their own and their family's health (Winickoff *et al.*, 2003; Jarvie and Malone, 2008; Hovell *et al.*, 2009; Abdullah *et al.*, 2005).

In modern neoliberal societies, such as the United Kingdom, public health discourses encourage people to 'define themselves in part by how well they succeed or fail in adopting healthy practices' (Crawford, 2006, p. 402). The growing emphasis on 'risky' lifestyles has led to greater scrutiny of parenting practice, especially the role of the mother, as women are 'exhorted to take precautions before, during and after pregnancy to enhance the optimum health and development of their children' (Lupton, 2011, p. 638). If a mother fails to take heed of 'expert' advice and does not instigate the recommended measures to protect her child from the very moment she contemplates having a baby, she can be considered irresponsible and morally suspect (Bell *et al.*, 2009; Lee *et al.*, 2010). In some instances, not confirming to expert advice has been likened to a form of child abuse (Field, 2010). As a result, Lupton goes on to argue that 'health conditions or problems or developmental delays in children are often attributed to their mothers failing to respond appropriately to expert advice' (p. 638).

'Doing' motherhood in a Western context is thus not only a politicised issue but a profoundly moral issue, too. There is a taken for granted assumption that mothers will strive to achieve the very best for their child, seeking out advice and information as appropriate and modelling their behaviour on culturally sensitive understandings of the 'right' way to parent (Faircloth, 2010; Shirani *et al.*, 2011). Mothers who do not or cannot implement these measures are seen as wilfully exposing their children to unnecessary risks and are subsequently depicted as morally deviant and problematic (Coxhead and Rhodes, 2006; Zivkovic *et al.*, 2010). Although there is greater scrutiny of mothers' action, fathers, as we go on to demonstrate, may also experience considerable pressure to parent in a particular way.

Intensive parenting thus encompasses a series of societal obligations that require parents (seen as responsible actors) to anticipate and mediate risks to family health while simultaneously managing potential risks to their performance of self and moral identify (Crawford, 2006). In this chapter we explore what it means to 'parent intensively' in relation to potential health 'risks' by first examining the challenges mother *and* fathers, and second, children encounter in attempting to realise dominant understandings of 'healthy' lifestyles and 'good' parenting.

Managing risk and 'choosing health'

The examples we draw on in this chapter explore parents and children's interpretations and reactions to the health 'risks' associated with smoking and alcohol (mis)use, as depicted in the numerous public health campaigns that have targeted problematic lifestyle issues in recent years (Fitzpatrick, 2001; Bunton *et al.*, 1995). Discussions about lifestyle 'choices' provide an interesting lens through which to explore the everyday interactions of family members and the doing of personal inter-relationships because these behaviours take place in the privacy of the home where they are not subject to state regulation but are nonetheless the focus of intense political scrutiny and moral judgement. As well as being something one does, both smoking and drinking are culturally symbolic and indicative of individual autonomy and the (potential) freedom to choose how one behaves (although the extent to which individuals continue to be able to exercise free choice is debatable). The imposition of various measures to control these activities has thus been associated with an attack on civil liberties and the creation of a 'nanny state' that seeks to control the personal and private choices of individuals (Thompson and Kumar, 2011).

Yet, at the same time, smoking, and to a lesser degree alcohol misuse, have in recent decades become marginalised and stigmatised activities and a marker of disadvantage, particularly as heavy smoking in many OECD countries has become a 'class issue', as a behaviour associated with people living on low-income in poorer areas of housing (Graham, 1993; Bell *et al.*, 2009). Parents who smoke and/or drink excessively are considered especially problematic due to the detrimental consequences for child health and well-being (Royal College of Physicians, 2010; Department of Health, 2010). As such, a parent who smokes, for example, may be the subject of harsh criticism and may be forced to justify their seemingly irresponsible behaviour through the construction of alternative narratives of morality (Holdsworth and Robinson, 2008).

Although evidence from the UK suggests that many parents respond positively to public health campaigns (Phillips *et al.*, 2007), a proportion do not align themselves with societal expectations of what parents 'ought' to do (Coxhead and Rhodes, 2006). Research offers various explanations for why many parents continue to engage in stigmatised behaviours, in spite of the health risks, and the difficulties parents may encounter in attempting to instigate 'safer' practices to protect their children's health. Although parents are often aware of health promotion campaigns, some parents, particularly those from lower socio-economic groups, living in constrained circumstances in disadvantaged areas, may find it more difficult to implement the suggested measures and may rely on their unhealthy 'choices' as a way of coping with the challenges and stresses of parenting with limited resources (Robinson and Kirkcaldy, 2007a). It has been suggested that this is related to the individualistic approach to health widely adopted by public health campaigns in the UK, which position often middle-class norms of idealised lifestyle behaviours as under the control of individuals and unrelated to external structural or economic factors (Lupton, 1995; Minkler, 1999; Graham, 1976).

Further, public health discourse often does not take into account that parents interpret 'risk' in various ways and some individuals may actively resist or deny public health messages or may articulate beliefs that contradict their practice (Thompson and Kumar, 2011; Bottorff *et al.*, 2006; Robinson and Kirkcaldy, 2007b). The evidence suggests that families do not simply accept 'expert' opinion but negotiate parenting practice in relation to their own beliefs, values, experiences and normative ideals, and that this is an ongoing and complex process (Finch and Mason, 1992; Smart, 2007). While some families interpret health 'risks' as self-evident and assimilate public health advice into their daily routines with little disruption, other families may find that members oppose changes to their lifestyle and adjustments may only be brought about via the enforcement of rules to control or prevent 'deviant' behaviours (Robinson *et al.*, 2011; Kegler *et al.*, 2007).

Here, we are interested in exploring how parents and children instigate and shape 'healthier' practices within the family and what this means for everyday parental interactions. To date, attention has focused on parents who continue to engage in risky behaviours in spite of the known health risks, highlighting the scrutiny and criticism these parents are subject to and the strategies parents employ to defend their 'deviant' behaviours and emphasise their moral standing to the moral majority (Holdsworth and Robinson, 2008; Douglas, 1994). Yet, less is known about the experiences of parents who want to put in place recommended measures to protect their child from harm (such as preventing people smoking within their home) but are unable to do so.

At the same time, children's awareness of and reactions to health 'risks', within the context of family relationships, remains largely absent from the current literature (although see Holdsworth and Robinson (2008) and Backett-Milburn and Harden (2004) for exceptions). These issues will also be discussed using the theory of 'socialisation-in-reverse' (Furedi, 2010) as a backdrop to explore the wider tension between the responsibilities of the state, parents and children. Socialisation-in-reverse suggests that the role of parents has become infantilised, with parents increasingly considered as incompetent role-models for children and in need of expert guidance, while simultaneously children are being given parenting duties in delivering expert messages from trusted sources (schools, health agencies) to their parents (Furedi, 2010; Colls and Evans, 2008).

We draw on data from two ethnographic studies that we conducted, one to explore tobacco use and the other alcohol among parents and children living in a range of family structures in the north-west of England.[1] The north-west is one of the largest and most densely populated regions in England, and is characterised by areas of both relative affluence and poverty. The region has the lowest life expectancies at birth in the UK, and in addition has particularly high rates of smoking and alcohol consumption among adults compared to other regions (Young and Sly, 2011). Also relevant to our discussion, the north-west has the highest proportions of households with single parents (Young and Sly, 2011) in England, and as legislation dealing with child custody in England recommends and promotes shared custody between parents, children of single parents are likely to spend time with another parent living elsewhere. Using a range of methods including observation, informal discussion, semi-structured and narrative interviews and focus groups we elicited a detailed understanding of parents and children's (differing) interpretations of (un)healthy lifestyles and the management of 'risk' in their day-to-day practice. We use two key concepts to structure the following discussion: the challenges parents may encounter in striving to maintain their identity as a 'good' parent; and children's interpretations and responses to dominant narratives of 'good' parenting and health. Using case studies we explore the divergent ways that family members (including children) attempt to 'parent intensively'.

Parenting, parenters and 'risk' management within the home

Public health discourse privileges an idealised version of parenting that emphasises parental responsibility and unified family decision making whereby parents are presumed to make joint 'choices' about family lifestyle based on what is in the best interests of their child. Moreover, the child is perceived to be largely passive in this process. In reality, parents may experience limited capacity to continuously control and monitor the environment in which their children reside and cannot modify and control for every form of 'risk' that their child may be subject to. During the collection of data we noticed that several parents experienced difficulties in trying to reconcile their own interpretation of 'good' parenting with the views and actions of another adult with whom they shared parenting or caring responsibilities. From this we deduced that 'risk' management in the home is particularly problematic due to the complexities of one parent 'regulating' the (un)healthy behaviours of another parent who resides within the same or a separate residence. Yet, there is little research that explores this issue in depth. It is our contention that often parents' parent in the way they are able to, not necessarily in the way that they want to due to the complexity of relationships and compromises that have to be made with another adult, and this has implications for their ability to manage health risks. This, in turn, shapes how parenting is perceived by others (including children) and indeed how parents judge themselves in an era of intensive parenting. On this basis, we ask: how do parents feel when they are prevented from fulfilling what they perceive to be as their motherly or fatherly 'duties'? What implications does this have for their practice as mothers and fathers in an era of intensive parenting? How does this impact on their relationships with their children? The following case study demonstrates that fathers are also actively involved in these processes, despite what current literature around 'intensive parenting' and 'mothering' might lead us to believe:

Shaun

Shaun is the father of three children of which only the eldest still lives with him, after he asked his partner Ruth to leave their home. Over the past ten years Shaun became increasingly aware of Ruth's 'secret drinking habit', finding stashes of alcohol which she initially blamed on their eldest daughter. Despite Shaun attempting to get her help and enlisting the help of voluntary organisations, she refused, and when his eldest daughter started to become withdrawn and dropping grades at school, he broke up with Ruth and asked her to leave saying that 'Being ill over the stress of it and seeing the children suffer I decided I wasn't going to have it anymore'. Ruth moved in with her parents taking their two younger children with her. Shaun remains estranged from his partner and younger children but feels like his eldest daughter is now beginning to recover from the experience. He claims that he is now appreciating how this has influenced his daughter's view of alcohol, 'in my own daughter's experience is that I think it's had a positive effect, the negative has ended up being a positive because now she's scared of alcohol, you know, she may drink but she will never be drunk if you like because she has seen the effect that it has had on close family'. Shaun no longer keeps alcohol in the house.

What this and the previous case study (Sonia) demonstrate is that while one parent may recognise the risks inherent in a particular behaviour and wish to protect their child from harm, they may find it difficult to do this when their views differ from other individuals with caregiver roles. Shaun, like Sonia in the previous case study, has had many discussions with his partner, using information from agencies to emphasise the severe implications of his partner's behaviour and to underline the responsibilities she ought to enact as a mother. Ruth's attempt to circumvent his intervention suggests that she interprets and negotiates a different set of risks in her parenting role. Shaun argues that because Ruth is the mother and primary caregiver she has additional rights, and as such Ruth does not regard the potential removal of her children as a risk in the same way a father (or secondary caregiver) might do. Indeed when Ruth leaves, she takes her two youngest daughters with her. Shaun wants to be a 'good parent' and protect his children from harm, but is relatively powerless to coerce or regulate his partner's behaviour. In the end he sacrifices custody of his youngest children to change the home environment, to protect his own health, and the well-being of his eldest daughter.

A common criticism of public health campaigns is that although messages highlight the measures parents should take to protect their children they seldom address the practical issues that parents may encounter when trying to implement these changes (Robinson, 2008; Robinson and Kirkcaldy, 2007a). Public health discourses emphasise individual choice and agency in risk management and frame individuals as rational and self-controlled agents who will make themselves aware of 'risks', will interpret risks 'correctly' and follow expert advice to mitigate potential harm to their health (Lupton, 1999; Thompson and Kumar, 2011; Robinson and Kirkcaldy, 2007b). A failure to act is presumed to stem from a lack of knowledge rather than a limited capacity to act, and is often dealt with by further initiatives and campaigns to raise awareness and encourage individuals to act in a culturally approved manner (see the UK's Department of Health most recent public strategy for an example (2010). Yet, as the case studies above have demonstrated, parents may have to negotiate parenting across multiple households requiring considerable trust in another adult's parenting practice and resulting in an inability to continually monitor all that a child may be 'at risk' from.

While we acknowledge that parents' lifestyle choice can have a significant and detrimental impact on childhood mortality and morbidity (Royal College of Physicians, 2010), and that parents can prevent or mitigate the harm caused to their child's health (Department of Health, 2010), we argue that parents seldom care for children as completely autonomous agents. Not only are parenting practices shaped by wider social structures including law, government agencies, education, healthcare and mass media, parents must also negotiate a complex network of inter-relationships that includes the beliefs of others who share parental or caring responsibilities (Finch and Mason, 1992; Smart and Neale, 1998). Moreover, these discussions take place within unequal and gendered power relationships that may restrict a parent's capacity to shape and control another adult's (un)healthy behaviours within the privacy of the home (Robinson *et al.*, 2011; Greaves *et al.*, 2007). Our research demonstrates that parenting is constrained by the actions of other adults (including another parent), who may or may not interpret health 'risks' in the same way and may resist lifestyle change within the home. Moreover, as we shall now show, children also play an active role in the transmission and discussion of public health messages within the family, and this may shape parental beliefs, behaviours and lifestyle practices.

Children as active agents in regulating parents' (un)healthy behaviours within the home

Within the intensive parenting literature there is an implicit assumption that while parents are actively challenged to fulfil an idealised model of parenthood (and childhood), children occupy a passive and vulnerable role (Caputo, 2007). We argue that this interpretation neglects children's awareness of dominant narratives of parenting and 'healthy' lifestyles that they can draw on in their everyday interactions, overlooking a child's ability to 'negotiate, resist and hold power' (Evans *et al.*, 2011). Perhaps one causal explanation of this oversight has been the focus on the health 'risks' for the foetus *in utero* (Shirani *et al.*, 2011) and children in early infancy (Faircloth, 2010), who are considered to be much more vulnerable and dependent than older children. It has been suggested elsewhere that the adult expectations of children are linked to chronological age (Such and Walker, 2004), with increasing competency (Mayall, 2001), and studies are now looking at children's agency and engagement with parenting from a broader age range (Francis, 2012; Backett-Milburn *et al.*, 2010).

In public health discourses children are not explicitly portrayed as passive, but as incapable and/or unwilling to make healthy decisions (Colls and Evans, 2008), or messengers of expert advice to parents (Colls and Evans, 2008; Furedi, 2010). In contrast, many of the children in our research articulated clear ideas about what 'good' parents should do in relation to common health 'risks'.

In the following excerpts from interviews with parents, and focus groups with children (age 13–14 years) around alcohol consumption and education, we aim to highlight their knowledge and awareness of dominant understandings of parenting and health and how these shape children's agency in responding to or resisting these discourses in relation to their everyday interactions. They demonstrated keen awareness of the ideal parent ideology, and applied this to expectations of what parents should or should not to, with one group of boys discussing:

> Yes because sometimes like you see like kids out until like at least 9.30 PM, when it's proper dark and I am not against that or nothing, but I just think why would your parents let you be out that late because your parents are meant to care.

Caring was a common theme discussed by the young people in this study, and supports other research that suggests that children expect parents to demonstrate their care by monitoring their whereabouts, and providing moral guidance (Backett-Milburn and Jackson, 2010). Discourses around the normative understanding of parents being absolutely responsible for children were articulated (Such and Walker, 2004), with one group of girls reiterating in their discussion that not only should adults provide information, but also an appropriate model of behaviour, saying that 'The adults are not setting a good example for the kids ... if they are drinking'.

Individual autonomy was also recognised, with children displaying awareness of their own role in maintaining and rejecting dominant parenting norms. 'Even ... when parents are there for you like, children don't want to listen. They just like run off', was the start of an intensive discussion in one focus group of girls, and was readily endorsed by other group members who responded, 'Sometimes you are not there for the parents. Whenever the parents need you, you are not there', and claimed, 'So it's both of their [parents and children] responsibilities really. Not just like one or the other it's both of them'. The recognition of responsibility was a key theme in the studies, and recognises the assertions by other research that responsibility is a meaningful part of children lives (Such and Walker, 2004), and that children engage what could often be termed as 'moral work' in maintaining and contributing to family relationships (Mayall, 2001).

Such and Walker (2004) have suggested that children are active in the construction of the moral self, and the children in the current study were also involved in constructing their parent's moral identity. One way this was achieved was in the differentiating of their own parents from 'other' parents. This process, often referred to as the 'generalised other' (Holdsworth and Morgan, 2007), was not only a way of protecting the integrity of their parents (Backett-Milburn and Jackson, 2010) but offered ways of differentiating between healthy and unhealthy selves (Crawford, 2006). One group of girls discussed their own parents' behaviour in relation to the actions of other parents: 'In [another town] ... some mums don't even care what the kids do, but most mums down here are dead protective of their kids'. Immediately following this comment, one girl in the group quickly remarked 'My mum is from here, but she lives in [next town] so that doesn't count', clearly making an attempt to ensure her own mother was not associated with the other 'bad' mothers from the next town. This wider 'othering' could be seen as a protective measure by which describing the deviant behaviour of different parents served to portray their own parents as good and decent.

While there is growing body of research examining parents' and children's perceptions of responsibility and agency (Mayall, 2001; Such and Walker, 2004), there is far less exploring how children may seek to actively regulate or influence their parents' behaviour, in particular lifestyle behaviours. Research has tended to explore children's agency in negotiating their *own* health and behaviour (Rawlins, 2009; Colls and Evans, 2008), not their role in influencing the behaviour of *others* and has typically focused on food choices and obesity (Backett-Milburn *et al.*, 2010; Colls and Evans, 2008; Curtis *et al.*, 2010;

Rawlins, 2009; Zivkovic *et al.*, 2010). For these researchers, obesity represents a contemporary moral panic, resulting in increased surveillance of children's bodies and inspection of parental responsibility and practices. However, we believe it may be useful to compare the obesity crisis to other 'deviant' vices such as tobacco and alcohol use, which have not only been subject to similar scrutiny (Bell *et al.*, 2009), but have experienced increasing levels of intervention (such as the Smokefree Legislation in England and measures criminalising pregnant women who drink in the US and Canada) not yet experienced in the field of obesity. The role of children in influencing smoking and/or drinking behaviour has been alluded to in some studies (Rawlins, 2009), but rarely discussed further (with the exception of Holdsworth and Robinson, 2008).

One way in which interventions in the field of alcohol and tobacco have been enacted in public policy in the UK has been the compulsory inclusion of informative messages in school education, in addition to increased spend on national media campaigns. This increased knowledge has created roles for children to deliver information (and interventions) to more responsible actors (parents) (Colls and Evans, 2008; Holdsworth and Robinson, 2008). This reflects what has been termed 'socialisation-in-reverse – a phenomenon where children are entrusted with the mission of socialising their elders' (Furedi, 2010: 89). Bridget is a 43-year-old mother of three, whose ex-husband had what she described as a 'drinking problem', and died shortly after they had separated. She described strategies to protect her children from his drinking behaviour, but recognised that, with increasing age, her children were more aware of the negative impact that alcohol had on their father's, and their own, lives. In an attempt to negate the visibility of drinking experienced in the household, Bridget does not drink often and will only drink small quantities if she does. Over the past few years, however, she has experienced a number of strokes. Immediately prior to these strokes she recalls that she had had a sip of, or a small alcoholic drink. When discussing that her eldest son linked the subsequent strokes to the alcohol and did not want her to drink, Bridget recalled 'if I said I'd like a drink I would get that stern face off him, what are you doing that for, you know 'cause he associated it with that'. Bridget believes that this not only influences her behaviour, but recognises that the child–adult relationship is something to be constantly negotiated (Solberg, 1997) and not simply a hierarchy of power (Evans *et al.*, 2011):

> Yeah I take note because at the same time I don't want my children to see, I don't want to see them in a state, I don't want them to see me in a state and I am trying to show them that you know I respect their wishes although I am the parent I am not always right and if it upsets them and it makes them feel uncomfortable then I wouldn't do that.

In summary the data above illustrates that children are not only aware but active in the construction of dominant discourses surrounding parenting and health. This supports other research which proposes that responsibilities are constantly in a state of negotiation in the home (Holdsworth and Robinson; 2008, Such and Walker, 2004), and affirms the criticisms directed towards viewing children as passive recipients in the intensive parenting and health discourses (de Castro, 2004). Children demonstrate an understanding of how public concerns about health contain specific moralities about how family life should be (Crawford, 2006), and in addition parents have been shown to respect and respond to children's anxieties over their lifestyle behaviours.

Conclusion

This chapter challenges two key assumptions about 'intensive' parenting; first, that parents have full control of risk management and health within the home, which neglects the complex relationships and behaviours that have to be negotiated between parents and wider family members; second, that children are passive agents in this process. As we have shown in this chapter, children are not only aware of the moral obligations implicit in intensive parenting and health discourses, but through socialisation-in-reverse are active in shaping them, too. As valuable agents in educating parents about health risks and appropriate lifestyles (Colls and Evans, 2008), we have shown how children can take an active role in promoting public health messages from educational sources and campaigns. The ethical considerations of using children in this way are unclear and there is little evidence about how children respond to the increased responsibility and pressure to 'police' their own parents and other family members, and research into more extreme examples of children playing a caring role (i.e. parentification), have shown that increased responsibility can have both a negative (Rothman *et al.*, 2010, Bancroft *et al.*, 2005) and positive impact (Backett-Milburn and Harden, 2004) on children.

We have also highlighted several barriers that parents may encounter when trying to follow public health advice and enact risk-aversive parenting. Far from being irresponsible, the parents we refer to experienced limited capacity to shape their child's home environment and protect them from known health risks (Robinson, 2008). Through this we can suggest that this limited agency is often linked to what parents see as something external, and out of their own control, something rarely addressed in public health discourses that focus on individual responsibility to manage risk (Lupton, 1995). This means that mothers, and fathers, may feel frustrated, inadequate and stigmatised if they are unable to emulate an image of health-conscious parenting. This may have detrimental consequences for parent–child relationships and individual well-being if parents consider themselves to be failing in their 'duty' to protect their children. Simply increasing the number of public health campaigns, a common strategy used to raise awareness and encourage individuals to act in response to a known health 'risk', will only reaffirm their ongoing failure to protect their children from harm, thereby increasing their guilt. Our participants did not lack knowledge as to how they should parent; rather they lacked the bargaining tools to bring about effective change to their children's health.

Acknowledgements

The research studies we discuss in this essay were funded by two separate grants from Liverpool Primary Care Trust, and from the Liverpool Institute for Health Inequalities Research. We acknowledge the significant contributions that Liverpool Primary Care Trust, Alder Hey NHS Children's Hospital, The Roy Castle Lung Cancer Foundation, the participating schools and the Liverpool Healthy School team made to this study. We are also extremely grateful to the families who gave their time to speak to us.

Note

1 For a more detailed discussion of the studies, please see:
   Hinton, D., Robinson, J., Peak, M. and Laverty, L. (2011) *Developing a Clinician-Led Smoking Intervention for Families and Carers of Children Attending Routine Outpatient Clinics at Alder Hey Children's NHS Foundation Trust*. Liverpool, HaCCRU, online, available at: www.liv.ac.uk/haccru/reports/HaCCRU%20Alder% 20Hey%20 SHS%20Intervention%20Report%20120.pdf.

References

Abdullah, A. S. M., Mak, Y. W., Loke, A. Y. and Lam, T.-H. 2005. Smoking cessation intervention in parents of young children: a randomised controlled trial. *Addiction*, 100, 1731–1740.

Backett-Milburn, K. and Harden, J. 2004. How children and their families construct and negotiate risk, safety and danger. *Childhood*, 11, 429–447.

Backett-Milburn, K. and Jackson, S. 2010. Children's concerns about their parents' health and well-being: researching with ChildLine Scotland. *Children and Society*, 26, 381–394.

Backett-Milburn, K., Wills, W., Roberts, M.-L. and Lawton, J. 2010. Food and family practices: teenagers, eating and domestic life in differing socio-economic circumstances. *Children's Geographies*, 8, 303–314.

Bancroft, A., Wilson, S., Cunningham-Burley, S., Masters, H. and Backett-Milburn, K. 2005. Children managing parental drug and alcohol misuse: challenging parent-child boundaries. In: L. McKie and S. Cunningham-Burley (eds) *Families in Society: Boundaries and Relationships*. Bristol: Policy Press.

Bell, K., McNaughton, D. and Salmon, A. 2009. Medicine, morality and mothering: public health discourses on foetal alcohol exposure, smoking around children and childhood overnutrition. *Critical Public Health*, 19, 155–170.

Bottorff, J. L., Oliffe, J., Kalaw, C., Carey, J. and Mroz, L. 2006. Men's constructions of smoking in the context of women's tobacco reduction during pregnancy and postpartum. *Social Science and Medicine*, 62, 3096–3108.

Bristow, J. 2009. *Standing up to Supernanny*, Exeter, Imprint Academic.

Bunton, R., Nettleton, S. and Burrows, R. 1995. *The Sociology of Health Promotion: Critical Analyses of Consumption, Lifestyle and Risk*, London, Routledge.

Caputo, V. 2007. She's from a 'good family'. *Childhood*, 14, 173–192.

Carsten, J. 2004. *After Kinship*, New York, Cambridge University Press.

Colls, R. and Evans, B. 2008. Embodying responsibility: children's health and supermarket initiatives. *Environment and Planning A*, 40, 615–631.

Coxhead, L. and Rhodes, T. 2006. Accounting for risk and responsibility associated with smoking among mothers of children with respiratory illness. *Sociology of Health and Illness*, 28, 98–121.

Crawford, R. 2006. Health as a meaningful social practice. *Health*, 10, 401–420.

Curtis, P., James, A. and Ellis, K. 2010. Children's snacking, children's food: food moralities and family life. *Children's Geographies*, 8, 291–302.

De Castro, L. R. 2004. Otherness in me, otherness in others. *Childhood*, 11, 469–493.

Department of Health. 2010. *Our Health and Wellbeing Today*. London, Department of Health.

Douglas, M. 1994. *Dominant Rationality and Risk Perception,* Occasional Paper No. 4. Polticial Economy Research Centre, University of Sheffield.

Douglas, S. and Meredith, M. 2004. *The Mommy Myth: The Idealisation of Motherhood and Why it has Undermined all Women*, New York, Free Press.

Evans, B., Colls, R. and Hörschelmann, K. 2011. 'Change4Life for your kids': embodied collectives and public health pedagogy. *Sport, Education and Society*, 16, 323–341.

Faircloth, C. R. 2010. 'If they want to risk the health and well-being of their child, that's up to them': long-term breastfeeding, risk and maternal identity. *Health, Risk and Society*, 12, 357–367.

Field, S. 2010. Don't take offence if we lecture you on how to stay alive and healthy. *Observer*, 8 August.

Finch, J. and Mason, J. 1992. *Negotiating Family Responsibilities*, London, Tavistock.

Fitzpatrick, M. 2001. *The Tyranny of Health: Doctors and the Regulation of Lifestyle*, London, Routledge.

Francis, A. 2012. Stigma in an era of medicalisation and anxious parenting: how proximity and culpability shape middle-class parents' experiences of disgrace. *Sociology of Health and Illness*, 34, 927–942.

Furedi, F. 2008. *Paranoid Parenting: Why Ignoring the Experts May be Best for Your Child*, London, Allen Lane.

Furedi, F. 2010. *Wasted: Why Education Isn't Educating*, London, Continuum.

Graham, H. 1976. Smoking in pregnancy: the attitudes of expectant mothers. *Social Science and Medicine* 10, 399–405.

Graham, H. 1993. *Hardship and Health in Women's Lives*, Hemel Hempstead, Harvester Wheatsheaf.

Greaves, L., Kalaw, C. and Bottorff, J. L. 2007. Case studies of power and control related to tobacco use during pregnancy. *Women's Health Issues*, 17, 325–332.

Hattery, A. 2001. *Women, Work and Family: Balancing and Weaving*, London, Sage.

Hays, S. 1996. *The Cultural Contradictions of Motherhood*, New Haven, CT, Yale University Press.

Hoffman, D. M. 2003. Childhood ideology in the United States: a comparative cultural view. *International Review of Education*, 49, 191–211.

Holdsworth, C. and Morgan, D. 2007. Revisiting the generalized other: an exploration. *Sociology*, 41, 401–417.

Holdsworth, C. and Robinson, J. E. 2008. 'I've never ever let anyone hold the kids while they've got ciggies': moral tales of maternal smoking practices. *Sociology of Health and Illness*, 30, 1086–1100.

Hovell, M. F., Zakarian, J. M., Matt, G. E., Liles, S., Jones, J.A., Hofstetter, C. R., Larson, S. N. and Benowitz, N. L. 2009. Counseling to reduce children's secondhand smoke exposure and help parents quit smoking: A controlled trial. *Nicotine and Tobacco Research*, 11, 1383–1394.

Jarvie, J. A. and Malone, R. E. 2008. Children's secondhand smoke exposure in private homes and cars: an ethical analysis. *American Journal of Public Health*, 98, 2140–2145.

Kegler, M. C., Escoffery, C., Groff, A., Butler, S. and Foreman, A. 2007. A qualitative study of how families decide to adopt household smoking restrictions. *Family and Community Health*, 30, 328–341 doi: 10.1097/01.FCH.0000290545.56199.c9.

Lee, E., Macvarish, J. and Bristow, J. 2010. Risk, health and parenting culture. *Health, Risk and Society*, 12, 293–300.

Lupton, D. 1995. *The Imperative of Health: Public Health and the Regulated Body*, London, Sage.

Lupton, D. 1999. *Risk*, London, Routledge.

Lupton, D. A. 2011. 'The best thing for the baby': Mothers' concepts and experiences related to promoting their infants' health and development. *Health, Risk and Society*, 13, 637–651.

Mayall, B. 2001. Understanding childhoods: a London study. In: L. Alanen and B. Mayall (eds) *Conceptualizing Child–Adult Relations.* London/New York: Routledge/Falmer.

Mead, M. 1962. A cultural anthropologist's approach to maternal deprivation. In: M. D. Ainsworth, R. G. Andry, R. G. Harlow, S. Lebovici, M. Mead, D. G. Prugh and B. Wooton (eds) *Deprivation of Maternal Care: A Reassessment of its Effects.* Geneva: World Health Organization.

Miller, T. 2005. *Making Sense of Motherhood: A Narrative Approach*, Cambridge, Cambridge University Press.

Minkler, M. 1999. Personal responsibility for health? a review of the arguments and the evidence at century's end. *Health Education and Behavior*, 26, 121–141.

Phillips, R., Amos, A., Ritchie, D., Cunningham-Burley, S. and Martin, C. 2007. Smoking in the home after the smoke-free legislation in Scotland: qualitative study. *British Medical Journal*, 335, 553.

Rawlins, E. 2009. Choosing health? Exploring children's eating practices at home and at school. *Antipode*, 41, 1084–1109.

Robinson, J. 2008. 'Trying my hardest': the hidden social costs of protecting children from environmental tobacco smoke. *International Review of Qualitative Research*, 1, 173–194.

Robinson, J. and Kirkcaldy, A. 2007a. Disadvantaged mothers, young children and smoking in the home: mothers' use of space within their homes. *Health and Place*, 13, 894–903.

Robinson, J. and Kirkcaldy, A. 2007b. 'You think that I'm smoking and they're not': why mothers still smoke in the home. *Social Science and Medicine*, 65, 641–652.

Robinson, J., Laverty, L. and Holdsworth, C. (2011) *Talking About Alcohol: Understanding Attitudes to Alcohol Consumption in Secondary School Communities in Liverpool.* Liverpool, HaCCRU Research Report, online, available at: www.liv.ac.uk/health-inequalities/Research/attitudes_to_alcohol_consumption.htm.

Robinson, J., Ritchie, D., Amos, A., Greaves, L. and Cunningham-Burley, S. 2011. Volunteered, negotiated, enforced: family politics and the regulation of home smoking. *Sociology of Health and Illness*, 33, 66–80.

Rothman, E. F., Bernstein, J. and Strunin, L. 2010. Why might adverse childhood experiences lead to underage drinking among US youth? Findings from an emergency department-based qualitative pilot study. *Substance Use and Misuse*, 45, 2281–2290.

Royal College of Physicians. 2010. *Passive Smoking and Children: A Report of the Tobacco Advisory Group of the Royal College of Physicians.* London: Royal College of Physicians.

Shirani, F., Henwood, K. and Coltart, C. 2011. Meeting the challenges of intensive parenting culture: gender, risk management and the moral parent. *Sociology*, 46, 25–40.

Smart, C. 2007. *Personal Life*, Cambridge, Polity Press.

Smart, C. and Neale, B. 1998. *Family Fragments?* Cambridge, Polity Press.

Solberg, A. 1997. Negotiating childhood: changing constructions of age for Norwegian children. In: A. James and A. Prout (eds) *Constructing and Reconstructing Childhood: Contemporary Issues in the Sociological Study of Childhood.* London/Washington, DC: Farmer Press.

Such, E. and Walker, R. 2004. Being responsible and responsible beings: children's understanding of responsibility. *Children and Society*, 18, 231–242.

Thompson, L. and Kumar, A. 2011. Responses to health promotion campaigns: resistance, denial and othering. *Critical Public Health*, 21, 105–117.

Warner, J. 2006. *Perfect Madness: Motherhood in the Age of Anxiety*, London, Vermilion.

Winickoff, J. P., Buckley, V. J., Palfrey, J. S., Perrin, J. M. and Rigotti, N. A. 2003. Intervention with parental smokers in an outpatient pediatric clinic using counseling and nicotine replacement. *Pediatrics*, 112, 1127–1133.

Young, R. and Sly, F. 2011. *Portrait of the North West*. London: Office of National Statistics.

Zivkovic, T., Warin, M., Davies, M. and Moore, V. 2010. In the name of the child. *Journal of Sociology*, 46, 375–392.

5 Problem parents?

Undocumented migrants in America's New South and the power dynamics of parenting advice

Nicole S. Berry

The idea that kin relations, such as those between a parent and child, can help explain and justify wider inequities has had popular appeal in both the past and the present. Oscar Lewis (1959) posited a 'culture of poverty', where he argued kin interactions essentially socialized poor Mexican children into a world view that subsequently perpetuated their own poverty in adulthood. More recently, Kurtz (2007) has invoked the kin practice of cross-cousin marriage in Middle Eastern societies to explain what others have argued is a war over global inequities (Le Billon, 2004; Walt, 2002). In Kurtz's view, cross-cousin marriage ensures a strong degree of insularity that isolates the Middle East from modernity and provokes terror in response. This essay focuses on a related kin narrative: the role of parent–child relations in making migrants to OECD[1] countries more vulnerable than the native born. More specifically, I use an ethnographic case study of undocumented Hispanic[2] families that settled in Durham, North Carolina, USA to explore the proposition that many immigrant families lack adequate parenting skills, which leads to problems for the families themselves, as well as for society in general.

The central tension of this chapter is my discomfort with ideologies that implicitly and explicitly focus on separating good from deficient parents without any reflection on or accounting for power relations. I see such ideologies as inherently dangerous to vulnerable communities. Perhaps no example speaks as strongly to the damage and injustice that such ideologies can produce as the legacy of forcibly removing indigenous children from their families to educate them in residential schools.[3] In hindsight, it is easy to understand how such misguided policies issued forth from a politics of colonization and domination that deemed the passing of indigenous cultures and modes of being from parent to child not only as backward, but as pernicious to a child's ability to lead a righteous life in White society. While perhaps extreme, this example helps sensitize us to how inequitable relations of power can easily become disguised in ideologies that purport to help disadvantaged children. It also reminds us of our moral responsibility to consider power relations that underwrite judgements of deficient parenting in non-dominant populations in OECD countries, lest these tragedies be repeated.

This chapter explores the self-perceived problem in the Durham Hispanic community of migrant families that fail – that is families that break apart much to the dismay of the parents. In these families, minors flee, sometimes letting their parents know where they are going, sometimes not. There has been a proliferation of parenting interventions for immigrant families to ameliorate and prevent the failures of families such as those in Durham (see for example Bjorknes, *et al.*, 2012; Gross, *et al.*, 2009; Murphy and Bryant, 2002; Renzaho and Vignjevic, 2011; and Jaysane-Darr this volume), and this approach is underwritten by dominant North America ideologies of expert-led, skills-based parenting that suggest parenting is a technical skill that can be learned. In this chapter, I question the efficacy of such approaches through an anthropologically inspired look at the Durham Hispanic community that emphasizes the importance of family and kin relations to parenting, rather than the skills of adults in a family. Ultimately, the case study highlights the role of structural constraints in family dissolution and in doing so clarifies the lack of potency of (poor) parenting skills as either an explanatory framework or underwriting a theory for intervention.

Exploring family experiences and kin relations in the undocumented Hispanic community also serves as an excellent means to draw out the contrasting kin ideologies involved in contemporary, dominant discourses of expert-led parenting. Juxtaposing these kin ideologies exposes how inequitable power relations can be embedded in contemporary parenting discourses. Far from being neutral, technical discourses of expert-led parenting whitewash the dangerous power dynamics inherent in current construction of 'good' parenting in OECD countries.

Expert-led, skills-based parenting

Before looking at the ethnographic case study at hand, in this section I review what I mean by expert-led, skills-based parenting. North American parenting is currently dominated by discourses shoring up the importance of expert knowledge in dictating parenting practice. Scholars have traced the importance of the role of the expert in modern parenting over the last century (Ehrenreich and English, 1978). Certainly the rise of the expert was tied to a push to professionalize domestic roles that women occupied. Where previous generations of new mothers learned their trade from informal networks, the 1930s saw the rise of mothering codified by experts as a technical trade that could and should be learned in environments like university 'practice houses' (Leinaweaver, 2012).

Contemporary experts on parenting are still perceived to possess important knowledge that parents need, and training parents is still an important mode of transferring this knowledge. Nevertheless, what it is that parents must learn is notably different from the past. A mother that Sharon Hays (1996: 115) interviewed offers an appropriate characterization of how the role of expert-led parenting has changed: 'parenting classes have only come up recently. Years ago, you know what they called parenting classes? Teaching somebody how to change a diaper. *That's* what they called parenting' [emphasis in original]. From this statement, we can understand that while in the past, parenting was an applied domain that corresponded to set tasks (for example, changing the diaper or preparing food), today's parenting classes have a different valence.

How might we characterize what it is that parents must learn from experts today? A partial answer to this question can certainly be found in some of the earliest anthropological work engaging scientific understandings of child development, that of Sara Harkness and Charles Super (1983). Harkness and Super draw our attention to the dominance of the 'antecedent-consequence' paradigm. Essentially, this paradigm is premised on the idea that aspects of child rearing at one point in time will impact children later in time. Sociologist Glenda Wall's (2010) recent work on the rise of contemporary discourses around brain development illustrates how the 'antecedent-consequence' paradigm is powerful for instantiating the importance of experts to those undertaking child rearing. Research has emphasized the need for parents to '[spend] ample, one-on-one quality time with children in order to stimulate brain development and future brain potential' (Wall, 2010: 254). In short, parents must learn how to provide 'quality time' that promotes brain stimulus early in a child's life to create 'brain potential' later in the child's life. Far from the know-how involved in changing a diaper, experts today possess evidence-based knowledge driven by research. Such knowledge is decidedly different from what is learned through experience. Not only are experts in Wall's case responsible for advising parents on how to best use their time, they are instrumental in producing technical understandings of what constitutes 'ample' time or 'quality' time.

It is difficult to resolve the contradictions between the importance of the antecedent–consequence paradigm in carving out the role of the expert with the recent shift in expert discourses on parenting that ostensibly endorses multiple parenting 'styles'. Today's parents can choose a variety of parenting styles, such as attachment (see chapters by Faircloth and Layne this volume), apparently distancing us from the idea that there is one right way to do things. Subsequently, the 'style' you use to discipline your child while engaging in one-on-one quality time is perceived by experts as fairly inconsequential. Yet the modes that constitute appropriate 'quality' during this time can not be heterogeneous, as they are derived from a uniform, expert-led research process (see Hoffman's chapter in this volume).

In addition to charting the course of lab-based science to contemporary discourses of parenting in North America, Wall also draws our attention to the ways that parents come into contact with this information. The increasing importance of esoteric knowledge to proper parenting has been accompanied by a cadre of experts who translate these findings. (Wall, 2010: 254) Parents come into contact with expert advice through a variety of mechanisms including informational pamphlets (Wall, 2001), magazines (Quirke, 2006), visits to the doctor's office (Bornstein and Cote, 2004), home visits, books, internet sources, television shows (see Jensen this volume) and of course, the parenting class.

In sum, when Hispanic families migrate to Durham, they find themselves ensconced in an environment that very much views parents' actions and choices as deterministic of children's success (or lack of it). What parents must to do secure their children's future is not necessarily intuitive, but can be learned. It is this ideology around parenting that supports the idea that imbuing migrant parents with expert knowledge is an important foundation for healthy migrant families.

Family dissolution in Durham

The 'New South'

While Hispanic migration to the United States has been an enduring phenomenon, Durham, North Carolina is part of what researchers call the 'New South', referring to a demographic transition underway in the south-eastern United States that is characterized by a dramatic increase in Hispanics. Traditional US receiving communities for Hispanic immigrants are in the West and Southwest. In comparison, states like Alabama, Georgia, as well as the Carolinas had been sparsely populated by Hispanic immigrants, and instead dominated by African American and Anglo populations. The situation in Durham is typical of this demographic transition. From 1990 to 2006, US census data shows that the Hispanic population increased 1,332 percent. In real terms this means that it has gone from about from 2,000 people to about 28,000 over those sixteen years.

One characteristic that marks many Hispanics in the 'New South' is their undocumented status, meaning that they lack legal permission to reside in the United States. Most of the Hispanics in Durham crossed the border between the US and Mexico illegally and as such do not have official papers that would allow them to work or reside in the US. While many people buy fake papers necessary to get a job, such as a social security card that allows them to pay taxes, others work under the table for cash.

Being undocumented in the US certainly creates vulnerabilities and stress. Legally, those who lack papers could be detained and deported at any moment should they come into contact with an Immigration and Customs Enforcement (ICE) officer.[4] For families in the Durham Hispanic community, this means that when anyone leaves the house, you are never certain that they will return home. Parents worry about what would happen to their children if one or both spouses were detained and deported. How would the family be reunited? Who would take care of the children? Being caught by ICE does not translate into a free trip home, but rather can result in people being lost for years within the privately run detention system in the US. Recent scandals (Pilkington, 2011) detail the impunity with which detention center guards have abused both male and female detainees, making the prospect of capture all the more terrifying.

Being undocumented in Durham created many barriers to accessing state services, namely health care.[5] The US health care system is privatized and notably expensive. Citizens access this system through employer-based insurance or, for those who are poorest, through state-sponsored insurance (Medicaid). In general, undocumented Hispanics in Durham tended to work in construction, cleaning, care giving, or as part of the flexible workforce that made up the service industry – none of which are jobs that offer health care. Despite the poverty many experienced, lack of citizenship disqualifies undocumented

Hispanics for Medicaid. Instead, for routine care, individuals relied on sliding-scale, fee-for-service clinics that had been established to cater to this population.

Finally, while prejudice and racism take a toll on ethnic minorities in the US, being undocumented and an ethnic minority heightened pressure on these Hispanics. Racism, that might otherwise be socially unacceptable, could be public when directed at Hispanics, as bigots took moral cover under the issue of legality of status. Prejudice against Hispanics could be, and continues to be, coded as action against criminals or free loaders.[6] In Durham, Hispanics of all ages felt this pressure on the street. Additionally, anti-immigration citizens groups tried to pressure undocumented Hispanics to leave through tactics like denying them drivers' licenses, which would make daily life difficult to impossible.

Research methods

During 2006 and 2007, I worked with six Hispanic women on a participatory action research (PAR) project to address the aforementioned issue of community members perceiving high rates of 'family dissolution'. What I mean by family dissolution is that teenagers who had not reached the age of majority were leaving their families and setting out on their own, without their parents' permission or approval. For parents, this constituted a personal tragedy, and they worried about the future fate of their children.

The following data concerning the conditions immigrant families lived in and how these conditions created challenges to family integrity were collected by myself and the women with whom I worked. We used the social networks of the research team to recruit a purposive sample of interviewees that included eight fathers, twenty-one mothers, thirteen adolescent boys, and eighteen adolescent girls, representing families that were considered by their neighbours to be doing well, those that were in trouble, and also those that had broken apart. As part of the PAR process, we analyzed the themes of the interviews as a group. To cross-check our interpretations and seek more input, we presented our findings to both teens' and women's groups at the local community-based organization that supported the Hispanic community.

Immigrant intentions, immigrant realities

The narratives of both adolescents and their parents were framed around an original intent to migrate to the US because it offered more opportunity. Certainly parents, who had made the decision to leave their home country, were able to easily articulate what that imagined opportunity looked like. First and foremost, they were excited about the possibility of their children getting a good education and learning English. The vast majority of these immigrants came from the Mexican countryside where there was very little economic or educational opportunity. Most had very low literacy and many had not completed much schooling. Second, while their children were being educated, parents would take advantage of work opportunities to save as much money as possible. With their children educated and savings accrued, many dreamed of returning to Mexico with their families to a more secure future. The question we tried to figure out though our conversations with community members was: What about migration was leading this quest for a secure family future into family dissolution?

Educational opportunity and the lack thereof

In talking with parents, the first thing we found was that their ideas about schooling were heavily based on experiences in Mexico. In their minds, the major barrier to completing high school was financial. Many reported that they themselves had given up their education to help their families financially or that their parents did not have enough money to send them to school. Parents that we talked to assumed that, like in Mexico, there was an inherent value in earning a high school diploma and that it would improve their own children's work options. Parents frequently criticized what they perceived as a lack of authority that characterized the school system in Durham in comparison to what they were used to in Mexico. This lack of authority was associated with a perceived inability to control children in the school. But they also characterized the expectation of parent involvement in school and education as signs of a weak school system – the need for parent help belied the school system's inability to educate the children itself.

The first thing that became apparent when we spoke to adolescents was that their experiences of schooling were radically misaligned with parents' original vision of educational opportunity. Though all children have a right to attend school regardless of their immigration status, the highest level that most undocumented adolescents could achieve would be a high school diploma. Undocumented Hispanic adolescents in Durham understood they would not be able to go to college. Tuition in the United States is incredibly expensive for most everyone, and non-citizens do not qualify for federal grants, government-sponsored, low-interest education loans or work study. Public colleges and universities try to make higher education more affordable through a tiered system whereby in-state residents are given preferential admission and a reduced tuition tariff. The North Carolina State Senate, however, passed a law that children of undocumented migrants are ineligible to receive in-state status, regardless of whether or not they completed all of their schooling in North Carolina.[7] This means that most Hispanic adolescents are forced to apply as international students, pay premium tuition fees, and compete for a very restricted number of scholarships given to the best and brightest from all over the world. In the end, the adolescents reported feeling frustrated that it did not matter what grades they got or how hard they worked; they could be just as smart as the kid they sat next to, but that kid could go on and they could not. What was the point of studying if they were not going to have any more job opportunities than their parents?

Undocumented Hispanic adolescents experienced racism in the school environment. The idea that they had no future was not just their own – everyone else at school knew it and treated them accordingly. Their adolescent peers let them know that they were not welcome, and over 14 percent of Hispanic high schoolers (compared to 4 percent for their peers) reported not going to school at least once during the past month because they were worried about their own safety (Durham County Schools, 2008). The potential for race to cause this insecurity is illustrated by one teenager's description of 'enemies' in high school, including one Black American who came up to him and said that he did not like 'Mexicans'. This adolescent felt this was a provocation and felt obligated to fight.

Teachers and administrators inflicted their own sorts of punishment. Most adolescents recognized that their relationships with their teachers was at least partially predicated on their own performance, but many claimed that teachers were primed not to like Hispanic immigrants and give them bad grades. Additionally, adults in the school environment reportedly approached students speaking Spanish and said things like, 'You can't speak in Spanish here, it's the US.' Many Hispanic adolescents said that they felt that adults at school were not encouraging them or investing in them. Consequently, they said that they felt they were being 'babysat'. Given how frequently adolescents we interviewed reported being demoralized by their schooling, it is not surprising that Hispanic students grades were significantly worse than their peers, and 34.3 percent of Hispanic high school students reported feeling 'sad or hopeless' for more than two weeks (compared to just 16.7 percent for their peers). Statistics for high school completion for foreign-born Hispanic students in North Carolina were dismal, with over 58 percent dropping out (NSHP Editor, 2005).

Working parents, endangered children

While conflicts over what, if anything, education was doing for adolescents' futures brewed, additional conflicts emerged within the household. Parents' own goals to work and save money could essentially translate into deep fissures within the family. Within this orientation, getting work, maintaining work and earning money were all prioritized. Undocumented Hispanics worked incredibly hard – it was not uncommon for a parent to work two or even three jobs.

Parents perceived a number of problems that working such intensive schedules created for them with regards to their children. Most notably, they had to deal with leaving their children at home alone when they perceived Durham as a particularly unsafe environment for children. Almost all interviewees commented that Durham was marked by significant amounts of delinquency including thievery and people drinking and taking drugs out on the street. Interviews were peppered with stories that signaled the amount of violence that went along with this delinquency, like getting in a fist fight at the SuperTarget store, families getting mugged by gang members near their own front door, people coming around 'looking for' a family member, or even getting shot or stabbed.

Race was also a significant theme in these stories. Many interviewees reported tensions with the Black community, and concern with Black gangs that operated in the area. Undocumented Hispanics had moved into or taken over many of the traditionally lower-rent housing areas, and many of the jobs that Blacks had performed before the demographic shift. Research conducted in the Durham area around the same time as this study showed the Hispanics in general felt much more akin to Whites than Black Americans, and living in mixed race neighbourhoods with Blacks created an even greater feeling of distance from them (McClain *et al.*, 2006). Indeed, McClain *et al.* (2006) argue that Hispanics brought their prejudice against Blacks with them when then migrated. Undocumented interviewees of all ages described incidence of feeling preyed upon by Blacks.

Not surprisingly, parents fretted about leaving their children alone at home while they worked. One mother told us that while she was at work, another Hispanic person who lived in her apartment complex had tried to recruit her children into a gang. The mother had made it clear to the children that they were never to leave the apartment or to open the door to anyone when she was not at home. The gang recruiter realized that the children were in the apartment alone and tried to get them to open the door, but to no avail. Eventually, s/he gave up that tactic and started writing notes to the children, trying to convince them to open the door. A different neighbor eventually alerted the mother, who then confronted her children to confirm the story. She was furious that the gang was trying to predate her children.

But there were also bureaucratic dangers involved in leaving children unattended at home while one worked. One day officials came to a Hispanic community center to talk about school opportunities for children and reminded the mostly female group of attendees that leaving a child under twelve in the house without an adult was grounds for Social Services to come and remove the child from the home. Were parents to be found negligent, they could lose guardianship of their children and children could be put into foster care.

Parents' work schedules also combined with other new aspects of the environment to challenge their ability to keep their children safe. Most families came from small villages where everyone knew everyone. It was far easier to know when your children were doing something that they should not – if you did not see them yourselves, then word would get back to you through a neighbor. But who was watching out for the children in Durham? Parents were also used to knowing their children's friends and the friends' families. Yet Durham was so large that they had no idea who their children's friends were. Someone who went to high school with your child did not even necessarily live in your neighborhood. This meant that parents would not know children's friends' parents either.

Hispanic parents coped with this situation by becoming very restrictive with their children and especially their daughters. Many adolescents reported living in a state of lock down, and were restricted from activities that their peers at school might consider normal. They were never allowed to go to the movies alone. They never did sleepovers. This was obviously a hot topic as many parents brought up their dislike of the concept – parents did not sleepover at friends' houses when they were growing up, and on top of it, they could not send their children off to spend the night in some unknown house. The only time that adolescents got to leave the house was on the weekend, and they would do so with the entire family. One girl's complaint about family outings was typical – she wanted to see the new *Pirates of the Caribbean* movie, but her parents made them go to a movie that was suitable for everyone, so she had to see a cartoon instead. For their part, parents resented adolescents' attempts to influence family activities instead of just enjoying what their parents considered as best for the whole family.

Immigration, kinship and parenting

The study of parent–child relationships has long history within anthropological scholarship on kinship (Strathern, 2011). Kinship studies have been instrumental in helping us understand how kin relationships create obligations and responsibilities among different members of family. Inevitably such relationships dictate who must do what for whom, as we see in Heather Montgomery's (2001) potent example of children who engage in sex work in Thailand. In her study, both Thai mothers and their children viewed children as indebted to their mothers for giving them life. The mothers of some of the kids insisted that their children engaged in sex work to pay them back. Some adolescent sex workers decided to become mothers themselves to escape that debt, gain more control over their resources, and become the person who is owed, rather than owing. In this section, I interpret the narratives and experiences above by looking at how members of families perceive their kin relationships as creating obligations, opportunities, goals and responsibilities. I then juxtapose these kinships scripts with those that characterize expert-led contemporary parenting.

The family members that we talked to emphasized the message that is replete in studies concerning migration to the US and elsewhere – parents frame their primary reason for migration in terms of future opportunities for their children (Dreby, 2006; Horton, 2008; McCarthy *et al.*, 2000; Pribilsky, 2001). This framing alone helps contextualize the heavy weight of the responsibility parent interviewees felt to improve their children's futures. Parent interviewees were very forthright in emphasizing that working to earn money was one of the primary ways that they fulfilled their obligations and responsibilities to their families, specifically to their children. As discussed above, parent interviewees perceived money as the primary barrier to successful schooling. Many parent interviewees held more than one job, and absence from the home was a norm. While the expert-led parenting framework also views parents as responsible for children's futures, the sorts of parental actions assumed to create future opportunities for children are decidedly different.[8] As discussed in the introduction to this volume, parents are assumed to need expert guidance to understand how to best fulfill their responsibilities, including dictates on the best use of parent time for good parenting.

Another aspect of child–parent relations in Durham concerns the authority and legitimacy of parents to make decisions for the good of their children. Parents we interviewed resented when their children questioned this authority, and in the case of the *Pirates of the Caribbean* dust-up, emphasized that children inappropriately tended to put their own desires over those of the family. Certainly expert-led parenting frameworks support the claim of parents to make decisions for the good of their children; however in the Durham parents' cases, the 'good' of the children was not determined by prioritizing children's needs over the needs of others in the family (be it siblings or parents) or over the family itself.

This example segues into another point emphasized in child–parent relations among undocumented immigrants in Durham: immigration is perceived by these families as what Leinaweaver (2008b) terms 'a family project'. Contemporary models of expert-led parenting are in tension with this goal, as they aim to produce independent and highly functioning individuals who can fledge from the nuclear family to create their own families (Wall, 2001). Yet both undocumented parents and children could articulate immigration as a project not of self, but one that would move the family to a different future. Family dissolution was therefore anathema to the whole point of immigrating, and this made it almost incomprehensible for parents.

Just as immigration mapped onto interviewee parents' perceptions of their obligations and opportunities vis-à-vis kinship, it also mapped onto their perceptions of children's obligations. In short, parents emphasized that children's main obligation was to do well in school. We asked parents at what age it was appropriate for children to start to work, or whether or not children should be involved in extra-curricular activities, and answers always came back around to connect to the issue of a child's grades in school. If a parent thought that working or doing other activities endangered grades, then they would say no, children should only study. Some parents hedged their answers: if a child can do these other things *and* do well in school it was fine, if they could not, they should just study. These answers emphasized that parents perceived other activities as ancillary. Indeed it was in questions around school that parents most frequently articulated their expectations of different roles: as one parent put it, their job was to work and bring home money, their children's job was to study, and the teacher's job was to guide their children's education. Again, it is difficult to find a corollary here in contemporary expert-led parenting as it is motivated by an implicit ideology of the child's needs superseding those of the parent (i.e. child-centered). In short, experts outline children's perceived needs so that parents can respond to them.

Expert-led, skills-based parenting is spun in a way that obscures these kin ideologies and instead treats parenting as if it is an independent and internal skill: like swimming, you can be trained to parent well and you can even get a certificate in it. Yet the analysis above has demonstrated how spurious this position actually is. Ideologies of kin relations are also intrinsic to expert-led, skills-based parenting. Unlike the Thai mothers who assume that their children owe them, expert-led parenting assumes that parents owe their children – that is that good parents are obligated to sacrifice for their children's futures. While migrant parents also tend to share the view that sacrifice to ensure greater opportunity for children in the future is a mark of good parenting, expert-led parenting conceptualizes children as individuals whose needs are separate from and superior to the priorities of the family. Thus, parental 'sacrifices' such as migrating and working two jobs fail to count as sacrifices for children. The decontextualized vision of expert-led, skills-based parenting creates an easy atmosphere to consider 'low income and immigrant parents [as] deficient in parenting skills and requir[ing] training to support their children's success' (Johnson, 2009: 259), a problematic that I take up in the next section.

Recontextualizing parenting problems

Considering the situation in Durham helps clarify how higher-level structures like law around immigration, poor access to care resources, unsafe environments, as well as palpable racism are influencing the lives of undocumented parents and their children. The example of Hispanic children in Durham schools attempting to get a good education helps us illustrate this point. There is no shortage of literature pointing to attempts to solve children's problems at school by intervening in parenting (Bjorknes *et al.*, 2012; Johnson, 2009; Norwood *et al.*, 1997; Peters, 2012). Yet in this case study, we can see a number of factors that are instrumental in creating problems in schooling that parents have absolutely no control over. Racism within the school system and among teachers and peers is certainly a major one. Lack of funding and perhaps lack of interest within the school system to actually teach 'illegal' children who arrive as non-English speakers is another. Laws that remove the rights of youth to access free or at least reasonably priced education is a third. Finally, undocumented immigrant families' own precarious societal positions that leave them without access to basic care (child care and health care) and in states of poverty, as well as working more than full time and not available in their own households, certainly contribute to parenting styles characterized by a perceived lack of involvement in their children's schools or after-school home lives.

My position is not that there are not bad parents, or better ways to interact with children; rather my discomfort here is with separating purported good parenting from bad parenting without reflecting upon or accounting for power relations. Expert-led parenting advice is regarded as both objective and neutral, particularly that concerning the development of the universal human mind. Yet an exploration of kin ideologies implicit in expert-led parenting shows that it is not neutral at all. Rather expert-led parenting emphasizes that parents contribute to the technical project of building autonomous individuals with the right skills who can successfully fledge from their families. And, as we can see in this case study at least, these values stand to clash with the 'family project' of immigration that is shaped by a relational view of self that prioritizes the family over the individual and emphasizes the reciprocal obligations and responsibilities of different family members. In other words, immigrant parents in OECD countries might not be deficient, but rather they might be acting on kin ideologies that are decidedly different from those espoused by parenting 'experts'. Immigrant families in OECD countries, particularly vulnerable families such as undocumented workers or refugees, are in no position to challenge dominant institutions in OECD countries (including schools, research, medical, and both government and non-government services). Presenting expert-led parenting advice as technical, scientifically correct information and ignoring or denying that is it also biased and value-laden creates clear situations where vulnerable families can be coerced or unfairly discriminated against.

If we do not recognize that expert-led parenting is laden with particular values, then discourses in OECD countries around poor parenting in immigrant households stand to shift blame onto immigrant families for their failures. Monture (1989: 11) details the 'vicious circle' created in Canada that continues to separate First Nations children from their families who are 'deemed so deficient that not even ... parental skill development would now help'. As we see in this example, references to parenting skill continue to locate the pathology within the family – for if the parents could develop good skills, then maybe this generation of children could be returned. Yet as this case study of undocumented immigrant families has demonstrated, marginal and vulnerable communities can be under such structural pressures, that it is difficult to imagine how any parenting intervention could make up for this. Suggesting so is to unfairly contribute to the burdens these families deal with.

Notes

1 I intentionally use the term 'OECD', which stands for the Organisation of Economic Co-operation and Development and represents the collection of the most economically privileged countries in the world. While the ethnographic material that I present in this paper comes from the US, I would argue that the dynamics I discuss regarding parenting arguably apply to a collection of economically enfranchised countries that currently struggle to deal with growing migrant populations. While OECD is perhaps cumbersome, it seems to fit the overall argument here that stresses how critiques of parenting can be used to reinstantiate and justify precisely the inequitable divides that the OECD represents.

2 I use the term 'Hispanic' throughout this paper as it was the term that people I worked with identified to describe themselves.

3 Kline (1992) provides a sobering look at the policies that led to so many First Nations children to be removed from their homes and placed in residential schools in Canada. Other OECD countries like Australia and the U.S. also share this ignominy.

4 Most local police do not have the jurisdiction or resources to enforce immigration laws. Nevertheless, since 2008, Durham County is a participant in the '287(g)' program, the details of which are laid out in a Memoranda of Understanding (MOU) signed with ICE and the Department of Homeland Security. The MOU stated that one police officer would be deputized to enforce immigration law for all suspects who were accused of a handful of different crimes, including gang membership, manufacturing identity papers and violent crimes. Nevertheless, many worry about media reports that giving ICE status to police has led to racial profiling and abuse of power.

5 See Willen (2005, 2011) for a nice exploration of migration and access to care as a global issue.

6 Many in the US argue that undocumented workers are criminal because they broke the law when they crossed the border, probably work without permission, and have participated in 'identity theft' by purchasing fake papers to work. The question of whether or not undocumented Hispanics cost a locality more in services than they contribute is

98   *N.S. Berry*

hotly contested. The idea that undocumented workers do not pay taxes is a fallacious one. Most states in the US have value added taxes at the point of purchase and property taxes that everyone pays, regardless of status. Workers paid under the table may escape income tax, but workers who have fake social security documents have taxes automatically removed from their wages like every other worker.

7 The DREAM Act, which sought to pathways to education and/or citizenship for undocumented children was recently shot down by congress. See Preston (2011) for coverage.

8 Leinaweaver (2008a) presents another excellent anthropological example that explores how the imperative of parents' responsibility can translate into diverse actions. In this case she describes parents' efforts to circulate children into the homes of better-off relatives or acquaintances in hopes that children's futures will improve.

References

Bjorknes, R., Kjobli, J., Manger, T. and Jakobsen, R. (2012) 'Parent training among ethnic minorities: parenting practices as mediators of change in child conduct problems', *Family Relations*, 61(1): 101–114.

Bornstein, M. H. and Cote, L. R. (2004) '"Who is sitting across from me?" Immigrant mothers' knowledge of parenting and children's development', *Pediatrics*, 114(5): E557–E564.

Dreby, J. (2006) 'Honor and virtue – Mexican parenting in the transnational context', *Gender and Society*, 20(1): 32–59.

Durham County Schools (2008) *Durham County Youth Risk Behavior Survey (YRBS) Results 2007*, Durham, NC: North Carolina Healthy Schools.

Ehrenreich, B. and English, D. (1978) *For Her Own Good: 150 Years of the Experts' Advice to Women*, Garden City, NY: Anchor Press.

Gross, D., Garvey, C., Julion, W., Fogg, L., Tucker, S. and Mokros, H. (2009) 'Efficacy of the Chicago Parent Program with low-income African American and Latino parents of young children', *Prevention Science*, 10(1): 54–65.

Harkness, S. and Super, C. M. (1983) 'The cultural construction of child development: A framework for the socialization of affect', *Ethos*, 11(4): 221–231.

Hays, S. (1996) *The Cultural Contradictions of Motherhood*, New Haven, CT: Yale University Press.

Horton, S. (2008) 'Consuming childhood: "Lost" and "ideal" childhoods as a motivation for migration', *Anthropological Quarterly*, 81(4): 925–943.

Johnson, L. R. (2009) 'Challenging "best practices" in family literacy and parent education programs: the development and enactment of mothering knowledge among Puerto Rican and Latina mothers in Chicago', *Anthropology and Education Quarterly*, 40(3): 257–276.

Kline, M. (1992) 'Child welfare law, "best interests of the child" ideology, and First Nations', *Osgoode Hall Law Journal*, 30(2): 375–426.

Kurtz, S. (2007) 'Marriage and the terror war' *National Review Online*, February 15, online, available at: www.nationalreview.com/articles/219989/marriage-and-terror-war/stanley-kurtz.

Le Billon, P. (2004) 'The Geopolitical economy of "resource wars"', *Geopolitics*, 9(1): 1–28.

Leinaweaver, J. B. (2008a) *The Circulation of Children: Kinship, Adoption, and Morality in Andean Peru*, Durham, NC: Duke University Press.

Leinaweaver, J. B. (2008b) 'Improving oneself: young people getting ahead in the Peruvian Andes', *Latin American Perspectives*, 35(4): 60–78.

Leinaweaver, J. B. (2012) 'Practice mothers', *Signs*, 38(2): 1–26.

Lewis, O. (1959) *Five Families: Mexican Case Studies in the Culture of Poverty*, New York: Basic Books.

McCarthy, J. R., Edwards, R. and Gillies, V. (2000) 'Moral tales of the child and the adult: Narratives of contemporary family lives under changing circumstances', *Sociology*, 34(4): 785–803.

McClain, P. D., Carter, N. M., DeFrancesco Soto, V. M., Lyle, M. L., Grynaviski, J. D., Nunnally, S. C., Scotto, T. J., Kendrick, J. A., Lackey, G. F. and Cotton, K. D. (2006) 'Racial distancing in a southern city: Latino immigrants' views of Black Americans', *Journal of Politics*, 68(3): 571–584.

Montgomery, H. (2001) 'Motherhood, fertility and ambivalence among young prostitutes in Thailand'. in S. Tremayne (ed.), *Managing Reproductive Life: Cross-Cultural Themes in Sexuality and Fertility*, New York: Berghahn Books.

Monture, P. A. (1989) 'A vicious circle: Child welfare and the First Nations', *Candian Journal of Women and Law*, 3(1): 1–17.

Murphy, S. M. and Bryant, D. (2002) 'The effect of cross-cultural dialogue on child welfare parenting classes: Anecdotal evidence in black and white', *Child Welfare*, 81(2): 385–405.

Norwood, P. M., Atkinson, S. E., Tellez, K. and Saldana, D. C. (1997) 'Contextualizing parent education programs in urban schools: The impact on minority parents and students', *Urban Education*, 32(3): 411–432.

NSHP Editor (2005) 'Pressure to earn money keeps Hispanic dropout rates high', *National Society for Hispanic Professionals* March 20, online, available at: www.nshp. org/education/pressure_to_earn_money_keeps_hispanic_dropout_rates_high [accessed January 25, 2008].

Peters, E. (2012) 'I blame the mother: Educating parents and the gendered nature of parenting orders', *Gender and Education*, 24(1): 119–130.

Pilkington, E. (2011) 'Sexual abuse of immigrant detainees rampant across US, lawyers warn: Civil rights group ACLU finds evidence of systemic assaults on women held in detention facilities across America', *Guardian*, October 19.

Preston, J. (2011) 'After a False Dawn, Anxiety for Illegal Immigrant Students', *New York Times*, February 8, online, available at: www.nytimes.com/2011/02/09/us/09immigration.html?_r=1 [accessed February 8, 2011].

Pribilsky, J. (2001) 'Nervios and "modern childhood": Migration and shifting contexts of child life in the Ecuadorian Andes', *Childhood*, 8(2): 251–273.

Quirke, L. (2006) ' "Keeping young minds sharp": Children's cognitive stimulation and the rise of parenting magazines, 1959–2003', *Canadian Review of Sociology/Revue canadienne de sociologie*, 43(4): 387–406.

Renzaho, A. M. N. and Vignjevic, S. (2011) 'The impact of a parenting intervention in Australia among migrants and refugees from Liberia, Sierra Leone, Congo, and Burundi: Results from the African Migrant Parenting Program', *Journal of Family Studies*, 17(1): 71–79.

Strathern, M. (2011) 'What is a parent?' *HAU: Journal of Ethnographic Theory*, 1(1): 245–278.

Wall, G. (2001) 'Moral constructions of motherhood in breastfeeding discourse', *Gender and Society*, 15(4): 592–610.

Wall, G. (2010) 'Mothers' experiences with intensive parenting and brain development discourse', *Women's Studies International Forum*, 33(3): 253–263.

Walt, S. M. (2002) 'Beyond bin Laden: Reshaping U.S. foreign policy', *International Security*, 26(3): 56–78.

Willen, S. S. (2005) 'Birthing "invisible" children: State power, NGO activism, and reproductive health among "illegal migrant" workers in Tel Aviv, Israel', *Journal of Middle East Women's Studies*, 1(2): 55–88.

Willen, S. S. (2011) 'Do "illegal" im/migrants have a right to health? engaging ethical theory as social practice at a Tel Aviv open clinic', *Medical Anthropology Quarterly*, 25(3): 303–330.

6 Nurturing Sudanese, producing Americans

Refugee parents and personhood

Anna Jaysane-Darr

Introduction

We are seated in a small kitchen which serves as the teachers' room during the regular school day. The director of the Sudanese[1] educational program, Judy, looks around at the room full of South Sudanese men and women and welcomes them to the first meeting of this session of the educational program: 'We think that parenting is the hardest job in the world.' She pauses as the group laughs and nods knowingly. 'But we also think it's the best job in the world.' The group is silent as she smiles at them expectantly. Judy's statement epitomizes the evolution of childrearing and family into the phenomenon known as 'parenting' and the expectation that parenting is a form of unpaid, but highly valuable labor performed primarily in the home. For the South Sudanese Assistance Organization (SSAO)[2] that arranges and runs this Saturday enrichment program for Sudanese children and parents, an underlying goal is to reprogram South Sudanese notions of childrearing, defined by community, kin, and lineage rights and obligations, to one defined by parental involvement, regimentation, nurturance, and outcomes measurable in educational achievement within the school system. For the South Sudanese, 'parenting,' as it is used in the discourse of the organizers, is akin to a foreign language, involving an interpretive framework for both parents' and children's behavior that fits imperfectly with their own. The group's puzzled silence at Judy's comment is just one of many moments of miscommunication over the course of the educational program sessions. This miscommunication involves several axes of childrearing behavior, including norms of emotional and physical interaction between parents and children, appropriate forms of discipline and comportment, the significance of ethnic identity, and ideologies of personhood, individualism, and sociocentrism.

The educational program, held in a suburban school outside of Boston, Massachusetts, has become the flagship of the SSAO's activities. 'I want to put our focus on the moms and the kids,' Judy, the director, told me. After years of giving grants to women and men for education, the SSAO began to worry that the children were not having enough success in school, and they endeavored to intervene in order to provide tutoring for older students, preschool experiences for young children, and science and art for elementary and middle school-aged children. The program is well loved by members of the Sudanese community, the white volunteers of all ages, and the organizers. By this measure, it is a great success. However, while the children move from activity to activity, the parents – primarily mothers – socialize in the kitchen. The organizers found this problematic, and sought to institute various activities to benefit the parents while the children are busy. They have tried numerous approaches to structuring the parents' time, and the approach salient here consisted of a series of guest speakers and structured discussions held with the parents while their children were 'at school,' as the children liked to call it.

In this chapter, I examine the SSAO educational program as it elucidates key elements of the South Sudanese experience of and response to reproductive and parenting discourses in the United States. In particular, I look at the unwieldy dialogues revealed during structured conversations between volunteers and South Sudanese parents and in encounters with invited speakers. These parents grapple with engaging in the kind of parenting practices deemed necessary to raise 'Dinka'[3] children, such as fostering respect and formality (Lienhardt 1961, Deng 1972), while also recognizing that they must appropriate some 'American' parenting practices in order for their children to succeed according to the standards held by American schools and other state institutions. For South Sudanese, American parenting practices are part of the cultural apparatus that they must understand and, perhaps, adopt in order to succeed in the American sociocultural context. Sudanese parents simultaneously resist these efforts to shape their parenting practices into something more 'American', and strive to understand and benefit from them.

This chapter shows how these workshops work to inculcate 'parenting' as a particular way of interacting with one's children and, in doing so, reify a middle-class American way of conceptualizing the individual child and its needs. In the discourse of the workshops, this kind of person – a fragile but confident, self-actualized person – is the most likely to succeed in school. Further, this chapter demonstrates to what degree Sudanese parents take up this mode of person-making in childhood. Ultimately, some of it will make an impact, especially as it is reinforced by children's television and other media. In the meantime, Sudanese parents compartmentalize what they encounter in these workshops. As I will show, beliefs about respect and formal shyness inform their responses and interactions with the visiting speakers and volunteers. Sudanese parents are eager to take knowledge about American schools and educational success and apply it within the school context. In the home and in Sudanese social contexts, a different set of childrearing priorities predominates, including babies' physical comfort and contentment and promoting respect and hospitality in growing children.

The workshop encounters described here will illustrate how Sudanese parents subtly restructure the program itself to make it more amenable to Sudanese concerns of reproducing ethnicity by raising good Dinka children. Indeed, analyses of the workshops and Sudanese childrearing reveal that Sudanese parents are engaged in a very different childrearing project than the one offered by the speakers and volunteers. Instead of focusing on the individual and internal development of a child, they seek to raise a new generation of South Sudanese, indexing national and ethnic identity through behavior, comportment, and speech.

Methods

This article is part of a larger research project that examines South Sudanese refugee ideas about and practices of reproduction and childrearing in the United States at a time when South Sudan itself was becoming a new nation. Thus, the larger project engages with how concerns about citizenship and national belonging are bound up with reproduction and childrearing. It draws on seventeen months of ethnographic fieldwork in the Massachusetts South Sudanese community, three months in 2009 and fourteen consecutive months in 2010 and 2011. The data presented here was primarily gathered at the SSAO Saturday educational program. I attended seventeen of these educational programs in 2010 and 2011, where I observed and participated in the parents' workshops. In addition, I observed meetings with volunteers at the SSAO community center, conducted semi-structured interviews with Sudanese parents of various ages, and participated in the daily lives of Sudanese families in their homes where I engaged in informal discussions regarding raising children and managing everyday life in the United States.

The civil war and its consequences

An estimated two million people died and 5.5 million were displaced both internally and externally over the course of the second civil war in Sudan (1983–2005). This brutal war, whose roots lay in British colonial practices of indirect rule as well as religious, racial, and economic conflicts, was contested between the Sudan People's Liberation Army (SPLA) and the northern army and paramilitary fighters, yet the impact was felt – as is often the case – primarily among civilians and children who were killed, enslaved, or displaced. The majority of the displaced remained inside of Sudan's national borders, many in internally displaced persons (IDP) camps around the cities and towns in the South. The Massachusetts South Sudanese community consists of former refugees who were resettled in the Boston area and later brought wives, children, and other family members to join them. The core of the Boston area community is a contingent of the so-called 'lost boys,' unaccompanied minors who attracted international media attention when tens of thousands of them arrived in Kenyan refugee camps in the early 1990s. About 4,000 of these young men were then resettled in the U.S. in the early 2000s. Within a few years the Massachusetts community expanded greatly, and now consists of single men, young couples with children, and a few extended families.

South Sudanese in Massachusetts bring with them experiences of loss, displacement, disease, and deprivation, which do impact their reproductive and childrearing practices. Although South Sudanese parents maintain transnational ties to family and homeland, as displaced young people, they are often isolated from kin and lineage groups, which feature prominently in South Sudanese Dinka social life, and have what they consider to be secondary knowledge of many 'traditional' cultural practices. A traditionally pastoral, patrilineal society, Dinka draw social identity from the web of kin and lineage relations that position a person in a family, and humans in a community. Although they have no cattle here, they still play a role in American marriages through bridewealth exchanges in South Sudan, although this is changing as more families turn to money as an adequate substitute (cf. Hutchinson 1996). Nevertheless, the very idea of exchanging cattle or currency in order to secure a marriage and rights to official paternity of a child indicates how the notion of a person is bound to both the herd (real or fictive) and to the lineage, as it can be traced back eight generations and projected forward eternally. As former refugees, these parents strive to assemble meaningful life worlds out of scraps of cultural practices gleaned from their community, institutions, popular media, and memory.

'Parenting' in the United States

'Parenting', as the process of raising children is known in the United States, is a relatively recent term. Although there have been, over the course of U.S. history, a number of evolutions in the dominant forms of child care, the notion of 'parenting' traces its origins to the 1950s, when middle-class women were subject to an ideological shift that returned them to the home and out of the workplace, and raising children became endowed with profound meaning and importance, even as women's abilities to perform childrearing successfully without expert guidance were placed in doubt (Coontz 1992). Child development experts, pediatricians, child-care manuals, behavioral specialists, all began to influence how American parents raised their children, and the main target of their efforts were women (Ehrenreich and English 1979). Over the course of the next fifty years, 'parenting' became increasingly regimented, time consuming, and supervised. According to Sharon Hays, the 'intensive mothering' that has resulted involves '[t]he idea that correct child rearing requires not only large quantities of money but also professional-level skills and copious amounts of physical, moral, mental, and emotional energy on the part of the individual mother' (Hays 1996: 4). Indeed, 'parenting,' as it is practiced in the middle class United States today requires skills, expertise, finances, and, in particular, large quantities of time and emotional investment (Douglas and Michaels 2004). The SSAO program for children and their parents draws its legitimacy from the pervasive parenting industry in the United States, and the parenting methods offered in the program combine elements of the child-oriented approaches exemplified by the 'attachment parenting' movement (Liedloff 1977; Sears 2003), and contemporary approaches variously called 'intensive,' 'helicopter,' or 'Tiger' mothering (Hays 1996; Nelson 2010; Chua 2011; Warner 2006).

The SSAO program is a striking instantiation of the 'culture of expertise' that increasingly governs family life in America and elsewhere (see Jensen, this volume, for a discussion of parenting pedagogy and the media). The parenting expert in its various forms – psychologists, pediatricians, books, and television – has come to be regarded as essential to successful parenting. Moreover, as Nikolas Rose (1999) argues, parents in the U.S. and Western Europe have internalized the lessons of parenting experts, conceptualizing their children as fragile, psychologically deep individuals who must maintain 'emotional stability' and must be raised by parents who have been 'professionalized' (Ramaekers and Suissa 2011):

> No longer does the socializing project have to be implanted by philanthropy or imposed under threat by courts and social workers [...] it inheres in each of us, maintained and reactivated constantly by the images that surround us – in advertising, on television, in newspapers, and magazines, in the baby books. No longer do experts have to reach the family by way of law or the coercive intrusion of social work. They interpellate us through the radio call-in, through the weekly magazine column, through the gentle advice of the health visitor, teacher or neighbor, and through the unceasing reflexive gaze of our own psychologically educated self-scrutiny.
>
> (Rose 1989: 213)

Furthermore, this 'new' parenting entails a particular way of understanding child development, one that is a 'linear-development story' (Ramaekers and Suissa 2011: 14), defined by its telos, a productive adult. Thus, that the expert would turn her progressive gaze on refugees is not surprising, nor is it especially new. In fact, immigrants to the U.S. have often been the targets of improvement campaigns over the past century, particularly by and toward women (Irving 2000). Sudanese parents have not absorbed this way of envisioning their children – yet. The SSAO program offers an explicit articulation of parenting as expert-driven, in which visiting speakers serve as the experts, and seeks to transform Sudanese parents into professionals, if not fluent in the language of child development and psychological needs, then at least 'good enough.'

Feeling special: teaching and learning individualism

One of the first parenting seminars I attended at the SSAO educational program focused on 'teaching our young children to read.' The visiting speaker, Debbie, who specialized in early literacy, stressed that 'this doesn't mean getting a very young child to actually read him or herself, but getting her ready to read when it's time by making books a wonderful part of her life.' She used modeling exercises to show us how parents could interact with their children over books. The Sudanese women in the audience were enthusiastic about participating in this manner. They would answer her questions, repeat things that she said, and participate in the modeling exercises. For example, Debbie asked the group if they knew the story of the three little pigs. One woman, Miriam, volunteered to tell it, but the story she told did not cohere with Debbie's plan. Miriam described the wolf as a featured character, while the pigs were easily eaten. Debbie interrupted her to say, 'Okay, there are different versions of the story' and began to tell the traditional version concerning the straw, sticks, and bricks. She told the story to suggest that by starting reading early, they are laying a strong ('brick') foundation for the child's life. To do so, she erected a wall out of large cardboard blocks.

This foundation aims to combine the advantages of early literacy with particular kinds of affective bonds forged around the pages of a book between parents and children, and among the children in a family. The kind of 'parenting' presented in Debbie's talk and the parents' program in general, advocated for particular kinds of displays of parental affect that would allegedly produce childhood self-esteem and suggested that in order for children to attain these levels of self-esteem they would need close physical contact, singular attention, and the 'freedom' to express themselves at will. In Debbie's presentation, these behaviors are implicitly and explicitly linked to future academic success.

When Debbie arrived at the program that day, she began by piling some twenty or thirty books around the table, and the Sudanese women began flipping through them, asking each other to hand them different books they spotted on the other side, and commenting on familiar texts. Parents, Debbie began as she mapped out the stages of child development on a large pad of white paper, should begin reading to their babies at birth. In early babyhood, she told us, parents should take their child on a 'picture walk' through the book by pointing to the pictures in the book and describing what is happening, without needing to consult the actual written words. As the baby gets older, parents should use the baby's finger to point to these items in the book. Later, they can use the finger to count things that appear in the book. As the baby becomes a young child, she will spontaneously point to things in the book. She will point to words, count items, rhyme with the book, and fill in familiar words in the story. This is important, Debbie explained, because early introduction of books familiarizes children with basic literary concepts, such as what a book is, what words and pictures are, how to hold a book, and how to read from left to right. This prepares children for preschool and kindergarten. More importantly, she said, when a parent sits closely with a child reading or looking at books, this teaches a child to associate books with 'comfort' and 'security' and, by extension, the child feels safe, secure, and relaxed with the parent. Furthermore, she explained, 'your kids know that you are busy,' but when a parents takes the time to sit with them and read a book, it makes the child feel 'loved' and 'important.' It is crucial, she explained, not to say, 'sit down and be quiet' to your children when reading a book, but to make it 'fun and enjoyable.'

Early literacy, in this American context, is credited not only with assisting in producing better educational outcomes in children, but also with producing particular outcomes in parent–child relations. 'Comfort,' 'security,' 'love,' feeling 'important,' and 'having fun' are emphasized in Debbie's talk. Debbie implies that her Sudanese listeners should reconceptualize their children as individuals with individual needs and desires. These individual needs and desires begin at birth, in this formulation, and early literacy can help to foster educational and developmental outcomes in each child.

Individualism and Sudanese personhood

For the Sudanese community gathered in the kitchen, there was attentive interest to ways they could bring about success for their children. They perceive through their experience with the SSAO, with the schools, and in programming like this, that there is a need to acquire some of these 'parenting' skills in order for their children to succeed educationally and economically. As one man, Jok, described in a different session, 'Sudanese are working multiple jobs, working very hard, just to put food on the table. Our kids need to get an education, or we are lost. We want our kids to do better than us.' Despite an interest in educational success, the Sudanese parents I came to know operated with a fundamentally different understanding of human infancy and childhood than the one Debbie espoused in her presentation. When Sudanese parents were given a chance to ask questions at the end of the presentation, it became evident that Sudanese expectations about infancy and childhood were colliding with Debbie's 'parenting' approach. Sudanese parents greatly desire babies, and are affectionate and loving with their infants, but they have a different orientation toward the needs and desires of their infants. Debbie advocates a configuration toward infants that emphasizes individuality and emergent agency, whereas Sudanese parents emphasize both physical needs and a status of babyhood. This expansive version of babyhood meant that Sudanese parents repeatedly asked Debbie to confirm the correct age for early literacy: it was difficult to believe the right answer was 'from birth'.

In contrast with the dominant American approach to personhood exemplified by Debbie's presentation, Sudanese mothers' interactions with their babies suggest that babies are treated as extensions of the mother's physical body (see Faircloth and O'Dougherty, this volume, for contrasting British, French, and Brazilian notions of parental selfhood). Newborn babies are kept very clean, washed frequently with very hot water and rubbed with oil. New mothers treat their own bodies with the same formula, and this method is described by Sudanese mothers as the best way for both to recover from the birth. Keeping babies that are awake in contact with the mother's body reinforces this connection, as well as near universal use of breastfeeding as both feeding and comfort for crying babies. Nyanriak, a young mother of one, would constantly hold her one-year-old baby girl. When she would get up to reach for the phone across the room, she kept the baby pinned to her knee. She did not use objects to distract her, instead using her own body and voice to comfort the baby. The close physical ties between mother and child described here also manifest in forms of address. Mothers are often called the name of their firstborn child with the prefix '*man*,' which means mother. For example, Nyanriak is often referred to as '*Man Yar.*'

Sudanese baby care practices de-emphasize individualized, agentive personhood and emphasize care for the baby's physical body, avoidance of crying, and an early sociocentricity. Sudanese mothers are highly affectionate with their infants. Babies are held almost constantly, kissed, hugged, checked for any source of discomfort, fed if hungry and comforted when crying, with a liberal use of pacifiers. These holding and feeding practices seek to avoid or eliminate crying in the baby. Babies are not allowed to cry for more than a few moments before the mother will begin using comforting techniques ranging from picking up to feeding with either the breast or a bottle (used in more public settings) to a pacifier. Babyhood, moreover, is seen as extending well into the second year. Infants and babies, until they are around two years old, are not addressed as true interlocutors or the bearers of personal desires. Babies are often not directly referred to by their names: *menh* or 'the baby' is used instead. Expectations of disciplined behavior are not introduced until around age two, and children are not expected to conform to childhood discipline until around age five. Thus, books, in this formulation, are efficacious only if they succeed in keeping a baby or toddler quiet and happy. Having baby books in the house is reasonable, but sitting down and reading to a baby positions that child in a very un-baby like posture: as an interlocutor. 'He is too young for the books,' one mother told me.

In contrast, 'specialness,' as described in Debbie's talk, serves as a vehicle for introducing particular ways of thinking about the individual. Indeed, instilling Sudanese parents with American parenting values brought with it the notions of sovereign individualism that partially define American personhood. Yet, as Kusserow (2004) notes in her study of preschool-aged children from three different social classes, the ideology of 'individualism' takes different forms in different American contexts. For upper-middle class preschool parents and teachers, 'individualism' meant that children were encouraged to be creative, assertive, and find their own singular way of expression in the world. For working class and poor families, however, 'individualism' meant that children were told that they should not be 'pushed around,' that they cannot 'trust anyone but themselves,' and they must be able to take care of themselves. Mental and physical toughness was encouraged to foster this sense of individualism. These differences serve to reproduce social classes through the socialization of individuals. The kind of individualism espoused by Debbie and the SSAO is one that relies both on creativity and self-expression, and having the resources available to enable these outcomes in their children.

Ideologies of individualism were further emphasized by another visiting speaker, Jonathan, a school principal from one of the wealthiest towns in the state. Jonathan told the group: 'You are responsible for your own children. Not the school. Not the community. You.' This formulation posits that parents situated in a nuclear family are exclusively responsible for the behaviors and outcomes of their children. South Sudanese parents constantly grappled with the nuclear family imperative. On the one hand, Sudanese parents do strive for a privacy that excludes those outside kin or fictive kin networks. On the other, these parents actively defined the workshop as a sociocentric space. Jonathan expressed frustration – what he called 'tough love' – at the movements in, out, and about the room as he spoke, suggesting that these parents and their children did not know how to play 'the game,' by which he meant the ways in which children must behave in school in order to succeed.

Sudanese parents, however, expected that their children would filter in and out of the room. A child would usually want something: food, drink, or a chance to sit on her mother's lap. The mothers matter-of-factly doled out whatever was needed, and were always willing to take the child to sit in the room with us for a while if she seemed like she needed it. Even if the mother stepped out for a minute, another mother would take that child to be comforted or fed. Some mothers sent their children to the educational program with other families, and in those cases, it was those mothers who provided the needed items.

Likewise, babies were passed around from woman to woman with little concern for the feelings of either the mother or the taker, regardless of ethnic affiliation or close friendship. Baby passing reflects important norms of hospitality, reciprocity, politeness, and respect that Sudanese mothers operate with, and it begins to instill qualities of hospitality and respect in the child. Sometimes a woman would get up and walk over to a mother to take her baby. She would then sit holding the baby, comforting it if it cried, fixing its clothes or its hair. At other points, a mother would stand up and deposit her baby in another woman's arms. Perhaps a little while later, a different mother might come over and pick up that baby. Baby passing and exchanging care in this manner not only conflicts with the primacy of the parent–child relationship as it is foregrounded in the American context (see Layne, this volume, and Dow, for the Scottish context), but it also restructures the parents' program itself to produce South Sudanese values in the children.

The SSAO educational program binds closeness and affection to notions of the specialness of each individual child, and places this specialness at the foundation of lifelong success measured in educational outcomes. Sudanese baby-care practices could not be construed as lacking affection, but the meanings behind these practices differ. Sudanese mothers love their babies, as both a representative of a lineage and as a part of themselves. Yet while babies are highly valued, they are not represented as individually special. Instead, babies are treated as an extension of their mother's physical body, and are culturally constructed as a physical body that must be cared for. Attempting to enact an Americanized parenting mode of thinking about baby- and toddlerhood proves awkward for South Sudanese parents, and it reinforces their awareness of their own marginalization in the education system and beyond.

Hospitality and respect

Twenty-five-year-old Amer, mother of one, said to me one day, 'Look, he does kudual!' and reached out her hand to her eight-month-old son. By this she didn't mean the greeting word *kudual*, which can mean 'hello,' but instead the act of greeting with a handclasp. She bent down to him where he sat in his high chair and reached out her hand to him. 'Kudual,' she said, and when he didn't respond immediately, she said it again, 'Kudual.' He reached out his chubby hand for hers and gently held it for a moment. At eight months, it was already important for a young baby to begin learning to appropriately greet another person. When a South Sudanese man or woman enters a room, he or she will walk around to every person in the room and clasp their hands. 'Kudual' is therefore a key element of socializing children. Amer's interaction with her son focuses our attention on the priorities of respect (*thek* in Dinka) and hospitality that Sudanese parents intend to engender in their children (cf. Lienhardt 1961; Deng 1972). These priorities are not just reflective of the expectations for children's behavior. They are deeply implicated in everyday life for Sudanese families, constitutive of their habitus, ranging from material culture in the home, to comportment, to linguistic practices. Furthermore, for families in the diaspora, these values serve to link their children to an ethnic identity and fashion their children as representatives of Dinka-ness.

In the SSAO education program, Sudanese participants reshaped the conversation to reflect these concerns about respectful and appropriate behavior in public and private. This interest in discipline was evident in Debbie's first visit, as the parents asked for strategies to control their children while reading. James, a Dinka elder, told Debbie, 'when my first child was born, I read to him a lot. When my second son was born, I read less. Now that there are three....' He laughed and gestured to indicate that he rarely reads to them. Others agreed, saying that multiple children make it difficult to maintain discipline. This was also an issue during Debbie's second visit, when parents asked how to get their children to behave as they prepared for school in the morning, and how to keep their children away from negative neighborhood influences. Concerns about children's behavior also reflect Sudanese views about hierarchy and authority, formed within the postcolonial context of war-torn Sudan. Not only are elders regarded as more authoritative, many Sudanese came to view teachers as also having final authority over their children, and in the U.S., parents want their children to conform to the expectations of their teachers without parental interference.

Parents struggle with adapting to an American context where the public sphere requires that parents constantly supervise their children's behavior. One day, I asked Margaret, a Sudanese mother of two, whether she was considering an offer from the SSAO to teach children at the educational program. She thought for a minute and said that she could not because Sudanese children in the U.S. are not well behaved. 'They don't listen,' she said. I suggested that American families are not very strict, either. She protested, 'American kids are much better than our kids! Sudanese kids always make huge messes everywhere they go and they don't listen.' For example, they set off the alarm at the church where the community gathered for Christmas prayers. She was very offended by these incidents. 'I want to see how Deng grows up, what will happen,' she said, 'I am watching him.' Margaret here engages in a kind of social scientific enquiry: how will her Sudanese child respond to the American context? If American children in America are well behaved and Sudanese children in Sudan are well behaved, is it just Sudanese children in America that are misbehaving? She hopes to observe her son to see whether he, too, will be affected by his American context.

Sudanese responses also indicate that anxieties about the behavior of children in public and private are partially driven by an emerging awareness of American racial and social inequalities that treat children's behavior unequally. Parents learn this through institutional interactions, particularly in the schools. Schools delineate these inequalities starkly: in the interest of educating both parents and children, school administrators and staff identify immigrant parents as in need of guidance. In response to Jonathan, Sudanese parents were not only concerned about how to interact with teachers; they were also eager to understand how to interact with other parents, and how their children should interact with their friends on 'play dates.' One woman spoke up with evident frustration: 'My son's friends invite him over to their house, but they don't want their child to come to my house. The parents, they come to my house and they check the fire alarm!' These concerns represent the intersection of cultural misunderstandings, such as how to communicate with people and what to expect of them, with their desire to allow their children the benefits of living in the United States. Whether they are detecting implicit racial discrimination or xenophobia, Sudanese parents perceive through these kinds of incidents that their children's social interactions are scrutinized and that they must control their behavior.

Becoming Dinka

For South Sudanese participants in the parents' program, the very notion of 'parenting' did not register clearly. Instead, members of the group immediately shifted the discussion to one about 'how being a parent is different in Sudan' and how this makes it difficult for them. There are multiple valences in this discursive shift. There is a discourse of complaint, embedded in the relationship of 'helper' and 'helpee' developed through the interactions of the Sudanese and the SSAO. There is also a refusal to divulge specific childrearing behaviors, in case they could be targeted by social services. Further, though, 'parenting' as a discrete set of practices does not exist. Instead, they choose to focus on their roles as parents and how hard it is in the U.S. to raise Dinka children. In the session described below, Judy wanted the group to discuss 'how parenting is done in "their culture."'

ABUK: Our kids don't like our traditional foods. All they want is pizza and chicken nuggets and the rest of the American foods.

NYANDENG: When my son sees the meals I prepare, he refuses them and just wants pizza.

JENNY [white volunteer]: All American parents have this problem! We want to prepare healthy meals for our kids, but our kids just want junk.

JOSEPH: I understand, chicken nuggets are good. I like them, and they're healthy.

This conversation is particularly indicative of the contradictions that constitute this parenting program that seeks to simultaneously shape and validate existent parenting behaviors. Judy and the SSAO do desire to make visible Sudanese and Dinka parenting practices, but ultimately they want South Sudanese parents to realize there is no one 'right' way to raise children in America despite facing similar parenting challenges. Jenny articulates that position when she says, 'All American parents have this problem!' These parents call into question this assertion when they suggest that, in fact, these foods are not undesirable based on their perceived nutritive value. Instead, their responses shed light on the importance of consuming foods considered ideal for Sudanese children to eat: their Sudanese foods that are lovingly prepared for friends and family. These mothers, in particular, take pride in the food they prepare, and consider cooking to be their most precious contribution to their family and an icon of ethnic identity. When their children reject these foods in favor of 'American' foods, it seems more than a simple choice to have junk food, as Jenny asserts. It is analogous, in their minds, to how their children reject Dinka. Here, some women tell Jenny and Bob, Jenny's husband, about language loss:

NYABOL: My daughter says, 'Dinka is *your* language and English is *my* language'.

AYUM: The kids understand Dinka, but they won't speak it.

BOB: Keep speaking Dinka to your kids. Bilingualism is a gift. They will eventually be proud of their language.

AKUR: When we were kids in Sudan, we were forced to speak Arabic in school but our parents still taught us Dinka at home. We all knew how to speak Dinka. But now when we speak Dinka, there are a lot of Arabic words too. The kids get confused about what is Dinka.

NYANDENG: Yes, and now we speak 'Dinglish.'

In this conversation, Jenny and Bob advocate for the importance of bilingualism, partially reinforced by recent research reported in the popular press that shows how bilingual children are 'smarter' and more successful in academic achievement (for example Cuda-Kroen 2011). However, the Sudanese women in the room are concerned with the politics of language – a different issue altogether, and a different set of childrearing priorities. The Dinka language was suppressed and infiltrated by Arabic in the unified Sudan under the rule of the north. Arabic stands in ideologically for northern domination in the south and the attacks by *murahiliin* during the second civil war. They regard Arabic as infecting their language, yet they are unable to completely purge themselves of it in order to communicate across ethnic lines and to accommodate concepts without Dinka equivalents. Mothers' concerns over their children's misunderstanding of Dinka reflect their feelings about Arabic. Dinka indexes an imagined, purified past, but it simultaneously indexes the future South Sudanese nation. Imbuing their children with Dinka links their children with both that past and the future. It is significant to note that the intermingling of Dinka and English in 'Dinglish' is not as much of a cause for concern, expressing the differing relations between the languages.

Furthermore, Dinka is seen as intimately connected with the raising of children and the mother–child relationship. I was told that Dinka makes sense to Dinka speakers only because it is taught to them by their mothers. Bob and Jenny drew on their experience as public school teachers to emphasize bilingualism as a 'gift' to their children that will ultimately benefit them as participants in the American educational system. For the Sudanese in the room, the Dinka language is more than a gift: it partially constitutes childrearing itself. Thus, the discursive shift South Sudanese parents make in these encounters with volunteers is not simply away from a notion of 'parenting' as an opportunity to raise creative, individualized, self-actualizing children, but toward the intersection of reproductive and childrearing practices with ethnic identity.

Conclusion

This chapter has described how 'parenting' as an American sociocultural practice becomes part of the effort to 'assimilate' refugee families. In fact, the intensive parenting practices espoused by the SSAO parenting program reinforce a socioeconomic hierarchy through the advocacy of middle-class values and the expectation of financial resources to manage them. While the program organizers strive to assert that 'there's no one right way' to raise children in America, their workshop sessions call this into question. The parenting approaches presented in the sessions suggest that in order for a child to succeed in mainstream America, both in education and in adult outcomes, he or she must embody an 'individual' with his or her own internal needs and desires. She or he has to have an individualized path through life, distinct from that of the parents, in which mistakes and successes primarily attach to his or her person. This child's life course is measurable by a series of standardized stages, particularly detailed in babyhood, but continuing through adulthood. The parents of this child must deploy extraordinary resources and time in the effort to correctly shape this child in order for him or her to succeed. In other words, the parenting methods advocated in the program seek to institute a new kind of personhood.

South Sudanese parents cannot achieve these standards of intensive parenting, and instead are at risk of being marginalized within the educational system. Yet, these parents are also comfortable applying a different set of priorities to childrearing in hopes of achieving a different set of outcomes. Some of these outcomes overlap – such as educational achievement – but others, like Dinka ethnic identity and South Sudanese national belonging, differ. In redefining the workshop both by controlling the space and through setting the terms of the discourse, South Sudanese in a sense graft their childrearing priorities on to the SSAO educational program. Parents foreground hospitality and respect within the program itself, and in their interactions with teachers, administrators, doctors, and social services.

New forms of belonging are also articulated through the education program that further complicate the SSAO's efforts. As Dinka elder James pointed out at another group session:

> The good thing about coming here [to the educational program], for the children, is that it's like looking in a mirror. For a lot of these kids, they go to schools where they look different from everyone else. In my kid's school, there is only one black child in each class – him. But when they come here, it's like looking in a mirror, and that's very important.

Here, he moves beyond any kind of concern with ethno-national belonging to a racial identity. The racial identity is an implicit acknowledgement of emplacement within a distinctly American socio-racial hierarchy. Even as it tries to transcend these hierarchies, the ideologies of parenting described in the educational program ultimately serve to reinforce them. Yet, the very acknowledgement of this socio-racial order helps to de-naturalize it. The program itself, as James suggests, allows the South Sudanese community to construct a place within which they can fasten ethnic identity to educational success, and, they hope, deploy it in support of the new South Sudanese nation-state.

Notes

1 Members of the South Sudanese community in Massachusetts primarily refer to themselves as 'Sudanese', despite the secession of South Sudan from the North in July 2011. I use the terms interchangeably to reflect their usage.
2 All names of participants and organizations have been changed. The SSAO is a not-for-profit organization located only in Massachusetts that serves the educational needs of the local South Sudanese refugee community.
3 The majority of South Sudanese living in Massachusetts are from the Dinka ethnic group, but there are also small numbers of other ethnic groups, including Nuer, Shilluk, Bari, and Mabaan.

References

Chua, A. 2011. *Battle Hymn of the Tiger Mother*, New York: Penguin.
Coontz, S. 1992. *The Way We Never Were*, New York: Basic Books.
Cuda-Kroen, G. 2011. 'Being bilingual might boost your brain power', *National Public Radio*, online, available at: www.npr.org/2011/04/04/135043787/being-bilingual-may-boost-your-brain-power.
Deng, F.M. 1972. *The Dinka of the Sudan*, New York: Holt Rinehart and Winston.
Douglas, S.J. and Michaels, M.W. 2004. *The Mommy Myth: The Idealization of Motherhood and How it has Undermined Women*, New York: Free Press.
Ehrenreich, B. and English, D. 1979. *For Her Own Good: 150 Years of Experts' Advice to Women*, Garden City, NY: Anchor Books.
Hays, S. 1996. *The Cultural Contradictions of Motherhood*, New Haven/London: Yale University Press.
Hutchinson, S.E. 1996. *Nuer Dilemmas: Coping with Money, War, and the State*, Berkeley: University of California Press.

Irving, K., 2000. *Immigrant Mothers: Narratives of Race and Naternity, 1890–1925*, Urbana: University of Illinois Press.

Kusserow, A. 2004. *American Individualisms: Child Rearing and Social Class in Three Neighborhoods*, New York: Palgrave Macmillan.

Liedloff, J. 1977. *The Continuum Concept*, New York: Knopf.

Lienhardt, G. 1961. *Divinity and Experience: The Religion of the Dinka*, Oxford: Clarendon Press.

Nelson, M. 2010. *Parenting Out of Control: Anxious Parents in Uncertain Times*, New York: New York University Press.

Ramaekers, S. and Suissa, J. 2011. *The Claims of Parenting: Reasons, Responsibility, and Society*, Dordrecht: Springer.

Rose, N.S. 1999. *Governing the Soul: The Shaping of the Private Self*, London/New York: Free Association Books.

Sears, W. 2003. *The Baby Book: Everything You Need to Know About Your Baby from Birth to Age Two* 2nd ed., Boston: Little, Brown.

Warner, J. 2006. *Perfect Madness: Motherhood in the Age of Anxiety*, New York: Riverhead.

Part III
Negotiating parenting culture

7 'Intensive motherhood' in comparative perspective

Feminism, full-term breastfeeding and attachment parenting in London and Paris

Charlotte Faircloth

Introduction

This chapter emerges from a research project involving networks of mothers – in London and Paris – who breastfeed their children to 'full term'. Typically, this would be up to the age of three or four, though ranged, in this case, between one and eight years old. As part of a philosophy of what is called 'attachment' parenting, other typical practices amongst this sample of mothers include breast-feeding 'on-cue', bed-sharing and 'baby-wearing'. The endorsement of 'full-term' breastfeeding provides a case-study by which to explore the recent 'intensification' of mothering. This is a trend identified by a range of scholars writing about parenting in contemporary Euro-American contexts (Douglas and Michaels 2004; Furedi 2002; Hays 1996; Lee 2007a, 2007b; Lee and Bristow 2009; Warner 2006), as well as beyond (this volume).

The data presented here reveal that the relationship between the dynamics of intimate relations and broader international trends is not straightforward: what is considered appropriate care is not cross-culturally stable. While it seems that 'inten-sive motherhood' is being exported from the US (and the UK) to other settings in a 'global ethics of care', its reception and interpretation is far from uniform. The argument is that whilst the endorsement of attachment parenting and long-term breastfeeding by some informants in London is a magnification of a more general-ised 'intensive parenting' culture in the UK, which encourages absorbed parenting on the part of mothers, the same mothering looks very different in Paris. In a culture where maternal–infant separation and autonomy is lauded as ideal, such as France, 'intensive' embodied care on the part of the mother is perceived as an impingement on female liberty, rather than a valid outlet for 'identity work' (see, for example, Badinter 2010). For this reason, 'attachment' parents in Paris struggle harder with marginality issues than their UK counterparts. The suggestion here, however, is that this parenting culture may itself be shifting towards the 'intensive' model. The chapter opens by providing a brief methodology of the study, before presenting findings, and offering a discussion of differing cultural perceptions around nature/culture, feminism and family life by way of conclusion.

Methodology

The research for this study involved long-term ethnographic fieldwork with women in *La Leche League International* (LLLI) groups, the world's foremost breastfeeding support organisation. The group was founded in 1956 in the United States by a group of seven mothers, to support all women who wanted to breast-feed their babies. It has now become a global organisation offering breastfeeding support through publications, telephone helplines and local meetings. Whilst it offers support for all women who want to breastfeed, it is known amongst the various breastfeeding support groups to be supportive of women who breastfeed for 'extended' periods, and has a significant proportion of members who practice 'attachment parenting'. This was a term coined by the Sears (the husband and wife paediatrician team) in the 1980s, and is a style of care which endorses long-term proximity between infant and care-taker (most typically, the mother).

Feeding, arguably the most conspicuously moralised element of mothering, was the focus of the study. Because of its vital importance for the survival and healthy development of infants, feeding is a highly scrutinised domain where mothers must counter any charges of practicing unusual, harmful or morally suspect feeding techniques (Murphy 1999). Strong feelings about feeding are derived from the fact that it operates as a 'signal issue' which boxes women off into different parenting 'camps' (Kukla 2005).

During 2006, and over the course eight months in London, and four months in Paris, participant observation at 18 local LLLI groups (ten in London, eight in Paris) was complemented by 39 semi-structured interviews and 48 question-naires with individual women across the two cities. In both cases, mothers were in the vast majority white, middle-aged (on average, 34), well-educated (to uni-versity level or equivalent) and married. More women in the Parisian sample than in the London sample were working full-time, as I discuss further below. Those that were identified as 'full-term' breastfeeders and 'attachment mothers' made up just over half of the sample in London, and just over a third in Paris, and it is their accounts I focus on here.[1] Certainly not all mothers in the organi-sation breastfeed to full term, though I engage particularly with the accounts of those who do, and with the values they promote and enact. In taking their feeding practices to one extreme of the spectrum, they magnify mainstream issues around motherhood and the construction of the self. These accounts do not represent official LLLI philosophy, but are rather particular women's under-standings of their breastfeeding experiences, equally influenced by broader philosophies of 'natural' or 'attachment' parenting.

The WHO states that breastfeeding in developed countries should be exclu-sive for six months and continue 'for up to two years, or beyond' in conjunction with other foods (2003). Along with other EU member states, this is endorsed by both the UK and French governments. Breastfeeding initiation rates at the time of research stood at 78 per cent and 69 per cent in Britain and France respec-tively,[2] with no formal statistics existing in either place for rates of breastfeeding at a year, or beyond. As I discuss below, these numbers reflect the shorter length of maternity leave women receive in France, which in turn informs (and is informed by) broader social attitudes towards women's social roles, feminism and childcare (Randall 2000). Whilst there were no statistics for the number of children breastfed beyond a year in the UK, by six months 75 per cent of children were totally weaned off breastmilk, and only 2 per cent of women breastfed exclusively for the recommended six months (Department of Health 2005). In each country then, women breastfeeding to full term are statistically non-conventional, inviting critical engagement with the 'accountability strategies' they undertake to explain why they do what they do (Strathern 2000).

Accountability – in the sense of rendering intelligible some aspect of our selves – 'is a distinctive and pervasive feature of what it is to be human' (Munro and Mouritsen 1996: 23). Indeed, many scholars have emphasised the role of language in the constitution of personhood, and have argued

> that human beings actually live out their lives as 'narratives', [and] that we make use of the stories of the self that our culture makes available to us to plan out our lives ... to account for events and give them significance, to accord ourselves an identity.
>
> (Rose 1999: xviii)

Typically, these mothers narrate their decision to continue breastfeeding as 'natural': 'evolutionarily appropriate', 'scientifically best' and 'what feels right in their hearts' (Faircloth 2009, 2010, 2011).

After Goffman (1959), attention to 'identity work' – in this case the narrative processes of self-making that mothers engage in as they raise their children – is part of an argument that for certain middle-class parents in the UK (and to a lesser extent in France), the word 'parent' has shifted from a noun denoting a relationship with a child (something you *are*), to a verb (something you *do*). 'Parenting' – as this volume explores – is now an occupation in which adults (particularly mothers) are expected to be emotionally absorbed and become personally fulfilled; it is also a growing site of interest to policy makers in the UK, understood as a solution to a wide range of social ills (Lee and Bristow 2009). The 'ideal' parenting promoted by these policy makers is financially, physically and emotionally intensive, and parents are encouraged to spend a large amount of time, energy and money in raising their children (Hays 1996). This 'intensive parenting' climate, I argue, has changed how parents experience their social role.

Intensive mothering

Writing about the UK, Lee and Bristow (2009) identify two major characteristics of the contemporary 'ideal' of intensive mothering; one, that mothering is defined as a practice that should be child-centred, and two, that mothers should pay attention to what is said by experts about their children. Each of these have instrumental effects with respect to knowledge and practice.

That a child's interests should be placed before the mother's is, perhaps, not to say anything remarkable – indeed, Mary Douglas has said that the 'absolute morality' of motherhood is that 'in all circumstances, babies take precedence over mothers' (1970: 25, in Murphy 1999: 200). But the way in which this injunction is realised is certainly novel. Hays notes that today, children are not to be excluded from adult leisure time, but 'listened to' and 'included'. Weekend activities, for example, should centre around maximising children's health and well-being, and mothers are expected to act as pseudo-teachers, optimising their children's intelligence through a range of extra-curricular activities (Hays 1996).

Indeed, the mother's role has expanded dramatically in recent years, not least because of the burgeoning interest in early infancy by psychologists in the 1950s. The interlocking 'myths,' as Furedi puts it (2002: 45), that experience during infancy determines the course of future development, and that parental intervention determines the future fate of a youngster, have had a profound effect on the way parents structure their relationships with their offspring. As he argues: 'By grossly underestimating the resilience of children, they intensify parental anxiety and encourage excessive interference in children's lives; by grossly exaggerating the degree of parental intervention required to ensure normal development, they make the task of parenting impossibly burdensome' (Furedi 2002: 45). In this framing, the agency of children themselves is reduced, at the same time that the effect of peers and social climate on child development is eclipsed through this focus on parents. Accordingly, a highly interventionist approach is legitimised on their part, and the importance of the parenting role increases in congruence.

The second aspect of intensive mothering – that mothers should refer to experts when caring for their child – is also intimately tied up with the expansion of the parental role. In *Paranoid Parenting* (2002) Furedi argues that parenting is increasingly considered too important a job to be left to parents themselves to deal with. Lee (2007b) suggests that this, in turn, binds mothering to the job of risk management, at once creating and fuelling the market for a plethora of experts who 'enable' mothers to avoid certain risks and optimise their children (whether that be judo teachers, osteopaths or psychologists – to use just some of Hays' examples). This outsourcing of authority has the potential to reduce parental confidence to the extent that all parents are tinged with some degree of paranoia, Furedi argues (2002).

Fashions in parenting are also best understood as barometers of wider cultural trends, which – in the UK, at least – have recently seen a growing validation of the 'natural' way of doing things in issues as diverse as what we eat, how we learn and how we treat illness. There is an enduring conviction in this position that 'nature' is a force to be trusted and respected, and with respect to parenting, deference to the 'natural' bond between mother and child, which attachment parenting certainly validates (paraphrased from Bobel 2002: 11, see Faircloth 2009). Based on a 'hominid blueprint' (Dettwyler 1995), which draws on evidence of primates and 'primitives' (whether in the fossil record or as represented by contemporary hunter–gatherer groups) attachment parenting is endorsed as both a traditional and 'adaptive' form of care (Sears and Sears 2001). The argument is that children have evolutionary expectations (such as an extended period of breastfeeding) that must be met if they are to mature into happy, healthy adults (see Faircloth 2009 for a full discussion: women clearly do not 'ape' all aspects of the hunter–gatherer lifestyle; a certain amount of cherry-picking goes on. See also Dow and Jiménez Sedano this volume).

The intention here is not to suggest that this 'new' parenting culture, evident in certain contexts in the UK or the US is somehow normative, stable or standard – indeed, there are many cultural specificities around codes of contact, notions of intimacy or ideas of equality that are peculiar to the UK, as this volume shows. What is more, there are many ways of caring for children 'intensively' (such as with methods which advocate strict timetabling of feeding, sleeping etc. and these are just as prevalent as the style of parenting I focus on here). The philosophy of 'attachment parenting' which validates attentive, embodied care for infants, offers women *one* set of norms by which to structure their 'identity work' in congruence with an over-arching framework of intensive mothering. There are points of congruence and points of departure with this framework, as I explore (Faircloth 2013).

A cross-cultural perspective: France

Whilst numerous scholars have fruitfully used the concept of 'Intensive Motherhood' in US and UK contexts, (Douglas and Michaels 2004; Furedi 2002; Hays 1996; Lee 2007a, 2007b; Lee and Bristow 2009) there has been less empirical work which looks at the impact of this ideology outside and across these settings – in part, the rationale behind this volume.

Famously, the French government has long had a policy aimed at boosting the country's population, at the same time as increasing the amount of women in the workforce (Randall 2000). The OECD (Organisation for Economic Co-operation and Development)[3] lists the fertility rate in France as 1.94, in contrast to the UK's 1.8. (These are both figures above the OECD average of 1.63).[4] In terms of female employment, 56.7 per cent of women of working age are employed in France, compared with 66.8 per cent in the UK. (The OECD average is 56.1 per cent, and this includes both full- and part-time workers.)

At the time of research, in the UK, a woman could typically expect 26 weeks (six months) of paid leave with five weeks additional unpaid leave if desired. (Women were not paid at full rate – it was calculated at 90 per cent for the initial six weeks and then at a flat rate, approximately 33 per cent of average wage, for 20 weeks.)[5] In France, women could take 16 weeks of (fully) paid leave, then being eligible for longer periods of unpaid leave. Since this is generally split on a four-week/12-week basis pre- and post birth, women are expected to return to work when their children are between ten weeks and three months old.[6] In the UK this point would typically be between five and six months. (Paternity leave at the time of research in both countries was two weeks, with only 25 per cent of this time paid in the UK.)

Crucially however, and unlike the UK, France has a system of heavily subsidised, easily available, affordable childcare. Municipal, cooperative and parental crèches exist, able to care for infants from the age of three months at rates that are close to free through a system of pay-back from social security. From the age of three (or two, in larger cities) children can attend pre-schools (*maternelles*) for eight hours a day, for free (with the option of a means-tested after-school and holiday club, available until 6.30 PM). By contrast, the average cost for a full-time nursery place for one child in London in 2005 was £197/week, or nearly £10,000/annum (Daycare Trust 2005). For French mothers, the need to 'juggle' careers around the demands of childcare following the end of maternity leave – practically and financially, at least – is mitigated.

So whilst I do not expand on it here, these data clearly chime with, or are the flip-side of the coin to, those presented by scholars working on cross-cultural variations in welfare regimes (Esping-Anderson 1999, being the classic example). Where childcare is seen as the responsibility of the family it will clearly chafe with a dual-earner family set-up, therefore precipitating the full-time breadwinner/part-time carer model, with all its usual gendered implications. In France where the state takes more responsibility for care, it is understood as a means of protecting parents' (and particularly mothers') independence, economic and otherwise. Drawing on Pfau-Effinger's work, Edwards (2002) therefore makes the point that even for women who *do* work under the first model, such as the UK, childcare is understood as a mother-substitute, again resonating with the anxieties propagated by an intensive mothering ideology explored here, and particularly pertinent to the infant feeding question.

Infant feeding in comparative perspective

Gelling with one permutation of the 'intensive' motherhood orthodoxy, new mothers in the UK can expect to hear a strong 'breast is best' message from a range of governmental and non-governmental agencies (Lee 2007a). This message to breastfeed exclusively for six months and 'for anything up to two years or beyond' (WHO 2003) is based on evidence from clinical studies which show benefits to infant (and maternal) health. This is largely due to the immunological character of breastmilk. Again however, whilst I do not elaborate on this here, it is arguable that these benefits have been overplayed by the policy and advocacy literature somewhat (Hoddinott *et al.* 2008; Faircloth 2013; Wolf 2011).

Current policy around infant feeding in the UK is best represented by UNICEF's Baby Friendly Initiative (BFI), a programme drawn up in 1992, and active in the UK since 1994, currently endorsed as the 'gold standard' of maternity care by NICE (the National Institute for Clinical Excellence) and the Department of Health. With the aim of addressing the infant feeding 'problem' by increasing the numbers of women who breastfeed, maternity facilities can be accredited as 'Baby Friendly' if they adopt the BFI's *10 Steps to Successful Breastfeeding*. This includes having a written breastfeeding policy that is routinely communicated to all staff, informing all pregnant women about the benefits of breastfeeding and helping women initiate breastfeeding soon after birth.[7] The tenth step of the programme aims to foster collaboration between hospitals and lay support groups (such as La Leche League International).

In France, breastfeeding is not, as yet, a public policy issue in the same way as in the UK, where it intersects with wider policy concerns such as health and social mobility. The *Baby Friendly Initiative* has been very slowly taken up in France – with Paris having no accredited hospitals (there were only five in the whole country by 2007; there were 51 in the UK at the same point).[8] The post of 'Lactation Consultant', increasingly found in hospitals in the UK, is not recognised in France, and the government has only recently taken up the adoption of breastfeeding advocacy campaigns. Indeed, breastfeeding exclusively for six months, in line with the WHO guidelines, was recommended for the first time by the Ministère de la Santé in its 2005 dossier.

Yet, in part because of EU commensuration and wider cultural shifts, it is true that breastfeeding is *beginning* to take more of a centre stage in health policy, reflected (and informed) by rising rates of initiation which increase each year – though this is, as Amelie, one of my interviewees, explains, a trend largely reserved for the educated classes:

> Breastfeeding has become very 'trendy' in the moneyed, well-educated classes, and I think that women choose it to be 'good mothers' ... [Yet] I live in an area with a very high amount of recent immigrants to France, and for them, the bottle is better because it is synonymous with being moneyed ('the breast is for poor people').
>
> (Amelie, 32, breastfeeding her two-month-old son, questionnaire response)

Sample

Where in the UK several breastfeeding support organisations exist (such as The Association of Breastfeeding Mothers, The National Childbirth Trust and La Leche League International) LLLI is the only national breastfeeding support organisation in France.[9] It therefore receives women from a more diverse range of backgrounds than in the UK. They are largely middle class (in the sense of being well-educated), but certainly not only those with an interest in attachment parenting or long-term breastfeeding (as is more typically the case in the UK).

The differing policies around employment and infant feeding were also reflected in my French sample. Whilst in my UK sample only one woman said that she was working full-time, and a third were working part-time; in France, a third were working full-time and a quarter part-time. So, although women were on average the same in many respects – married (around eight out of ten in each case); similarly aged (33 years old in France compared with 35 years old in the UK) and sharing a high level of education (with the overwhelming majority having university level qualifications) the key difference was that *many more* women with young children were working outside of the home in the French sample.

In my responses, it was also clear that I had two fairly distinct sets of respondents in my French sample, in a more pronounced fashion than in the UK. More women came along to meetings when their babies were under three months old in France (nine out of ten, on average) than in the UK (just under half), indicating an interest in breastfeeding largely within the brackets of maternity leave rather than 'long' term as would be desirable according to attachment parents. Based on my coding, just over a third of mothers answering the questionnaire fell into the 'attachment mother' definition (compared with just over half in London). They constituted themselves as a marginal in relation to French society at large, framing their answers to my questions with complaints about their own marginality, in more pronounced but ways familiar to those I encountered in the UK.

French-parenting: non-intensive motherhood?

The American author, Warner (2006), has written about her experience of motherhood in Paris (and for a more recent, similar take, see Druckerman 2012). She argues that unlike her native US (and, I suggest, the UK) motherhood was far less intensive – it was just not such a 'big deal' in France, and certainly not something women would consider their primary source of what I term 'identity work.' This is corroborated by findings from this research. Just one example of this would be the differences in responses to a question in the questionnaire: where 11 out of 25 UK women listed their 'profession' as a mother, only one in the sample of 19 women did this in France. There was far less fetishisation about the role of 'mother' in general; women were less effusive about the 'wonders' of motherhood in their answers. This was reflected by one word answers to, for example, 'Why was it important for you to feed your child at the breast?' in contrast to long essays from the UK or from attachment mothers in France.

It is certainly the case that there does not (yet) exist an industry surrounding parenting as there does in the UK. (Searching 'parenting' in the Google UK site generates 85,100,000 hits; *parentage* in Google France gets just 1,660,000.)[10] 'Parenting' has also not become a policy buzzword. As Warner explains, this lack of 'support' for parents is double-edged, in that at the same time that it collapses choice, it also reduces anxiety and accountability:

> Guilt just wasn't in the air. It wasn't considered a natural consequence of working motherhood. ... The general French conviction that one should live a 'balanced' life was especially true for mothers – particularly, I would say, for stay-at-home mothers, who were otherwise considered at risk of falling into excessive child-centeredness. And that, the French believed, was wrong. Obsessive. Inappropriate. Just plain weird.
>
> (Warner 2006: 10–11)

Indeed, the argument might be that where there is less plurality about infant care (mothers in general must go back to work earlier, limiting their ability to – for example – breastfeed to full-term and parent in an 'attachment' fashion), less 'identity work' is required about one's decisions, as a form of accountability. By the same logic, those that do, say, breastfeed to full-term require even more 'identity work' than their UK counterparts.

In her work in France, Wolfenstein (1955, with Margaret Mead) notes that for the Parisian parents she studied (in the 1950s) childhood was not about fun but about *preparation*. This is, she argues, almost in direct contrast to her native America, where 'childhood is a very nearly ideal time, a time for enjoyment, an end in itself' (1955: 115). In France, she says, '[c]hildhood is a period of proba-tion, when everything is a means to an end; it is unenviable from the vantage point of adulthood' (ibid.). The child in France would not be expected to disrupt adult life, and should certainly not be the main preoccupation of adult conversa-tion, for example (Wolfenstein 1955: 114).

This is reiterated in more recent research by Suizzo, published in *Ethos* (2004). In her article 'Mother–Child Relationships in France', she uses a cultural models framework to argue for two distinctive features of the French parenting. One was that mothers wanted their children to be '*debrouillard*', a term difficult to translate into English but which broadly means being prepared and therefore enabled to achieve one's personal goals. The second more pertinent feature was a pervasive worry about mothers being enslaved (*esclavage*) to their children who could easily become infant kings (*l'enfant-roi*). As she explains:

> [*Esclavage*] is the idea that mothers can become dependent on, even subor-dinate to, their children. This notion is quite different from the much more pervasive concern among parents in individualist cultures that children may become overly dependent on their mother. Mother-enslavement was described as a loss of personal freedom with very negative consequences for the mother.
>
> (Suizzo 2004: 317)

The fear about enslavement means French parents

> prefer more distal relations, maintaining separate beds and bedrooms for their infants, and engaging in less body contact, in part because they believe that separateness fosters independence in children … French parents also avoid prolonged body contact, such as co-sleeping, holding, and carrying babies. … These findings point to a concern with fostering independence.
>
> (Suizzo 2004: 296)

Weaning would be a good example of ensuring distal relations are maintained, as Louise from my French sample (not an 'attachment mother') makes plain:

CHARLOTTE: Can you tell me what breastfeeding represents, to you?
LOUISE: [28, just weaned her six-month-old daughter] … it was the

'fusioned' aspect most of all, between mother and baby. Privileging all of the senses; touch, smell. In fact, I had a lot of trouble separating myself. So after six months it was a good moment to stop being so close to her.

There is an implication here that although breastfeeding is enjoyable (for both the mother and the child), being 'close' for too long is undesirable. Suizzo argues that these ideas come through the ideas of the influential thinker Rousseau, who wrote:

The first tears of children are prayers. If one is not careful, they soon become orders. Children begin by getting themselves assisted; they end by getting themselves served. Thus, from their own weakness, which is in the first place the source of the feeling of their dependence, is subsequently born the idea of empire and domination.

(Rousseau 1979: 66 in Suizzo 2004: 317)

Another mother in the sample echoed the view that for the French there was a concern about women becoming '*mères fusionelles*':

There is a massive misunderstanding around babies who breastfeed often, and for a long time … it is also difficult to breastfeed for longer than four to six months without being seen as a *mère fusionelle* who is not able to separate from her baby.

(Sandrine, 28, five- and two-and-a-half-year-old sons, no longer breastfed)

Warner notes, for example, that for mothers who do stay at home (and are not in paid employment) it is considered important to maintain a 'sense of self' by using childcare on a regular basis for fear of becoming too tied to one's children.

It's natural? Feminism and (long-term) breastfeeding in France

To understand why the 'intensive motherhood' orthodoxy (and validations of personal liberty and/or emotionally absorbing parenting) are more or less salient in London or Paris a broader cultural perspective is required.

I suggest that there is currently a more 'embedded' attitude towards the place of nature in France, in opposition to the growing fetishisation of nature as something desirable to 'get back in touch with' currently prevalent in the UK, and so in vogue in parenting fashions (Faircloth 2009). True, Rousseau counselled women to 'look to the animals' in his campaign against wet-nursing in eighteenth century France (Badinter 1981; Blaffer Hrdy 2000). But it would be fair to argue that this injunction has been rebuked over the last two centuries with a legacy of the Enlightenment which stresses human separation from nature and, in turn, other animals. As Nicole, a La Leche League leader with whom I discussed these issues puts it:

CHARLOTTE: You said that in France there is not a 'breastfeeding culture'
— why?

NICOLE [LLLI LEADER]: I think that in England there was always, at least for
the last century and a half, a culture of returning to nature, proximity
with nature, with one's choices, with people – there is a conscience about
children that is much more ancient. In France, there was, by contrast, a
'hygienist' culture, with a very strict order, 'puéri-culture' centres [like
health-visiting centres], which set the rules: 'One must do it like this, and
like that.' It's something that's very evident.... It really harmed breastfeeding, and it's an approach that has never really been discredited. It
just didn't fit with breastfeeding, where you can't be 'controlled by the
rod,' in such a rigid way.

The 1970s 'return to nature' which saw feminist movements (including LLL)
blossom in the UK was not replicated in France (although Badinter suggests that
the same roots were present, if not as elaborated, 2010). Indeed, 'being close to
nature' as something desirable is a relatively new phenomenon in France, one
which, I argue, is a 'culture on the make' for a privileged section of society (and
it is worth restating here that I was working in London and Paris which, as urban
capitals, cannot be said to represent Britain and France in any straightforward
way. Indeed, any nostalgia for 'nature' might be said to be a product of these
very settings and middle-class contexts). This was even evident in the sorts of
food present, brought along by mothers to the meetings. Whilst in the UK there
was typically organic bread, cheese and vegetables, in France it was normal to
see packaged and processed foods – although there is a growing market for
'organic' (*biologique*) food in France which may well start to feature in much
the same way as the UK.

For many women, the idea of being 'a mammal' was one reason mothers in
France were put off breastfeeding – unlike in the US or the UK, where this discourse is frequently drawn upon in advocacy literature as a way of encouraging
women to breastfeed: 'Breastfeeding seems like an animal act, uncivilised'
(Sophie, 25, breastfeeding her three-month-old daughter, questionnaire
response). This ambivalence about our status as mammals was seen to be part of
the country's different history of both the Enlightenment, and of feminism, as
Nicole expounds:

CHARLOTTE: There is also the fact that people think of breastfeeding as
'*esclavage*'...

NICOLE [LLLI LEADER]: Yes, I agree, [French] feminism was constructed
outside of and *against* motherhood. The battle of feminism was: equal
salaries between men and women, for abortion to defend the sexual
liberty of women ... but not at all in favour of motherhood, absolutely

not! Whereas in other countries, such as Scandinavia, feminism was constructed *with* motherhood. Moreover, the majority of French feminists
didn't have children ... like it was a liberty not to have children. Revenge
against nature, yes, that's it, a controlling of nature. To be free was to get
out of that condition.

Speaking about a friend who did not breastfeed her child, Louise explains again that
her reasoning is a product of a feminist inclination which does not encourage
women to adjust to the 'rhythm' of their children, but rather, the other way round:

CHARLOTTE: Why do you think your friend didn't want to breastfeed?
LOUISE [28, just weaned her six-month-old daughter]: In '68 there was a
big revolution, the liberation of women and all that ... so in our parents'
generation there weren't many feminists who breastfed. And even now
there is an image of the modern woman: ...she goes everywhere, does
everything, she works and she is not dependent on anyone and above all
not to her children. When one breastfeeds, one has another rhythm, one
is obliged to adapt to the rhythm of the child...

CHARLOTTE: It's interesting, the distinction between motherhood and
womanhood...
LOUISE: When one looks at northern societies [such as Scandinavia], it's
different, women don't get posed the same question [to breastfeed or
not]: they breastfeed. If they do not breastfeed they are not considered
good mothers. Whereas in France, it's the opposite, it's the woman who
breastfeeds who is thought of badly, and who is thought 'strange'. ...
One must go back to work early ... I took holiday, and after, I had
holiday to use up ... like that I was able to [breastfeed] for five months.
In short, one has to fight to be able to breastfeed, you have to find combi-
nations that work.

Many women in the French sample were therefore conscious that for mothers in
France, using either formula or expressed milk, rather than feeding directly from
the breast, made sense according to these cultural norms about bodies and
dependency:

It can appear more practical to bottle-feed [with expressed milk] as one can
better manage the rhythm of the feeds; the woman is not strictly tied to her
baby (for me, the idea of expressing milk with a pump is pretty distasteful,
so I sometimes time where I will be with breastfeeding, not wanting to or
not able to take the baby out everywhere – cinemas and theatres etc). The
body of a woman who breastfeeds becomes totally maternal, and that can
change the relationship one has with one's partner (especially if the breastfeeding is long-term).[11]

(Diane, 32, breastfeeding her five-month-old daughter,
questionnaire response)

In a more pronounced way than in the UK it was clear that many women in the French sample were concerned about preserving their 'corps erotique' (as opposed to their 'corps maternelle', as Diane put it later) as representative both of their autonomy and as part of their commitment to relationships with their partners. Indeed intensive (attachment) parenting can intersect with couple relationships in a problematic way, which Layne (this volume) observes in her case-study of a single-mother-by-choice.

Overall, then, for my French informants, there was an association between feminism and the work of de Beauvoir (unlike the UK responses which drew on cultural feminist trends, as Nicole explains above). Her work *The Second Sex* describes how female physiology renders women subservient to the requirement of the species to procreate, in ways vastly more costly than those accrued to men. Her view of breastfeeding was indeed as some sort of enslavement. As Layne and Aengst note:

> [s]he celebrates human society which exerts mastery over nature: '[h]uman society is an antiphysis – in a sense it is against nature; it does not passively submit to the presence of nature but rather takes over the control of nature on its own behalf' (1989: 53).
>
> (Layne and Aengst 2010: 73)

So, breastfeeding at all is seen to be against the ethic of 'French' feminism. Breastfeeding 'to full term' makes one even more marginal.

Shifting orthodoxies

Yet there are counter-currents to this. Recently, Badinter, the author and philosopher, has argued that the traditional French model of motherhood is under threat from a rising orthodoxy of 'Good Motherhood' (of the kind familiar to many British women) which champions 'natural' practices such as long-term breastfeeding, using washable nappies and cooking organic food, and impels women to take a considerable periods of time off work to look after children (2010). Indeed, an article appearing in *Elle* magazine, entitled 'The end of Feminism? What happens when super-woman returns to the house,' featured two of my informants, describing their feminism in a language reminiscent of 'attachment mothers' in London.[12]

> Stephanie, 34 years old, in a couple, one child: I never 'found' myself in feminism. There are fundamental differences between men and women. Motherhood is an essential one. I intend to be a mother as much as a woman. I have the chance to work at home, so my son, who is nearly three years old, has never been looked after [by anyone else]. There is a rhythm with the rest of the world. I breastfed him for a long time, and until the age

of one he was always by my side, in a scarf next to me. Yet, I have an active life; I am a journalist and a translator and I work in public associations. But to work should not be synonymous with separation from one's child. I do not want to impose that on him. Moreover, I did not register him at school: I like the idea of him being free in his activities.

Like attachment parents elsewhere, and in line with an 'intensive motherhood' orthodoxy, women practicing attachment parenting in France speak about being emotionally absorbed and personally fulfilled through their parenting practices – which in turn form the basis of their 'identity work.' Yet their approach to parenting, which relies heavily on a validation of nature as opposed to culture, is not, in general, endorsed in broader French culture (or philosophers such as Bad-inter), which validates the Enlightenment legacy of humanism and domination over nature. They are therefore not seen to be helping the traditional feminist cause – quite the reverse.

Yet like the UK, attachment mothers in France considered themselves to be 'beacons' who were 'spreading the light' about attachment parenting, in distinc-tion to mainstream patterns of care. Indeed, women who practice attachment parenting in France have a commitment to the cause that was even stronger than those I met in the UK, perhaps as a result of their exacerbated non-conventionality. Typically, and to a greater extent than in the UK, they spoke of their marginalisation. This mother (who was French, but currently living in London) noted:

> My friends in Paris think I am totally mad for not wanting an epidural during the birth, and for breastfeeding for five months – if only they knew I might do it for five years! They say to me that I pick him up too much when he cries and that *il faut frustrer le bébé* – I don't know how you would trans-late that, but it basically means I am making a rod for my own back by making a clingy baby, or 'you must frustrate the baby.'
>
> (Audrey, 35, breastfeeding her newborn son)

Conclusion

What is interesting in this discussion is how the experiences of French and British women who practice attachment parenting challenge the prevailing norms in each country. We see that the length of maternity leave routinely given to women, the importance of work outside of the home for self-realisation and notions of individual autonomy combine to have a substantial impact on how women go about narrating their experiences of parenting. Where in the UK, attachment mothering might be said to be an intensification of the prevail-ing climate of 'intensive motherhood' (a prevailing climate for the middle classes, at least), in France, attachment mothering goes against this grain. Indeed, in a culture where maternal–infant separation and autonomy is lauded as ideal, intensive, embodied care on the part of the mother is perceived as an impingement on female liberty, rather than as a valid outlet for her 'identity work'. Yet – as evidenced by the rapid growth of mothering boutiques, magazines and clubs many of my 'attachment' informants frequented – it seems that the climate in France is on the cusp of a change, in which case, women there will start to face a similar but exacerbated cultural contradiction between their working and domestic lives.

Whilst Badinter's analysis of shifting orthodoxies is useful, it does not highlight the struggle of many French women who would like to spend more time with their children in the early months – attachment parents or otherwise – and who resent the social pressure to return to work. What she does show, however, is how this 'struggle' is itself a result of these very shifts, which, I suggest, appear to be turning towards a validation of intensive, 'natural' mothering. How each group of women negotiate these shifts: one with a generous system of childcare (in France), the other with a long length of maternity leave (in the UK), will undoubtedly be a source of feminist interest for some time to come. As she says, 'The majority of French women reconcile maternity with professional life. Many of them work full-time when they have a child. They are resisting the model of the perfect mother, but for how long?'[13]

Notes

1 These are women who practice an 'attachment parenting' philosophy in addition to being members of LLLI. Classification is based on statistics and responses derived from the questionnaire – that is, those women breastfeeding their children beyond a year – as well as the author's observations at groups meetings and interviews.

2 These statistics should be read cautiously. 'Initiation' means that the baby is put to the breast once. By one week in the UK, over a third of women are not breastfeeding, and by six weeks, that figure is well over half (Department of Health 2005). These were the rates correct at the time of research from the Department of Health and Ministère de la Santé surveys (Ministère de la Santé 2005). The most recent report available in France (2002) however, puts the rate of initiation at 52 per cent, with an average duration of ten weeks. Formerly available at: www.sante.gouv.fr/htm/pointsur/nutrition/allaitement.pdf [accessed 23 April 2009].

3 An organisation based in France with 30 member countries, including France, Germany, Italy, Japan, New Zealand, Australia, the UK and the United States, committed to democracy and the market economy.

4 The following statistics are taken from the data set at: http://stats.oecd.org/ wbos/default.aspx?DatasetCode=LFS_D [accessed 2 December 2008].

5 This was the case at the time of research; recent (2008) measures have extended standard maternity leave to one year. Online, available at: www.gov.uk/maternity-leave [accessed 2 December 2008].

6 These are the national, standardised rates of maternity leave. Some women – particularly in the UK sample – had more generous maternity packages. Women also have the option of taking extended periods of unpaid leave.

7 www.babyfriendly.org.uk/page.asp?page=213 [accessed 26 February 2009].

8 www.lllfrance.org/Promotion-et-protection-de-l-allaitement/LInitiative-Hopital-Ami-des-Bebes.html [accessed 23 April 2009].

9 Save Solidarilait, which is more strictly a campaigning organisation.

10 Indeed, the word 'parenting' as a description of a genre of literature is in debate, which is an interesting social comment in itself. Some informants would use *parentalité* (the

state of being a parent – which renders 400,000 hits on Google.fr) in place of *parentage* [accessed 23 April 2009].
11 Indeed, although I do not discuss this here, there was a far higher prevalence of mothers who fed their babies with expressed milk in my French sample, and it was clear that women in my French sample struggled more with the 'contradiction between the erotic and the maternal bodies' (as one informant put it).
12 'Quand Superwoman rentre à la maison', online, available at: www.elle.fr/elle/societe/les-enquetes/quand-superwoman-rentre-a-la-maison/la-fin-du-feminisme/(gid)/740943 [accessed 23 April 2009].
13 Online, available at: www.guardian.co.uk/world/2010/feb/12/france-feminism-elisabeth-badinter [accessed 11 March 2010].

References

Badinter, E. (1981) *The Myth of Motherhood: A Historical View of the Maternal Instinct*, trans. Roger De Garis, London: Souvenir Press.
Badinter, E. (2010) *Le Conflit; le femme et la mere*, Paris: Flammarion.
Blaffer Hrdy, S. (2000) *Mother Nature: Maternal Instincts and the Shaping of the Species*, London: Vintage.
Bobel, C. (2002) *The Paradox of Natural Mothering*, Philadelphia: Temple University Press.
Daycare Trust (2005) *Childcare Costs Surveys* online, available at: www.daycaretrust.org.uk/pages/childcare-costs-surveys.html [accessed 6 September 2012].
Department of Health (2005) *Infant Feeding Survey 2005*, London: Department of Health.
Dettwyler, K. (1995) 'A time to wean: a hominid blueprint for the natural age of weaning', in P. Stuart-Macadam and K. Dettwyler (eds) *Breastfeeding: Bio-cultural Perspectives*, New York: Aldine de Gruyter, pp. 167–217.
Douglas, S. and Michaels, M. (2004) *The Mommy Myth: The Idealization of Motherhood and How it has Undermined All Women*, New York: Free Press.
Druckerman, P. (2012) *Bringing up Bébé. One American Mother Discovers the Wisdom of French Parenting*, London/New York: Penguin Books.
Edwards, R. (2002) 'Conceptualising relationships between home and school in children's lives', in R. Edwards. (ed.) *Children, Home and School: Regulation, Autonomy or Connection?* London: Routledge Falmer.
Esping-Anderson, G. (1999) *Social Foundations of Post-industrial Economics*, Oxford: Oxford University Press.
Faircloth, C. (2009) '"Culture means nothing to me": Thoughts on nature/culture in narratives of "full-term" breastfeeding', *Cambridge Anthropology*, 28(2): 63–85.
Faircloth, C. (2010) 'What science says is best: Parenting practices, scientific authority and maternal identity', *Sociological Research Online* Special Section on 'Changing Parenting Culture', 15(4)4, online, available at: www.socresonline.org.uk/15/4/4.html (accessed 6 September 2012).
Faircloth, C. (2011) 'It feels right in my heart: Affect as accountability in narratives of attachment', *The Sociological Review*, 59(2): 283–302, online, available at: http://onlinelibrary.wiley.com/doi/10.1111/j.1467-954X.2011.02004.x/abstract [accessed 6 September 2012].
Faircloth, C. (2013) *Militant Lactivism? Infant Care and Maternal Identity Work in the UK and France*, Oxford/New York: Berghahn Books.

Furedi, F. (2002) *Paranoid Parenting: Why Ignoring the Experts May be Best for Your Child*, Chicago: Chicago Review Press.

Goffman, E. (1959) *The Presentation of Self in Everyday Life*, New York: Doubleday.

Hays, S. (1996) *The Cultural Contradictions of Motherhood*, New Haven/London: Yale University Press.

Hoddinott, P. Tappin, D. and Wright, C. (2008) 'Clinical Review: Breastfeeding,' *British Medical Journal.* April, 336: 881–887.

Kukla, R. (2005) *Mass Hysteria, Medicine, Culture and Women's Bodies*, New York: Rowman and Littlefield.

Layne, L.L. and Aegnst, J. (2010) '"The need to bleed?" A feminist technology assessment of menstrual-suppressing birth control pills'. in L.L. Layne, S.L. Vostral and K. Boyer (eds) *Feminist Technology*, Urbana/Chicago/Springfield: University of Illinois Press.

Lee, E. (2007a) 'Health, morality, and infant feeding: British mothers' experiences of formula milk use in the early weeks,' *Sociology of Health and Illness*, 29(7): 1075–1090.

Lee, E. (2007b) 'Infant feeding in risk society,' *Health, Risk and Society*, 9(3): 295–309.

Lee, E. and Bristow, J. (2009) 'Rules for feeding babies', in S. Day Sclater, F. Ebtehaj, E. Jackson and M. Richards (eds) *Regulating Autonomy: Sex, Reproduction and Family*, Oxford: Hart, pp. 73–91.

Ministèe de la Santé (Ministère des Solidarités, de la Santé et de la Famille) (2005) *Allaitement Maternel: Les Bénéfices pour la Santé de l'Enfant et de sa Mere.* Les Synthèses du Programme.

Murphy, E. (1999) '"Breast is best": Infant feeding decisions and maternal deviance', *Sociology of Health and Illness*, 21(2): 187–208.

Munro, R. and Mouritsen, J. (eds) (1996) *Accountability: Power, Ethos and the Technologies of Managing*, London: International Thomson Business Press.

Randall, V. (2000) *The Politics of Childcare in Britain*, Oxford: Oxford University Press.

Rose, N. (1999) *Governing the Soul: The Shaping of the Private Self*, 2nd edition, London: Routledge.

Sears, W. and Sears, M. (2001) *The Attachment Parenting Book, A Commonsense Guide to Understanding and Nurturing Your Baby*, London: Little, Brown.

Strathern, M. (ed.) (2000) *Audit Cultures: Anthropological Studies in Accountability, Ethics and the Academy*, London: Routledge.

Suizzo, M.-A. (2004) 'Mother–child relationships in France: Balancing autonomy and affiliation in everyday interactions', *Ethos*, 32(3): 293–323.

UNICEF (2006) *The Baby Friendly Initiative*, online, available at: www.unicef.org.uk/BabyFriendly/About-Baby-Friendly/Breastfeeding-in-the-UK [accessed 3 December 2006].

Warner, J. (2006) *Perfect Madness, Motherhood in the Age of Anxiety*, London: Vermilion.

WHO (2003) *Global Strategy on Infant and Young Child Feeding*, Geneva: WHO.

Wolf, J. (2011) *Is Breast Best? Taking on the Breastfeeding Experts and the New High Stakes of Motherhood*, New York/London: New York University Press.

Wolfenstein, M. (1955) 'French parents take their children to the park', in M. Mead and M. Wolfenstein, *Childhood in Contemporary Cultures*, London: University of Chicago Press, pp. 99–117.

8 Intensive mothering of Ethiopian adoptive children in Flanders, Belgium

Katrien De Graeve and Chia Longman

Introduction

> SANDRA: The only thing I found really difficult when we were waiting for
> our Eyob, that was that my other children have been breastfed and that I
> wouldn't be able to give that to my adoptive child. [...] So, I spoke to a
> doctor who said that he had seen it before in his practice [women who
> induced breast milk without recently giving birth]. And I had done it
> [breastfed] for so many years, so I knew I could do it. And because his
> mother had died, Eyob lived off the people and the neighbours who had a
> baby; there he could drink from the mothers. When he was here in
> Belgium he even walked up to someone he saw with a pram. [...]
> Because he thought: 'There's food'. It took less than three weeks before
> the milk production set in and then I was perfectly happy that I could
> give him the same as my other children. [...] And he did breastfeed for I
> think three years. But for me that was really very important and maybe it
> sounds very absurd, but I'm still really glad for it. [...] As far as attach-
> ment goes it was really important to me.[1]

The above fragment is taken from an in-depth interview with the parents of both
biological and adoptive children in the framework of a qualitative research
project on the experiences of Belgian adoptive children from Ethiopia. Sandra's
account of the importance of breastfeeding in rearing her children is a fascinating example of the intertwining of 'intensive mothering' practices (Hays 1996:
50–54) with biologizing discourses. The narrative shows how adoptive parents
tend to stress an equivalence between adoptive and biological bonds. But at the
same time it shows how they mobilize biology in a myriad of new ways (Carsten
2000: 12). It strikes a chord with Hayden's (1995) examples of the strategies
used by lesbian co-mothers to equalize their claims to the child, for instance by
one partner injecting the donor's sperm in the other partner's vagina. Sandra sees
breastfeeding as both essential to the maternal bond as well as easily exchangea-
ble – any pair of breasts will do. Breastfeeding, which is generally seen together
with child bearing as the essential prerequisite for mother–child bonds, is essentialized, being seen as necessary for a healthy mother–child relation. Yet it is

simultaneously de-essentialized as an act that bodily connects rather than essentially defines mother and child. Hence the interview fragment attests to the complex and often ambivalent ways contemporary transnational adoptive parenting practices are both pulled to biological or genetic models as well as have the ability to go beyond these and create openness to other forms of kinship beyond essentialisms.

From a feminist perspective, some authors have heralded adoption as a radical anti-essentialist feminist act through its potential to eliminate the 'umbilical mythology' (Bordo 2005: 234). Yet, such a stance has, we believe, rightly been criticized because it overemphasizes the class and race privileges of only a small group of women to be able to engage in the kind of mothering relations they choose. Adoptive parenthood may indeed contain the potential to transcend essentialist conceptions of identity toward a more 'nomadic' conception that leaves room for difference and transitions (Braidotti 2011). Yet its embeddedness in prevailing parenting and kinship ideologies puts considerable constraints on its empowering ability.

The focus of this chapter is on the way intensive mothering is implemented and experienced in the context of the non-biological and transracial kin ties of transnational adoptive families.[2] First, it shows that intensive mothering is invoked to justify the transfer of poor African children to affluent families in OECD countries and how feelings of indebtedness inform the parents' charity work. Second, it discusses how intensive mothering ideology is pushed to extremes in adoption circles by dramatizing adoptive parenthood and conceptualizing it as in need of extraordinary measures. Biocentric discourses that continue to dominate kinship ideology in OECD countries problematize the non-biological adoptive family. They construct adoptive children as highly susceptible to identity crises and psychological dysfunction. Adoptive parents, and especially mothers are encouraged to become 'semi-professional parents' (Buysse and Vandenbroeck 2010) in order to anticipate these problems caused by the child's deviance from what is perceived as the norm. Adherence to the 'autonomous responsible family', defined by Rose (1999) as 'a machine held together by the vectors of desire, [that] can only function through the desires that members have for one another' (Rose 1999: 206) fuels a perceived need within adoption circles to problematize the adoptive children's attachment to the adoptive family (and vice versa). This leads to a further intensification of the parenting work, and at the same time tends to reduce all problems surrounding the adoptive child that may show up in society to personal dysfunction and maladjustment. As such, the family comes to be seen as the locus of disciplining or domesticating difference and the source of, as well as the solution to, a multitude of social troubles, such as social exclusion and racism.

This study of intensive parenting practices in the realm of Belgian–Ethiopian adoption can further our understanding of the dynamics that shape contemporary ideas on parenting in general and on the parenting of adoptive children in particular. By addressing the specific ways intensive mothering ideologies are lived within non-biological kin-ties, we hope to provide new insights into the construction of ideologically charged parental identities and furthermore, show the ambiguities that spring from the essentialized understandings of kinship and gendered, racialized identities and inequalities.

Methods

The chapter draws on an ethnographic study of cultural practices of adoption and qualitative interviews with Belgian parents who have adopted children from Ethiopia. The fieldwork was carried out from 2008 to 2011 in the region of Flanders, which is the northern, predominantly Flemish speaking part of Belgium.[3] Approximately fifty-five (including prospective) adoptive mothers and fathers were interviewed, about ten of whom on a regular basis, and (unrecorded) conversations with parents and social workers involved in the adoption procedure were conducted. An additional thirty participant observation sessions were carried out during adoptive parents' information sessions and festive and charity events. The main author's experiences of being an adoptive mother of a child from Ethiopia for about ten years facilitated entering the field and constituted an important source of practical knowledge.

The study participants come from diverse backgrounds (working in diverse professions, living in both cities and rural areas, unbelieving or Catholic), yet are predominantly middle-class, (highly) educated, white, heterosexual and married. A minority of the mothers were single at the time of the interviews or engaged in a lesbian relationship. The motives for adopting a child varied, from infertility to illness, to the wish to 'help an orphaned child'. Their number of children ranged from one to six and several families had both children by birth and by adoption. Their children's age varied from a few months to twenty-five years old, although the majority of the families had small children. All families followed a stringent adoption procedure prescribed by the Belgian Federal and Flemish community authorities. This includes preparation courses and social investigation. All the parents in this study adopted through a state recognized adoption agency.

Intensive mothering ideologies and charity work

> SOPHIE: In the end, whatever way you look at it, you're helping kids. I'm not saying that was our primary motivation, but you're doing that anyway. People then discuss: 'Is it a good thing to take a child out of its country? But then I think: 'What is best for a child?' To grow up in an orphanage without a family, or grow up somewhere with one? Then, I believe, the choice is easily made.

Sophie, who is an adoptive mother of an Ethiopian-born sibling pair, phrases what many parents expressed during the interviews. Most parents did not portray themselves explicitly as benefactors, yet their narratives are flavoured with rescue elements. Although a few parents confided that no one will ever know if adoption made their child happier, most parents emphasize that without adoption their child would have lived in orphanages. Some parents indicated that their child may have died or would have been forced to live in the streets, deprived of protection and care.

Intensive mothering ideologies that naturalize the nuclear family as the prime locus of childrearing and that problematize every other context in which children can be raised, turn transnational adoption into a viable, albeit not an ideal option. Adopters construct children in 'underdeveloped' parts of the world as innocent victims in need of the help of affluent middle-class people, who are capable of being intensive and loving parents. Yet the children's biological parents, who are in an increasing number of cases alive and known (at least by the Ethiopian authorities), are deemed less rescuable by the adopters.[4] Adoptive parents' legitimizing narratives depict the birth parents of their children as too poor to take up parenting roles appropriately. As such they strip birth parents of their parenting capabilities or, within an intensive mothering ideological vein, construct them as altruistic carers who make the ultimate sacrifice of giving up their child to offer it a better life. Hans, for example, makes use of this kind of discourse when he tries to frame his daughter's abandonment. He and his wife Lisa adopted a five-year-old girl whose biological mother, according to the files, was too poor to keep the child after her husband died.

> HANS: We think it is a very altruistic decision of that mother. If it's true what they told us, then she really chooses life for her daughter, counter to her own self-interest. Because in Africa, having children is still a form of social security, of course.

Adoptive parenthood (and the intensive parenting practice that goes with it) is part of the adoptive parents' construction of themselves as what counts as 'good' citizens, by fulfilling the middle class obligation of raising a family, and acting as sympathetic, philanthropic and broadminded human beings.

Yet this obviously does not challenge the status quo of exclusion and unequal (global) power relations that frame the adoption industry in the first place. On the contrary, interpretations of 'the best interest of the child' current in OECD countries that naturalize and universalize the middle-class heterosexual nuclear family have been used to legitimize and to regulate the neo-colonial transfer of poor 'Third World' children to affluent and intensive parenting 'First World' families.[5] Furthermore, transnational adoption is cloaked in a language of charity and philanthropy while structural imbalances between demand and supply carry the risk of making the practices of transnational adoption self-perpetuating (Högbacka 2008: 314). They may even pave the way to illegal baby markets and child trafficking (Brysk 2004: 166; Nelson 2006: 89). Adoptive children are caught up in the imbalanced global exchange that tends to turn children into globally traded objects (Leifsen 2004: 192). It makes them part of the flow of resources that are extracted from the former colonized world to supply the former colonizers' needs (see e.g. Eng 2003; Hübinette 2006).

Although relatively little public criticism has been voiced about transnational adoption in Belgium, several parents in the study expressed their discomfort with the unjust conditions which are at the root of transnational adoption and which disturb their rescue narratives. This discomfort leads up to what Jacobson (2008: 31) calls a 'taboo on rescue', urging parents to minimize the role of humanitarian impulses in their decision to adopt and emphasize their own 'selfish' desire to have children as their primary motivation. But the minimizing of their own role as rescuer or benefactor is also in line with what Hays (1996: 167) specifies as two central elements of the larger cultural model of intensive mothering, notably (1) the image of a mother as unselfish nurturer and (2) the ideology of the sacred child. Adopters emphasize the yearning to parent and to engage in an unconditional loving relationship with a child and protect the assumed right of children to be raised in the warmth of a family (without expecting any gratitude). They construct themselves as intensive caring parents who are just performing their duty and who do not pursue reward or recognition for their perceived good deeds.

In spite of, or perhaps as a result of the rescue taboo, most adopters indicate that adoption somehow triggers an increased involvement in charity work. A strikingly high proportion of the adoptive parents in this study say they financially support one or more (mostly Ethiopian) children through child sponsorship organizations, or donate money to other charity organizations working in Ethiopia or elsewhere. Furthermore, several adoptive parents have even set up or actively participate in non-profit organizations supporting projects in Ethiopia and invest a considerable amount of time in organizing money-raising events and/or in following up the projects they sustain. Several of these parents assert they engage in this kind of work because 'it's the kids' country and you want to do something back'. Feelings of indebtedness to the country that has provided them with a child and pity for the children 'left behind' seem to precipitate their thirst for action. The charity work shows how the adoptive parents' ethics of care is intertwined with the idea of the child as a gift and feelings of personal responsibility for structural global inequalities. Moreover, by doing charity work adoptive parents 'tap into a wider transnational flow of meanings, goods and practices that are firmly associated with transmigrant populations' (Willing 2010: 218). The parents perform culture and charity work in relation to a country in which they were not born and did not grow up in, but to which they feel connected through their children's migration. This bears a lot of striking similarities to the identity practices of transmigrants, who 'maintain connections, build institutions, conduct transactions, and influence local and national events in the countries from which they emigrated' (Schiller *et al.* 1995: 48).

Some of the parents also emphasize the importance of the charity work for their adopted children. John, an adoptive father of three children, for instance, describes the charity project he and his wife Anne-Marie have set up in Ethiopia as a 'gate' their children are free to use to re-connect to their birth country whenever they feel the need. As such, the charity work the parents perform can be seen as 'caregiving for identity' (Kershaw 2010) and part of the intensive parenting work that seems to push parenting beyond the intimate sphere of the family. These activities are usually described as pleasant and the feeling of doing something good as satisfactory. However, in some cases the charity work can become too demanding, threatening the familial health and stability and urging parents to back down. John and Anne-Marie, for instance, decided to withdraw their active membership of the non-profit organization they once founded. For several years, they invested a huge amount of time and energy in this project, yet they felt compelled to end their involvement after one of their children was diagnosed with a severe mental health disorder. As they felt that their child's particular needs demanded all their attention they both decided to pass on the management of their organization to other people.

> ANNE-MARIE: We will turn our heart into stone, and [resign]. But I will regret that the rest of my life, I know it. But what I will never regret is that ultimately we have chosen for our family here. That's also a commitment we made.

The example shows that the parents' charity efforts are closely interwoven with their intensive parenting work. Their rescue fantasies attest to the way global inequalities slip into the adoptive parents' everyday life and how they both justify and challenge imaginations of adoptive parenthood.

Dramatized adoptive parenthood

The transformation of childhood driven by modern psychological theories on child development, into a special and crucial period of life in which the foundations of a (sound) human personality are laid, has changed the conception of motherhood into a serious responsibility that requires total and exclusive devotion (Glenn 1994: 14; Hays 1996; Rose 1999: 145; Furedi 2008: 48). Hence, mothering an adoptive child, whose early development may have lacked intensive care, is deemed extraordinary difficult. It is seen as 'having to try to put right' the (irreparable) damage that may have been caused by the lack of what is considered appropriate care. Moreover, in an era where 'the mundane tasks of mothering', as Rose (1999: 161) points out, 'came to be rewritten as emanations of a natural and essential state of love', adoptive motherhood is somehow seen as an oxymoron (Park 2006: 203). The lack of the bodily connection to the child that grounds a traditional conception of motherhood (Park 2006: 206) urges adoptive parents, driven by dominant cultural images of parenting, to feel *more* in need of education and support. The growing authority of psychological explanations for behaviour creates and naturalizes criteria of normality, and as a consequence, problematizes those who deviate.

Misalignments between expectation and reality, Rose (1999: 132) argues, create a constant need for expertise and guidance in the difficult task of producing normality. In Belgium, as in many other countries, this need is met by a lengthy, highly regulated and state controlled judicial procedure, providing for a number of compulsory and voluntary courses. Adoptive parents are usually eager to follow the courses. Most of them even engage in additional reading or in

Internet discussion groups on the subject. As a matter of fact, fieldwork shows that it is mainly the (prospective) mothers, encouraged by 'intensive mothering expectations' (Johnston and Swanson 2006: 510) who invest a lot of time and energy in the gathering of expert knowledge and turn themselves into 'semi-professional parents' (Buysse and Vandenbroeck 2010) who feel prepared for the supposedly arduous task of raising adopted children. As Anagnost (2000: 396) argues, women seem to be more in need of the circulation of signs that endorses their subject position as 'mother in the making'. Adoption challenges the 'natural' division of labour. Due to the adoption procedure, adoptive fathers are usually more actively involved in the process of becoming a parent than in pregnancy and delivery. Yet, mothers still seem to bear most of the responsibility for children (Wall and Arnold 2007: 510; Doucet 2009: 105) and parenthood seems to figure more prominently in women's identity constructions than in that of men.

In addition to 'official' adoption expertise that is provided by two state recognized adoption preparation centres in Flanders, a number of professionals (predominantly psychologists and paediatricians) present themselves as adoption experts and attract a lot of adopters into their practice or give lectures to an audience of adopters. But also peer-mentoring and testimonies of experienced adoptive parents are generally seen as highly informative by other adopters. The general tenor of adoption expertise in Flanders is that adoptive parenting requires extraordinary measures. As the adoptive parents lack a 'natural' biological bond with their adoptive children, and adoptive children are snatched from the presumed 'natural' union with their biological mothers, the adoptive parenting task tends to be dramatized and wrapped in a language of emergency, pathologization and exceptionality.

Strikingly, whereas ties with birth mothers are constructed as natural and indissoluble, adoptive parents and professionals usually allot a far less crucial role to the rupture with the biological father for the child's psychological health. What is more, birthfathers are in some cases (in official reports or as part of the adoptive parents' imaginations) narrated as untrustworthy, irresponsible and even violent. One adoptive mother for example confided that the official report mentioned rape as justification of relinquishment, a fact that she found very difficult to fit in the adoption story she was going to tell her child. Some adoptive parents in the study claimed to wonder if the biological father even knows he has a child and widowed fathers' decisions to relinquish their children are considered quite understandable.

Middle-class adoptive fathers in OECD countries seem to see themselves as loving, attentive parents, actively involved and concerned with the rearing of their children. Yet biological fathers in the metaphorical South who live in poverty are not attributed a similar connection to their children and seem to figure less prominently in the adoptive families' adoption narratives than birthmothers do. This kind of stance resonates with feminist postcolonial insights into the way in which in contemporary colonial discourse in OECD countries 'black men' are often stereotypically sexualized as oppressors of subjugated black women – and in this case black children – to be saved by white 'civilized' men (Abu-Lughod 2002). It also reflects work in gender and development that points at complex historicised masculinity constructions of 'lazy' African men (Whitehead 2000; Chant and Gutmann Matthew 2002).

The striking emphasis in adoption circles on children's attachment within the adoptive family, rather than on belonging and inclusion in society stems from the 'familialization of society' (Rose 1999: 128) and the ideological separation of home and world that goes with the intensive mothering ideology (Hays 1996: 34). It is believed that if belonging on a familial level can be obtained, belonging on a broader societal level will automatically follow, and that when problems arise, their causes must also be found in the bosom of the family. More than one adoption professional involved in the process of educating and supporting adoptive parents in Flanders claimed that attachment, and not racism, was the real issue for adopted children. Experiences of racialization tend to be trivialized and minimized, whereas the skills of being able to adequately cope with racism and exclusion are emphasized. As such, racism tends to be assessed as the adoptee's responsibility.

Our data analysis shows that various ideas on how best to increase the child's attachment to its new family circulate among adoptive parents and professionals supporting the parents, including the idea that adoptive children must be kept 'in quarantine' during the first months after arrival. A few years ago, this idea was launched in Flanders by Dr Gillis, a paediatrician who established a medical centre for adoption and tropical paediatrics in a small town hospital. He gives advice to the many adoptive parents who come to his clinic and provides them with an eleven-page report of a training he attended in an adoption study centre in Canada (Gillis 2005). He is also regularly asked for lectures organized by adoption agencies and an adoptive parents advocacy group. He recommends that during the first months, adoptive children should enjoy the exclusive care and supervision of the adoptive parents (in practice, mostly the mothers), while grandparents, siblings or close friends are not supposed to touch or even have eye contact with the child. Although these directions are questioned and criticized by several other adoption professionals as well as by parents, and are characterized as rather extreme (and sometimes even strongly rejected), the underlying idea of parental exclusivity is far less contested. The directions are clearly influenced by widespread attachment parenting theories that start from the idea, as Layne (this volume) explains; 'that children are hard-wired to bond with one primary caregiver'. Moreover, a culture of paranoid parenting (Furedi 2008: 25) tends to positively sanction excessive parental supervision. Therefore, and as the data suggests, the 'quarantine' concept is slowly trickling into Flemish adoption circles.

Several of the parents interviewed who adopted rather recently told they had applied the guidelines, though in varying degrees of intensity. They, for example, asked friends and acquaintances to postpone their visit by a couple of months, or prohibited grandparents to touch their newly arrived grandchild. Yet this intense emphasis on exclusivity threatens to further problematize the multiple parenthood that is at the heart of adoption. By considering the adoptive relation as the only one that is 'decisive for the child's sociality' (Leifsen 2004: 193), several potentially significant others are implicitly made unimportant and previous social connections (as with birth parents or caretaking persons) are symbolically dismantled during the 'quarantine' period in which children are disciplined in (exclusively) loving their new carers.

(Re-)forging relations

Nevertheless, previous relationships of the child with biological parents or other caretakers may be narratively (and in some cases also effectively) rekindled as soon as the child is found ready for it. The paradox for adoptive children of being assigned exclusively adoptive kinship in a society that values blood ties as 'indissoluble bonds of love and solidarity' (Ouellette and Belleau 2001: 27) incites parents (as part of their intensive parenting work) to search for ways of reconstructing and archiving the children's origin story. Testimonies of adult adoptees worldwide of their painful identity struggles have induced an emphasis in prevailing adoption discourse and practice on biological and cultural roots. Origin stories and the authenticity they are believed to entail are part of a discourse of identity that is understood as essential for knowing oneself (Yngvesson and Mahoney 2000: 101). The impossibility of ever knowing about adoptive children's birth origins and therefore, it is claimed, of ever fully knowing oneself, is assumed to heavily complicate adoptive children's identity work.

Therefore, parents search for material with which they can construct a pre-adoption memory for their child and archive objects that refer to the child's early existence (such as its baptismal cord, clothes and photographs) or record the child's stories of its pre-adoption life. Ria, a single mother who adopted a girl at the age of eight, narrates:

> RIA: I find it a pity that she tends to forget many things about her life in Ethiopia. That's why I have written down things she told me about her family. About her grandma she told me that they often had to fetch water with the donkeys by the river and that her grandma had cow manure and goats. And that there was a party once and that family of hers went to live in Sudan. Yes those kinds of things she told me.

Contacts with biological siblings or orphanage friends of the adopted children are valued and maintained, and (if some information is available) biological family members living in Ethiopia are tracked down. However, as many of the adopted children from Ethiopia have been abandoned anonymously, in these cases bonds with the birth family seem to be permanently cut through.

Engaging in Ethiopian culture and 'fascination with the imagined "birth culture"' (Volkman 2003: 29) seems to be part of the parenting work that attempts to remediate potential identity problems (De Graeve forthcoming). As Volkman (2003: 29) argues for her research on US–China adoption, it probably

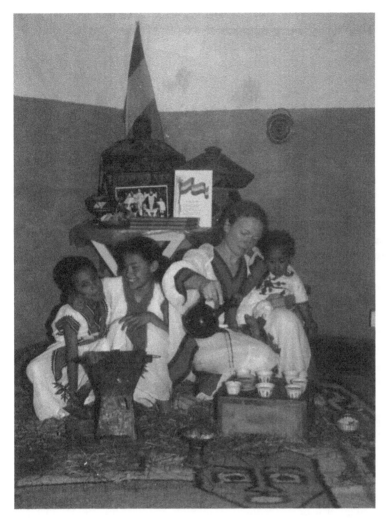

Figure 8.1 Card announcing the adoption of a sibling pair (reproduced with permission).

'represent[s] displaced longings for origins and absent birth mothers'. However, what is striking is that the cultural origins of adopted children are particularly rendered important – as Marre (2007: 82) demonstrates in her comparison of intraracial and transracial adoption – when the child is racially different from its adoptive parents. This tends to confirm that cultural identity is at least partly considered as a product of biology. Pieter, the adoptive father of a baby from Ethiopia, referred to the child's skin colour to explain his interest in Ethiopian culture: 'I mean, the child does have a background, doesn't he? We will not be able to hide it, will we? When we put the hands on the table, I mean, you won't be able to hide that…' Several parents asserted that they had searched for god-parents as a way of providing their children with positive role models. These stories also exemplify parents' explorations of alternative kinship configurations. Elise and Victor, for instance, invited two men and two women to become the godparents of their son, named Eskeder, who was adopted at age five. One of the godparents was a black friend who lost her mother when she was four.

> ELISE: She is someone who, first, lost her parents at an early age, and who, secondly, chose to leave her family and culture behind – even though in her case, it was a voluntary decision – and then she came here. She has a partner here, she is married here, and, normally, she's going to stay here. So I do think that if Eskeder ever struggles with issues like these, she might be someone who can help him and that is something we thought was really important.

Godparents were also given an important role in the support of adopted children in the narratives of some of the single mothers in this study, who also seemed to search for compensation for the absence of another, male partner. Ria, for instance, provided her daughter, who had a Muslim birthfather and a Christian birthmother, with three godfathers.

> RIA: They are no godfathers in the Christian sense, but male role models that I wanted to give to her. One of her godfathers is Muslim. She liked that, and then she was asking: 'Am I a Muslim or a Christian?' And I said: 'You can choose what you are.'

Narrative processes of self-making

Adoptive parents, instead of being passive receivers of expert knowledge, do not conform blindly to expert recommendations but as active agents 'subject such recommendations to evaluation and questioning, operating as an informed con-sumer' (Faircloth 2009: 15). Analogous to Faircloth's findings (2009: 17) in her research on long-term breastfeeding, by making childrearing choices that are informed by both scientific and affective arguments, adoptive parents put 'their authority in congruence with wider social trends'. At the same time, by referring to expert knowledge, they justify decisions that are socially less accepted. The following text from an adoption announcement card for an Ethiopian-born baby exemplifies the parents' negotiation of their childrearing strategies. The parents involved used the announcement card to inform family and friends about the unusual measures they planned to take.

> In his short life, Warre has not yet been able to really attach to someone. […] We want to give Warre time and space to attach to us. Adoption experts advise us to reserve feeding and nursing, but also hugging, sitting on some-one's lap and eye contact exclusively for the parents during the first months.

By adhering to these guidelines, we hope to give Warre a safe basis for his further development.

Interviews showed that parents act in relation to all others involved in the child's education, for example childcare workers or schoolteachers but also grandparents or other family members, as educated semi-professionals who are best-informed about and sensitive to the child's needs and feel eligible enough to instruct them on how the child must be approached. Their childrearing decisions and parenting practices turn out to be an important part of the parents' 'narrative processes of self-making' (Faircloth 2009: 15, chapter this volume). Making certain choices, or distancing themselves from parental identities that do not fit them, plays a part in parents' constructions of themselves as the kind of parent they want to be (see also Jensen's chapter, this volume, for a discussion of parenting as an opportunity for social distinction). As such, the semi-professional care as well as the charitable or cultural work they perform on behalf of their children also changes themselves and intertwines with the construction of their own identities as informed conscious parents and/or non-racist, tolerant and open-minded citizens.

Although the exceptionalization of adoptive parenthood can play an important part in the parents' identity construction as hardworking, concerned and self-sacrificing parents, we can raise the question whether the characterization of adoptive parenting as an extremely difficult enterprise turns out all that positive for the child's identity development. For it tends to reinforce images of the adoptive child as different, deviant and difficult to handle and as such, to reproduce differences instead of normalizing them. Parents stress 'the equality and equivalence of their family arrangements' and aim at providing the child with a more positive sense of identity, for example, by means of culture work. Yet on the other hand, they run the risk of marking the child as different by dramatizing its non-normativity and confirming the normative conceptions of kinship and ethnic identity. Hence while 'difference' is absorbed into the intimate space of the familial, it seems to be simultaneously reinscribed (Anagnost 2000: 390).

Concluding remarks

This chapter has described some Belgian parents' experiences of intensive mothering ideology in a context of unequal global relations, leading to the utmost dramatization of transnationally adoptive kinship. Our study has interpreted the intensive adoptive parenting practices as a broad set of actions (ranging from the mundane everyday caring tasks over the study and application of specialized expert knowledge to the engagement in charity or cultural work), entrenched in prevailing ideologies that ultimately tend to essentialize (global) configurations of difference and inequality. With this analysis we hope to have contributed to a further understanding of the ideologically charged parenting practices and their transformative potentials as well as possible constraints in realizing more inclusivity for all parties involved.

This chapter challenges over-optimistic representations of adoption as an anti-essentialist act (see e.g. Bordo 2005). It argues that the dramatization of the adoptive parenting work tends to further underline adoptive children's and adoptive families' deviance from the aspired norm. Because of the articulation of the parenting work with ideas that define the 'true' needs of children in terms of exclusive parent–child bonds, it carries the risk of reinforcing essentialisms that parents seek to disavow and of further problematizing the plurality that is inherent in adoption. Furthermore, the intensive parenting practice conforms to and reproduces the middle-class and upper-working-class imperative that constructs motherhood as central to femininity and parenting as a civic duty while risking overlooking the reproductive rights of less privileged women and men (Cuthbert *et al.* 2009: 395, 412).

Yet, this chapter also recognizes the potential to unsettle essentialist understandings of kinship and belonging. It acknowledges that the 'transgressive act' of transnational adoption opens possibilities to re-imagine identities and citizenship (Watkins 2006: 269) and offers alternative conceptualizations of parenting and kinship. By charity and culture work, by their daily negotiations of and searching for alternative family forms, parents explore how their non-biological family can take shape in the context of profound global inequalities.

Notes

1 All interviews were carried out in Flemish. Excerpts are translated from Flemish to English. Names of parents or children are changed to assure confidentiality.
2 We use the term 'intensive mothering' to refer to the ideological complex as described by Sharon Hays (1996), whereas we prefer to use the term 'parenting' to speak of the practices that are discussed in this chapter. Both adoptive mothers and fathers in this study have strong childrearing ideas and in most cases appear to be intensely involved in the parenting work, which covers a whole array of tasks however often differentiated along traditional gendered lines. So, we do use the term 'parenting', however, without ignoring the differences in maternal and paternal practices or denying the historical and lived reality of women being disproportionally responsible for childcare (Ruddick 1997: 216).
3 Flemish is a variant of the Dutch language.
4 Until 2005, children that were made available for adoption in Ethiopia were orphans (children who had lost both parents) or foundlings (children whose parents were unknown by the Ethiopian authorities). Since 2005 also children who have been officially given up by their parents are sent abroad for adoption.
5 For another discussion of the way parenting can be co-opted to obscure structured inequity see Berry's chapter, this volume.

References

Abu-Lughod, L. (2002) 'Do Muslim women really need saving? Anthropological reflections on cultural relativism and its Others', *American Anthropologist*, 104: 783–790.
Anagnost, A. (2000) 'Scenes of misrecognition: Maternal citizenship in the age of transnational adoption', *Positions-East Asia Cultures Critique*, 8: 389–421.
Bordo, S. (2005) 'Adoption', *Hypatia*, 20: 230–237.

Braidotti, R. (2011) *Nomadic Theory: The Portable Rosi Braidotti*, New York: Columbia University Press.

Brysk, A. (2004) 'Children across borders: Patrimony, property or persons?' in A. Brysk and G. Shafir (eds) *People out of Place: Globalization, Human Rights, and the Citizenship Gap*, New York: Routledge.

Buysse, A. and Vandenbroeck, M. (2010) 'Focusgroepenonderzoek "nazorg adoptie"', Universiteit Gent & Steunpunt Nazorg Adoptie.

Carsten, J. (2000) 'Introduction: Cultures of relatedness', in J. Carsten (ed.) *Cultures of Relatedness: New Approaches to the Study of Kinship*, Cambridge: Cambridge University Press.

Chant, S. and Gutmann Matthew, C. (2002) '"Men-streaming" gender? Questions for gender and development policy in the twenty-first century', *Progress in Development Studies*, 2: 269–282.

Cuthbert, D., Murphy, K. and Quartly, M. (2009). 'Adoption and feminism: Towards framing a feminist response to contemporary developments in adoption', *Australian Feminist Studies*, 24: 395–419.

De Graeve, K. (forthcoming) 'Festive gatherings and culture work in Flemish-Ethiopian adoptive families', *European Journal for Cultural Studies*.

Doucet, A. (2009) 'Gender equality and gender differences: Parenting, habitus, and embodiment', *Canadian Review of Sociology/Revue Canadienne de Sociologie*, 46: 103–121.

Eng, D.L. (2003) 'Transnational adoption and queer diasporas', *Social Text*, 21: 1–37.

Faircloth, C. (2009) 'Mothering as identity-work: Long-term breastfeeding and intensive motherhood,' *Anthropology News*, 50: 15–17.

Furedi, F. (2008) *Paranoid Parenting: Why Ignoring the Experts may be Best for your Child*, London: Continuum.

Gillis, P. (2005) 'Verslag van het symposium: "Le monde est ailleurs", "L'enfant adopté et sa famille", Hôpital Universitaire St-Justin, Montreal, Canada: 13–17 juni 2005', unpublished manuscript.

Glenn, E.N. (1994) 'Social constructions of mothering: A thematic overview', in E.N. Glenn, G. Chang and L.R. Forcey (eds) *Mothering: Ideology, Experience, and Agency*, New York: Routledge.

Hayden, C.P. (1995) 'Gender, genetics, and generation: Reformulating biology in lesbian kinship', *Cultural Anthropology*, 10: 41–63.

Hays, S. (1996) *The Cultural Contradictions of Motherhood*, New Haven, CT: Yale University Press.

Högbacka, R. (2008) 'The quest for a child of one's own: Parents, markets and transnational adoption', *Journal of Comparative Family Studies*, 39: 311–330.

Hübinette, T. (2006) 'From orphan trains to babylifts. Colonial trafficking, empire building, and social engineering', in J.J. Trenka, J. Sudbury and S.Y. Shin (eds) *Outsiders Within: Writing on Transracial Adoption*, Cambridge, MA.: South End Press.

Jacobson, H. (2008) *Culture Keeping: White Mothers, International Adoption, and the Negotiation of Family Difference*, Nashville, TN: Vanderbilt University Press.

Johnston, D.D. and Swanson, D.H. (2006) 'Constructing the "good mother": The experience of mothering ideologies by work status', *Sex Roles*, 54: 509–519.

Kershaw, P. (2010) 'Caregiving for identity is political: Implications for citizenship theory', *Citizenship Studies*, 14: 395–410.

Leifsen, E. (2004) 'Person, relation and value. The economy of circulating Ecuadorian children in international adoption', in F. Bowie (ed.) *Cross-Cultural Approaches to Adoption*, London: Routledge.

Marre, D. (2007) 'I want her to learn her language and maintain her culture: Transnational adoptive families' views of "cultural origins"', in P. Wade (ed.) *Race, Ethnicity and Nation: Perspectives from Kinship and Genetics*, New York: Berghahn Books.

Nelson, K.P. (2006) 'Shopping for children in the international marketplace', in J.J. Trenka, J. Sudbury and S.Y. Shin (eds) *Outsiders Within: Writing on Transracial Adoption*, Cambridge, MA: South End Press.

Ouellette, F.-R. and Belleau, H. (2001) *Family and Social Integration of Children Adopted Internationally: A Review of the Literature*, Montreal: INRS-Université du Quebec.

Park, S.M. (2006) 'Adoptive maternal bodies: A queer paradigm for rethinking mothering?' *Hypatia*, 21: 201–227.

Rose, N. (1999) *Governing the Soul: The Shaping of the Private Self*, London: Free Association Books.

Ruddick, S. (1997) 'The idea of fatherhood', in L.H. Nelson (ed.) *Feminism and Families*, New York: Routledge, pp. 205–220.

Schiller, N.G., Basch, L. and Cristina Szanton, B. (1995) 'From immigrant to transmigrant: Theorizing transnational migration', *Anthropological Quarterly*, 68: 48–63.

Volkman, T.A. (2003) 'Embodying Chinese culture: Transnational adoption in North America', *Social Text*, 21: 29–55.

Wall, G. and Arnold, S. (2007) 'How involved is involved fathering? An exploration of the contemporary culture of fatherhood', *Gender and Society*, 21: 508–527.

Watkins, M. (2006) 'Adoption and identity: Nomadic possibilities for reconceiving the self', in K. Wegar, (ed.) *Adoptive Families in a Diverse Society*, New Brunswick, NJ: Rutgers University Press.

Whitehead, A. (2000) 'Continuities and discontinuities in political constructions of the working man in rural sub-Saharan Africa: The "Lazy Man" in African Agriculture', *European Journal of Development Research*, 12: 23–52.

Willing, I.W. (2010). 'Transnational adoption and construction of identity and belonging: A qualitative study of Australian parents and children adopted from overseas', unpublished thesis, University of Queensland.

Yngvesson, B. and Mahoney, M.A. (2000) '"As one should, ought and wants to be": Belonging and authenticity in identity narratives', *Theory, Culture and Society*, 17: 77–109.

9 'Staying with the baby'

Intensive mothering and social mobility in Santiago de Chile

Marjorie Murray

Introduction

Several of the current trends of intensive parenting that have been identified in Euro–American contexts and described in different chapters in this volume have arrived in Chile, a context in which 'child-centredness' and 'intensive mothering' are inherent to the ideology of motherhood and kinship. In this chapter, I explore the ways in which a group of women in Santiago de Chile interpret, negotiate and reject recent pedagogies of intensive parenting ideologies coming from private, public and medical entities. Specifically, I focus on the stories of a group of women belonging to a segment of the population that forms a 'first generation outside of poverty' in Santiago. I argue that, for them, several intensive mothering mandates, encouraged by the state and by private practice, reinforce their sense of being good mothers. However, these do not satisfy another inherent feature of their intensive mothering expectations: social mobility aspirations in a neoliberal system. The study of their mothering aims and practices grounds both intensive mothering and existing kinship literature on mothering in Chile. This chapter provides a case-study of the appropriation and experienced contradictions of a global trend in a specific context that questions the 'newness' in the new intensive parenting.

I start by introducing the methods of the study. I then provide data about the economic and political context of this case-study and describe the current Chilean government policies directed specifically at early mothering. The main results will be presented in two sections. I first focus on relevant aspects of a type of child-centredness that can already be identified in the prenatal period and which combines rooted and recent tendencies in pregnancy care and mothering, with particular attention to women's relationship with the medical systems. I then present the specific kind of 'intensiveness', regarding these women's mothering, as observed in 'staying with the baby', during the first year. Their routines in 'intensive mothering' and 'child-centredness' question the newness of intensive parenting, understood as a recent ideological movement taking place in contexts such as the UK and USA (Hays 1996; Kukla 2008; Faircloth 2010, this volume). I suggest that their 'intensiveness' cannot be separated from long-term rationales surrounding mothering in Chile, so that recent intensive parenting discourses are appropriated and negotiated along existing values of mothering. At the same time, their intensive early mothering style cannot be separated from a strong aim of social mobility for their families.

Mothering at the edge

During 2010–2011, as part of a wider research project,[1] I studied the process of becoming a mother in a heterogeneous group of sixteen mothers with diverse income and education levels, and living in different areas in Santiago de Chile. Following an ethnographic approach that would illuminate the processes of growing children and mothers (Miller 1997), I first met my informants during their third trimester of pregnancy and visited them on a monthly basis, mostly at their homes – the environment in which both baby and mother spent most of their time – until the babies reached one year of age.[2] In this year of change, I paid specific attention to the 'taken-for-granted', everyday lives or *habitus* (Bourdieu 1977) of the informants considering material culture as constitutive, expressive and framing of selves and relationships (Miller 1987; Latour 1993). From this perspective, I became acquainted with these mothers' expectations, fears and involvement with other relevant relations during this period.

Santiago is a heavily stratified and segregated city,[3] and it did not take long to confirm that class and income differences create parallel cosmologies for these families. At the same time, I encountered a widespread awareness and interest in ascendant social mobility – change in one's position in this hierarchical social structure (Torche and Wormald 2004) – for informants and their children[4] which, I will argue, is constitutive of their sense of motherhood. Taking into consideration the incommensurable differences between social classes, in this chapter I focus specifically on a group of seven upwardly mobile women belonging to lower-middle-income families. Six of these women achieved a secondary school level of education and were employed full-time in such roles as secretary, chemical laboratory technician and pharmacy clerk, at the time they became pregnant. The seventh woman was finishing her technical studies and working part-time in a supermarket. All of these women live on a monthly family income of between 260,000 and 500,000 pesos (US$500 and US$1,000 approximately)[5] meaning that they have overcome the 'poverty line' and, as such, belong to the lower-middle class of Santiago.[6] More importantly, all of them were aware of having experienced at least a modest improvement in their socio-economic situation or material comfort compared to their own childhood, either through increased income (two salaries) or new access to consumption by means of commercial debt (see Han 2011), in line with the Chilean macro-social and economic changes in the last decades. During the time of fieldwork they were all involved in stable relationships: four were living with their partners independently; three were living as *allegados*,[7] in the maternal home; only two were married.

Early mothering in Chile: economic and political context

Chilean society has experienced social and economic processes marked by the consolidation of a neoliberal system during the Pinochet dictatorship (1973–1988) and the Concertación governments (centre-left coalition which governed from 1989 to 2010). On the one hand, socio-demographic indicators show important advances. The number of people living under the poverty line decreased from 38.4 per cent in 1990 to 15.1 per cent in 2009 (PNUD 2010). During these decades, graduation rates for secondary education increased from 46 per cent in 1995 to 68 per cent in 2011 (OECD 2011: 55), while the proportion of the population made up of students between eighteen and twenty-four years of age increased from 16 per cent in 1992 to 34 per cent in 2006 (OECD and World Bank 2009: 2). On the other hand, this model, with its privatization and consumer-oriented agenda, provides access to a range of consumer goods, and new levels of commercial debt, to a range of population groups beyond the traditional middle-classes (Moulian 1998; Han 2011).[8] In this context, thousands of families have experienced a redirection of their aspirations and demands: from the demand for 'access' to education to an expectation of 'quality' of education in a fairer system;[9] from demanding a solution to housing problems to solving problematic and unfair indebtedness with retailers; from combating undernourishment in children to dealing with overweight children.

Along with the consolidation of neoliberal values and macroeconomic growth, the governments of the Concertación and, more recently, of President Piñera (centre-right) have implemented and reinforced relevant social policies aiming at overcoming social inequality. During the government of President Michelle Bachelet – a paediatrician – several social security laws were implemented in the name of 'social protection', including an unemployment insurance system[10] and a system of state-paid treatment of a list of diseases. One of the emblematic policies during her government was *Chile Crece Contigo* (Chile Grows with You, from now onwards ChCC), brought about by a 2009 national law. This policy epitomizes a new kind of state involvement in early parenting[11] devoted to undermining various social inequalities 'since the beginning of life',[12] with the help of expert support.

ChCC is a good example of state-led reflexivity around how people 'parent' (see introduction to this volume) – an enterprise that is too important and difficult to be left up to parents alone (Furedi 2008). The programme consists of

> a system of integral infant protection whose mission is to accompany, protect and support integrally every child and their families through actions and services that are universal [for every child] and by focalizing special support on those who are more vulnerable: it adapts to the specific needs.
>
> (Chile Crece Contigo 2010)

Following well-established medical and psychological theories, mostly inspired by attachment theories and developmental psychology (see Unicef 2001; Wall

2010), this programme promises to secure opportunities for new citizens[13] by attacking biological, psychological and social inequalities 'since the beginning of life' (Silva and Molina 2010: 20). Even though the identities of the source authors of the theories behind these policies are not made explicit, it is clearly the work of people like Bowlby (1969, 1973, 1980) that inspires its specific priorities in line with 'attachment parenting' (Faircloth, this volume). The state allies with the newly born citizens, providing them with tools to confront a possibly adverse environment and its negative effects on development, performance in education, conduct problems, and reproduction of poverty. The programme encourages women to participate in several workshops (on preparation for childbirth, early stimulation, massages for babies, and childrearing tips). Women receive music CDs during the perinatal period to enhance the child's language development. Every child born in a public hospital receives an *ajuar* or layette worth US$400 which includes a cradle, clothes, a diaper bag and a 'secure attachment set' consisting of nursing pillow, sling-type baby carrier and a booklet on secure attachment. Several posters promoting long-term breastfeeding are placed in public hospitals and surgeries. Health and education professionals celebrate this law, which has indeed become inspiration for similar programmes in other countries in the region.[14] Women seem to appreciate this support to parenting. In tune with this enthusiasm, in 2011 the congress approved an extension of fully paid maternity leave, from three to six months for working mothers, consolidating a national commitment to promote attachment and breastfeeding as the most beneficial approach for mother and baby.[15]

In the following sections I show how my informants easily related to and followed some of the intensive mothering principles that ChCC encourages, which are, in many respects, congruent with the long-term kinship values of the devotional, self-sacrificial mother. I will also discuss a rather different set of practices, considered important in constructing the maternal and child selves, aimed at a more prosperous future and increased social mobility. The extensive consumption of private healthcare is one of them.

Pregnancy, child-centredness and the consumption of medicine

Once my informants heard they were pregnant, a set of strategies or 'technologies of motherhood' (Ragoné and Twine 2000) came into play in such a way that by the time of birth their self-identification with the role of the devotional, self-sacrificial mother (Mayblin 2012; Göknar this volume) and a sense of 'child-centeredness' (Hoffman 2000b) were already quite developed. A range of discourses and practices regarding the 'miracle of the baby', the new 'maternal self' of the mother and the sacrifices she would incur were ubiquitous, in line with previous research on motherhood in Santiago, where discourses such as 'children are the joy of a home'; 'a couple is empty without children'; 'women without children are selfish, abnormal and not even real women'; 'children are the eternal companions to their mothers, life without them is empty and lonely' abound (e.g. Mattelart and Matterlat 1968; Godoy and Reynaldos 1984: 240–243).

From an early stage, these women started doing 'everything they can for their children', and following medical authority appeared a useful tool for reassuring them they were doing a good job. They all systematically attended the medical appointments in their local surgeries and followed prescriptions when required. For example, three informants who were overweight at the time they became pregnant managed to lose weight following the food intake indications from physicians and midwives, an achievement they probably never would have reached for themselves (two of them regained their weight after birth). These informants felt that the public-health system did not offer enough medical advice and support. So, although they did not give up the public system appointments, they were proud to tell me 'me atiendo particular' – 'I go to private practice' – where they found what they believe is the medical quality their family deserved – and they paid for it.[16] For them, 'the best for their children' during pregnancy included double checkups combining public and private medical appointments, several elective sonograms and, hopefully, giving birth in private clinics (see Murray (2012) on the stratification of birth preparation and outcome).

Melanie, a twenty-one-year-old woman, pregnant with her first baby and with the lowest income in the group, told me: 'these [private medical appointments] are a supplement plus. Everything is special and much more comfortable here. You don't have to wait and they provide you with all the necessary information'.[17] Certainly, these women seek a sympathetic doctor (not a nurse!) who will understand them and will provide the information they may require. However, the use of private practice exceeds medical requirements. Private healthcare is provided in relatively smart establishments, meaning that patrons feel more of a need to 'dress up for the occasion', thus lending a sense of dignity to both mother and child. The whole event inspires feelings of prosperity and a 'better future' for Melanie and her child, reinforcing her sense of herself as a caring mother who knows the right path to take.[18] In accordance, the preparation for birth consisted significantly of finding the right place for child delivery. Saving money and selecting their best possible option for the birth relieved these mothers from what they perceived to be a 'second-class' birth in public hospitals where hygiene problems and mistreatment abound.[19]

These informants certainly welcomed the public concern with pregnancy and mother–child attachment, and could relate easily to the expert advice provided. They were happy to receive the ChCC CDs and books, and two of the women actually followed the exercises and enjoyed playing the music CD to the baby. However, it was generally felt that the public programme could hardly compete with the benefits of private practice checkups or of giving birth in a private clinic. Their priorities are not contradictory with what ChCC recommends during pregnancy: a concern with and love for their babies, caring for them and socializing them to the relevant others.[20] Actually, it is in the name of this concern and love for their babies that these women buy into these practices.

For example, sonograms[21] play an important role in enhancing the mother's emotional feelings towards the baby. The examination itself, and the acquisition of the images on CDs or printouts for further contemplation, constitute devices for creating excitement or '*emoción*' towards the baby's existence, certainly reinforcing the mother's relationship with the baby, and the baby's socialization within the network of family and friends. As a gynaecologist explained: 'this exam calls everyone's attention … they bring children, mothers, grannies and, increasingly, partners to the exam'. Three informants placed their fourth or fifth sonogram (most had monthly sonograms) on display on their living-room shelves. They also uploaded various sonograms to their Facebook sites. These sonograms stayed on display during the rest of fieldwork and were considered keepsakes of this early stage in the baby's life.

During pregnancy these informants had already developed a sense of (or objectified) the baby's individuality, attributing to them likes and dislikes. For example, Kelly identified her baby's taste in food based on movements inside the womb: 'she likes chocolate much more than other sweets'. They all anticipated the arrival of a fully demanding child that by no means should be detached from their mother for at least one year. From the point of view of ChCC expectations these women were doing a good job in providing love and care to the baby from conception onwards. Much more controversial and class specific is the fact that this group of women anticipated the arrival of 'a pampered, spoilt child' (*regaloneado, fundido*[22]), which they considered a virtue, indicative of a family that can afford to spoil a child with infinite love, cuddles and goods. Melanie suggested 'I think that my partner will be selfish, he will want to keep the baby to himself and keep the rest [of family members who also want to hold and cuddle the baby] away'.

Dafne's expectations regarding her baby in the womb also evince her somewhat ambivalent desires:

> Anais [Dafne's three-year-old daughter], selects everything she wants for her room, she is like independent. I always taught her to be like that, since she was little she could select her clothes, manifest her taste. She is stubborn, but it is because of me, because I have told her to choose, because I don't want her to suffer if sometimes she needs me; I want her to be much more independent [than me]. This is the way we want to teach her little sister, but I doubt it will work, because she will be spoilt by everyone around here.

Dafne wants her baby to become an 'independent' person, meaning mainly someone with a personality and the knowledge to face adversity. At the same time, she does not hide her desire to develop a protective relationship that results in everlasting closeness, though she does not want her child to suffer if sometimes she is not there to help. These discourses escape two stereotypical dichotomies regarding childrearing. The first dichotomy is that of childrearing practices as either individualistic or collectivist (Hoffman 2000b; Jaysane-Darr this volume). In this case, the individual is highly valued and the relationship is set during pregnancy with the aid of anticipatory sacrificial discourses and 'technologies', such as the use of medical appointments and sonograms. In this relationship, 'independence' and 'interdependence' (Raeff 2010) – the second dichotomy – are administered cautiously, in contrast with a developmental psychology that aims at autonomy and independence (Hoffman 2000b) and that sees the foetus (and the baby) in terms of 'a project'. Gender and religious background in this context remain fundamental clues for an understanding of this specific way of understanding the child, one that allows perceiving the existence of the baby as a miracle, and motherhood as an enchanted experience. I turn to these in the concluding section of this chapter.

'Staying with the baby': principal routines during the first year

In our first meetings two weeks after they had given birth, my informants were adjusting to their new routines, breastfeeding and getting a few hours of sleep. Having a healthy baby by their side was everything that mattered and the variable experiences of birth delivery were considered irrelevant (Murray 2012). They were all certain that they needed to 'stay with the baby' for the longest possible time at any cost, and struggled with the idea of returning to work in the near future. Chilean women's reluctance to engage in formal work – particularly that of those with small children – has been documented (Lehmann 2003; Acosta *et al.* 2007). However, these women's disdain for formal work outside the home, understood as a sign of being a good mother, surpassed any expectations; at this early stage, two women gave up work after giving birth and two others started to plan how to get fired from their jobs, hopefully getting monetary compensation after a year of planned absence, in which they would obtain several medical leaves that would make employers disappointed and reluctant to keep their contracts.

This need to 'stay with the baby' had no limits. An extreme case is that of Camila, who was hoping that her baby displayed some symptoms of reflux when she was born just so that she could postpone her return to work and stay with the baby for longer. Physicians in the public and private health systems – strong defendants of long-term breastfeeding and attachment – became important allies of these women. By making use of the well-known practice of medical leave for mothers in the case of 'serious illness of the child under a year of age',[23] as well as other leaves for depression, these informants were able to stay at home for at least one year (Murray 2011). Kelly and Ignacia's accounts show how the fight for leave legitimates them as good mothers.

> I told the doctor that I was working and that I didn't want to go back because I did not have anyone to leave the baby with. In the end, she herself told me 'okay, here is your medical leave'. I cried, I cried for real. She told me she would provide licences only until he is six months. The first ones were for bronchitis, and now for reflux.
>
> (Kelly, 30)

even in the public system I have been given a whole month of medical leave, but this will be over soon, because they are very strict now with leaves. I'll need a private one. I am now looking for a good paediatrician, one which will give me the next licences until he is one year old. I need a doctor that will allow me to stay longer with my son.

(Ignacia, 28)

These were typical narratives to reaffirm their sense of being good mothers, a sense in which staying with the baby during the first year is a moral duty.

In what follows I further explore what 'staying with the baby' means and what the main practices involve. I suggest that rooted ideals of motherhood in this context are reinforced and redefined together with expert-led, imported ideals of intensive mothering.

During the first year of their babies' lives, these mothers consolidated their fundamental role as nurturers and experts in the needs of every child. Primarily, they committed to maintaining physical proximity to the baby, and to staying alert to the baby's needs (conceived principally in terms of physiological and metabolic needs and the capacity to identify the baby's discomfort or sources of pain). These concerns differed from those of middle-class, university-trained informants, who were interested in developmental processes, stimulation and pedagogic practices, including sleeping arrangements from an early stage, in tune with pedagogical ideologies of motherhood observed in the middle-classes in the USA (Hays 1996; Weisner 1999; Hoffman 2000a) and elsewhere (O'Dougherty, this volume).[24] In line with policy makers' guidelines, medical mandates and Chilean high rates of breastfeeding – 97 per cent of mothers breastfeed and 60 per cent still breastfeed when the baby is twelve months old (Atalah 2006) – all informants attempted exclusive breastfeeding for six months, while one received a prescription of complementary formula milk because her baby was not gaining enough weight. All of them considered breastfeeding as central to their mothering discourses (see O'Dougherty, this volume, for a similar observation in Brazil), and were aware of its benefits: it is 'the best food for the baby', 'cheap' and 'helps with bonding'. In contrast to other contexts, in which breastfeeding is a contested practice (e.g. Faircloth, this volume), for these women breastfeeding consists mostly of a 'taken-for-granted', uncontested moral duty of the 'good mother', which happens also to be supported by physicians and the state under the ideals of nurturance and attachment as the most beneficial for the mother–infant dyad. By the end of the year, five informants were still breastfeeding, (which they viewed as a moment *'de regaloneo'* – 'for spoiling' – the baby and themselves) and used breastfeeding for calming the baby at night or during our meetings. As Melanie put it, 'this is a space just for the two of us, I don't want to give it up'.

These women found hardly any limits for physical proximity and cuddling with their babies, while relative co-sleeping (usually after breastfeeding) was also usual during the first year. Home routines and duties were performed while maintaining physical closeness with the child. Most mornings began with a session of TV-watching with the baby, in bed. Later, they performed housework and cooking, placing the baby in a strategic place where they could secure eye contact.[25] For example, Kelly and Camila placed the baby in the centre of the living room in a baby chair or baby walker. Rocío placed the baby in a corner where she could have a panoramic view of the house's rooms. For these women, their babies are their main company during the day, so even if they were not committed to having verbal communication with the baby, they often talked to them and they naturally included the baby in conversations, either speaking as if they were the baby – for example, saying 'hello' or 'thanks for visiting' – or addressing them as adults, while they rarely questioned their understanding capacity or accommodated speech (Snow 1990).

Further important activities, such as family visiting and paediatric health checkups, are also constitutive of this year devoted to 'staying with the baby'. These women have a routine of visiting and receiving visits from extended family – principally from those living nearby – and, to a lesser extent, from a limited number of friends, in the privacy of their households. For example, Kelly's father visited her every other day after work to have tea with his grandsons and daughter. Camila visited her mother every Wednesday before and after church service. Valentina stayed at her mother's place every time her husband worked the night shift. Ignacia welcomed her younger teenage sisters most afternoons after school. The strength of these family ties stands in contrast with the avoidance of the street, neighbours and other acquaintances, all of whom are kept outside of the social picture and considered as potentially dangerous.[26]

Just as they had during their pregnancies, they combined the monthly '*control del niño sano*' – 'healthy child checkups' – in the public system with private practice appointments, also on a monthly basis, for at least the first few months. They argued that in the public system children are not examined thoroughly and that it is only in private practice that they find the time, patience and information they require. Dafne claimed: 'I didn't like the public check-up; they only weighed and measured her. That was it. The private doctor examined in detail: eyes, ears and tonsils'. The comfort of private practice in this case fulfils the mothers' concern with examining and scanning the baby. They want to receive advice and supportive validation of their skills and they find this ally in the paediatrician. They also attend public checkups under the motto 'the more the better' (especially now that they receive books and CDs and are offered breast-feeding and massaging workshops through ChCC). They silently contrast the information they receive in the two systems, twice every month. They like to hear that their baby is fine and that they are doing a good job.

These women committed to a kind of intensive mothering during the first year that, in some aspects, resembles the international mandates of intensive mothering, specifically attachment mothering practices (Faircloth this volume), while contrasting with other tendencies in which extreme closeness is rejected (e.g. Suizzo 2004 for the French case; LeVine and Norman 2001 for the US). Most of these first-year practices are 'taken-for-granted' normative imperatives of the 'good mother'. Reflexivity and creativeness are much more focused on other kinds of important duties of the 'good mother', such as the combination of private and public medical care and advice.[27]

These mothers' sense of 'staying with the baby' follows a rather different path in the history of parenting than that usually described within the feminist literature (Badinter 1982; Ariès 1962), which claims that intensive parenting and child-centredness comprise a relatively recent ideology taking place in Western contexts, such as the UK and France (Kukla 2008; Faircloth 2010, this volume) or the USA (Hays 1996). These women's rooted parenting practices and their current challenges, and even contradictions, require contextualization within a specific understanding of the maternal and child's selves. It is from there that one can understand their negotiations in changing scenarios.

Intensive mothering in context

Crucial differences between tendencies in international models of intensive parenting and the approach of the women in this study reside in women's aims, the meaning of the mother–child relationship, and the sense of what it means to be a good mother. The women discussed in this chapter work for a close relationship with their child for life, contrasting with the kind of parenting culture aimed at preparing parents and children for a child's maturity at age eighteen. This intensive mother–child relationship reflects the intersection of long-term mothering priorities that involve child-centredness, kinship and religion, usually associated with *marianismo*, with more recent expert-led advice on mothering, political economy, and recent changes to Chilean socio-demographic structure. This intersection also involves these women's social mobility aspirations, which are often contradictory with their mothering practices. I reflect upon these intersections and their contradiction with social mobility aspirations by way of conclusion.

Rather than just devotion to the Virgin Mary, *marianismo* consists of a cult to feminine spiritual and moral superiority, one which, in turn, leads to abnegation or 'the infinite capacity of sacrifice and humility' (Paz 1959; Stevens 1977; Morandé 1984; Montecino 2010). Mothers not only embody the tender, nurturing, self-sacrificial being that devotes her love (and life) to children in ways that have been the focus for feminist critique (e.g. Warner 1985; Göknar this volume), they are also considered pillars of society (culture); men (for reasons that exceed the scope of this chapter) have remained external, peripheral, even ephemeral (nature) (Montecino 2010). In this picture, womanhood is one with motherhood, while manhood relates to childhood (Montecino 2010: 3). It is a context in which the ideology of the stable nuclear family of the male breadwinner and the soft housewife is limited mostly to the privileged classes. In this context, acknowledging the existence of the baby is synonymous with incomparable fulfilment, to the extent of 'enchantment' – a miracle that consecrates the child and mother. This resembles Mayblin's (2012) point regarding two possible ways of understanding and experiencing mother's love within Western ontology. According to Mayblin (2012) within Christian ontology mother's love may operate mainly in two ways. Some societies or groups[28] approach maternal love as metaphorical, that is, as somehow 'analogous' to divine love. Other groups, including her informants in a Catholic town in Northern Brazil – and certainly this group of women in Santiago de Chile – perceive mother's love as a metonymical conduit of divine grace, one that even overcomes the nature–culture dichotomy (Mayblin 2012).

For these women self-identification with motherhood at an early stage is expectable, while the awareness of this lifelong, inalienable bond makes all sacrifices for the baby worthwhile. Its achievement takes place by means of the objectification of this needy subject capable of expressing demands requiring a devotee through practice. The aid of a range of tools (including the already mentioned medical appointments and sonograms, among several others) are constitutive to such recognition.

The prioritization of the mother–child relationship is clear in these women's discourses and practices from an early stage. As Melanie put it, the child 'is the only thing that really belongs to you'. Certainly, a lifetime of material scarcity and family conflicts influenced her scepticism towards possessions and other people. This defensive attitude includes her partner: 'now that I have the girl he can pack up and leave if he ever wants to'. She has somehow secured (divine) grace and company for life through motherhood, making every effort worthwhile. Furthermore, every woman in this group mentioned their preference for baby girls at some point in the research. They believed girls to be more 'vulnerable', 'dependent' and more likely to become a friend in the long term. 'I like girls better because they are more attached to their mothers than boys. Boys are too independent and difficult to handle' (Valentina). Rocío (aged thirty-two) constantly highlighted the fact that her daughter is needier and more pampered than her son: 'she is *fundida* (pampered) ... I think all girls are like that'.[29]

The *marianismo* thesis illuminates the concrete stories in which these women negotiate[30] 'intensive mothering' standards. Further understanding of the situation that these women confront, however, requires consideration of the encounter between this frame for understanding motherhood, their sense of the child's self and body, and their social and economic aspirations: a mix that seems to result in a dangerous short-circuit along the lines of social reproduction.

These women commit to early mothering under the imperatives of physical presence, in line with a fragility that both empowers the mother – as the one able to protect and provide the baby with all the necessary care – and threatens her with the prospect of what may happen to her child in her absence. They consider the child as not only vulnerable but porous, liable to be affected by anything he or she is exposed to in a way that is more akin to magic contagion than developmental cognitive processes; mixing with strangers beyond the front door or risking a unknown individuals' involvement in child rearing may be disastrous. By the same token, these women value a crafted or engineered exposure of the child to what they believe to be the positive qualities of a nice neighbourhood, a 'quality school' or a private practice doctor.

At this early stage in mothering, the porosity attributed to the child and the corresponding responsibility of the mother regarding the orchestration of exposure in the long term intersects dramatically a neoliberal logic of purchase (of such exposure), which is also constitutive of these women's dreams of social mobility and 'better opportunities'. Paradoxically, these women's intensive mothering style and sense of child-centredness may undermine their very goal of social mobility that is constitutive of their mothering project.

At the beginning of this chapter I suggested that these women have experienced at least a slight improvement in their socio-economic situation. They also envision social mobility and their children to 'be more than myself' (*que sean más que uno*), as an attainable goal achieved by means of traversing what once were rigid class and symbolic boundaries. To raise children who will 'be more' than themselves is as important in their self-definition as good mothers as their aims of company and mutual dependency for life. Unlike the middle-class mothers involved in this research, these women's reflexivity regarding the idea of the good mother centres on their social mobility goals, while the mandates of 'new' intensive mothering – specifically attachment mothering – come somehow naturally to them. The specific efforts encouraged by experts inspired by attachment theories, including long-term breastfeeding and co-presence, are certainly welcome as easily attainable goals that reinforce these women's self-understanding as good mothers. However, the crucial contradictions and difficulties they confront are of a different kind. It is unclear, for example, how these women will negotiate the dual exigencies of staying with their children while also generating income that fulfils challenging economic expectations. This is a puzzle that merits further research into the experience of mothering in this context. The configuration of the sources of satisfaction and frustration in the longer term remains uncertain.

Notes

1 FONDECYT Iniciación en Investigación (2010–2013) 'Motherhood and Early Childhood in Chile Today: A Study of Mother–Infant Dyads from an Ethnographic Perspective' No. 11100432. Funded by Consejo Nacional de Ciencia y Tecnología CONICYT.

2 I also interviewed several professionals involved in the process, including gynecologists, midwives, pediatricians and nursery professionals working in public and private practice.

3 Segregation in Santiago follows the national trend. For example, in Chile over 50 per cent of couples share the same educational level, compared to 30 per cent of couples in the UK (Valenzuela and Duryea 2011). Having a university degree instantly situates a person in the richest 20 per cent of the population (Beyer 2000).

4 The only exceptions to these social mobility aspirations came in the case of two upper-middle-class informants.

5 The income measurement of poverty in Chile marks 65,000 pesos (US$130) per person per month as the limit between poor and non-poor.

6 They belong to the second and third income quintile (INE 2008).

7 In Chile, *allegamiento* is the name given to the housing arrangement in which a nuclear family (*allegados*) share the same home with a host family, usually one of the couple's parents.

8 Between 2004 and 2005 alone, household indebtedness increased by 21 per cent, a startling amount considering that household income increased by only 9 per cent during this period (Banco Central de Chile 2005: 38) and that income gaps have decreased only very slightly, in a country with a huge income gap (OECD 2011).

9 The students' movement and riots during 2011 show Chilean citizens' awareness of old and new social inequalities.

10 Benefits include money, healthcare, a family allowance and support in being reincorporated into the workforce through a national employment office and training scholarships.

11 Chilean governments have a long history of involvement in parenting, traditionally focused specifically on the actions leading to the reduction of infant mortality (Jiménez 2009) and health and nurturing improvement (Chile Crece Contigo 2010).

12 The beginning of life refers here to life in the womb, although the point during the gestation period of gestation at which life is posited to begin is not specified.

13 The programme is coordinated by the ministry of Social Development, and coordinates the work of the Ministries of Health, Education, Work, Women's National Service and Councils.

14 For example, Uruguay has recently launched a programme 'Uruguay Crece Contigo'.

15 Policies aiming at the encouragement of women's participation in the workforce (another serious problem for the overcoming of social inequality) have never been as popular. The building and coordination of public and private daycare and kindergarten appear to be a rather partial solution for participation in the workforce for women who argue strongly that they 'do not have anyone to leave the child with' in surveys.

16 The Chilean health system has developed a system of co-payment in which patients may attend private practice paying a ten-dollar fee for a medical appointment.

17 Melanie's and other women's statements resemble the critiques of public healthcare in other contexts (e.g. Lazarus 1994 in the USA) in which women are critical of the public system's fragmentation and desire a 'continuity of treatment' with one professional with whom they could hopefully develop a personal relationship.

18 Han (2011) develops a similar argument of anticipation of prosperity through debt by low-income families in Santiago.

19 This bad reputation has been highlighted with the recent proliferation of private clinics committed to this 'market'. In their advertising campaigns, happier and better looking (whiter) women give birth in an aseptic and friendlier environment where women may feel proud to welcome visits to the newly born. These clinics and the kind of delivery they offer place these women at the edge of different fantasies of womanhood, femininity and, metonymically, of the newborn baby.

20 See website www.crececontigo.gob.cl/categoria/desarrollo-infantil/gestacion.

21 See Georges 1996, Gammeltoft 2007 and Taylor 2008 for comparative accounts on the use of sonograms in different countries.

22 'Regaloneado', 'fundido' do not have a negative connotation. In Santiago, the word 'fundido' is common among lower and some lower-middle-class contexts, but not used in middle and upper-middle-class contexts.

23 www.dt.gob.cl/consultas/1613/w3-article-60111.html.

24 O'Dougherty (this volume) reminds us of the class differences in mothering in Latin-American countries.

25 Dafne said 'Maite [her three-month-old baby] is always looking at me, checking out whether I'm with her or not'. She wants to highlight how 'awake' ('despierta') her baby is, meaning smart and alert, yet her agency focuses specifically on the mother.

26 These divisions have been widely acknowledged in Latin American countries. For example, Da Matta (1985) in the Brazilian distinction between house and street, and Valenzuela and Cousiño (2000) who analyse the Chilean case using the sociological analysis of 'trust'. See also Berry, this volume.

27 Other important activities consisted of starting a savings plan (at home or in a bank), with paid education for their children in mind.

28 Mayblin refers to the implications of the understanding of god mainly as a divine
    absence creator and to human–divine continuation within the world.
29 Further research should address the situation of isolation that these claims evoke.
30 It does not suffice for an understanding of how mothering and class interweave.

Bibliography

Acosta, E., Perticara, M. and Ramos, C., 2007. *Oferta laboral Femenina y Cuidado Infan-
    til*. Santiago: Banco Interamericano de Desarrollo.
Ariès, P., 1962. *Centuries of Childhood*. New York: Vintage Books.
Atalah, E., 2006. Situación actual de la lactancia en Chile. *Medwave*, 6(5), online, availa-
    ble   at: www.mednet.cl/link.cgi/Medwave/Cursos/pediatraynutricion06/1/   3528
    [accessed 25 January 2012].
Badinter, E., 1982. *The Myth of Motherhood: An Historical View of the Maternal Instinct*.
    London: Souvenir Press.
Banco Central de Chile, 2005. *Informe de Estabilidad Financiera, Segundo Semestre
    2005*. Santiago.
Beyer, H. 2000. Educación y desigualdad de ingresos: Una nueva mirada. *Centro de Estu-
    dios Públicos*, 77, pp. 97–130.
Bourdieu, P., 1977. *Outline of a Theory of Practice*. Cambridge: Cambridge University
    Press.
Bowlby, J., 1969. *Attachment*. London: Hogarth Press.
Bowlby, J., 1973. *Separation: Anxiety and Anger*. London: Hogarth Press.
Bowlby, J., 1980. *Loss: Sadness & Depression*. London: Hogarth Press.
Chile Crece Contigo, 2010. ¿Qué es el sistema Chile Crece Contigo? Online, available at:
    www.crececontigo.cl [accessed 28 February 2012].
Da Matta, R., 1985. *A Casa e a Rua*. São Paulo: Editora Brasiliense.
Faircloth, C., 2010. 'If they want to risk the health and wellbeing of their child, that's up
    to them': Long-term breastfeeding, risk and maternal identity. *Health, Risk and Society*,
    12(4), pp. 357–367.
Furedi, F., 2008. *Paranoid Parenting: Why Ignoring the Experts May be Best for your
    Child*. 3rd ed. London: Continuum.
Gammeltoft, T., 2007. Sonography and sociality: obstetrical ultrasound imaging in urban
    Vietnam. *Medical Anthropology Quarterly*, 21(2), pp. 133–153.
Georges, E., 1996. Fetal ultrasound imaging and the production of authoritative know-
    ledge in Greece. *Medical Anthropology Quarterly*, 10(2), pp. 157–175.
Godoy, M. and Reynaldos, C., 1984. *Una aproximación psicológica a la maternidad en
    estrato social bajo*. Licenciate Thesis. Santiago: Pontificia Universidad Católica de
    Chile.
Han, C., 2011. Symptoms of Another Life: Time, Possibilities, and Domestic Relations in
    Chile's Credit Economy. *Cultural Antropology*, 26(1), 7–32.
Hays, S., 1996. *The Cultural Contradictions of Motherhood*. London: Yale University
    Press.
Hoffman, D., 2000a. Childhood ideology in the United States: a comparative cultural
    view. *International Review of Education*, 49(1–2), pp. 191–211.
Hoffman, D., 2000b. Pedagogies of the self in American and Japanese early childhood
    education: A critical conceptual analysis. *The Elementary School Journal*, 101(2),
    pp. 193–208.
INE, 2008. *Resultados de encuesta de presupuestos familiares*. Santiago: INE.

Jiménez, J., 2009. *Angelitos Salvados*. Santiago: Uqbar Editores.

Kukla, R., 2008. Measuring mothering. *International Journal of Feminist Approaches to Bioethics*, 1(1), pp. 67–90.

Latour, B., 1993. *We Have Never Been Modern*. Cambridge: Harvard University Press.

Lazarus, E., 1994. What do women want? Issues of choice, control, and class in pregnancy and childbirth. *Medical Anthropology Quarterly*, 8(1), pp. 25–46.

Lehmann, C., 2003. Mujer, Trabajo y Familia: Realidad, Percepciones y Desafíos. *Puntos de Referencia*, 269. Santiago: Centro de Estudios Públicos.

LeVine, R. and Norman, K., 2001. The infant's acquisition of culture: early attachment re-examined from an anthropological perspective. In: C.C. Moore and H.F. Mathews (eds) *The Psychology of Cultural Experience*. New York: Cambridge University Press.

Mattelart, A. and Mattelart, M., 1968. *La Mujer Chilena en una Nueva Sociedad. Un Estudio Exploratorio Acerca de la Situación e Imagen de la Mujer en Chile*. Santiago: Editorial Pacífico.

Mayblin, M., 2012. The madness of mothers: agape Love and the maternal myth in northeast Brazil. *American Anthropologist*, 114(2), pp. 240–252.

Miller, D., 1987. *Material Culture and Mass Consumption*. Oxford: Blackwell.

Miller, D., 1997. How infants grow mothers in North London. *Theory Culture and Society*, 14(4), pp. 67–88.

Montecino, S., 2010. *Madres y Huachos. Alegorías del Mestizaje Chileno*. 5th ed. Santiago: Catalonia.

Morandé, P., 1984. *Cultura y Modernización en América Latina: Ensayo Sociológico Acerca de la Crisis del Desarrollismo y de su Superación*. Santiago: Universidad Católica de Chile.

Moulian, T., 1998. *El Consumo me Consume*. Santiago: LOM.

Murray, M., 2011. Negotiating with paediatricians in times of contradictory authoritative knowledge: early mothering and 'fraudulent' health licences in Chile. In: *Symposium Health Behaviours, Therapy Culture and Criticism, Intervention*. Cambridge, 28 June.

Murray, M. 2012. Childbirth in Santiago de Chile: stratification, intervention and child centeredness. *Medical Anthropology Quarterly*, 26(3), pp. 319–337.

OECD, 2011. *Growing Income Inequality in OECD Countries: What Drives it and How Can Policy Tackle it?* PDF available online at: www.oecd.org/dataoecd/32/20/47723414.pdf [accessed 28 February 2012].

OECD and World Bank, 2009. *Tertiary Education in Chile: Reviews of National Policies for Education*. PDF available online at: https://files.nyu.edu/ft237/ public/OECD09_tertiary_education_chile.pdf [accessed 1 March 2012].

Paz, O., 1959. *El laberinto de la soledad*. México: FCE.

PNUD, 2010. *Reducción de la pobreza en Chile* [online]. Santiago: PNUD. Available at: www.pnud.cl/areas/ReduccionPobreza/datos-pobreza-en-Chile.asp [accessed 28 February 2012].

Raeff, C., 2010. Independence and interdependence in children's developmental experiences. *Child Development Perspectives*, 4(1), pp. 31–36.

Ragoné, H. and Twine, F.W., 2000. Ideologies and technologies of motherhood: race, class, sexuality, nationalism. London: Routledge.

Silva, V. and Molina, H., 2010. *Cuatro años creciendo juntos. Memoria de la Instalación del Sistema de Protección Integral a la Infancia Chile Crece Contigo 2006–2010*. Santiago: Chile Crece Contigo. PDF available online at: http://cesfamsi.files.wordpress.com/2010/04/memoria-chile-crece-contigo.pdf [accessed 25 June 2012].

Snow, C., 1990. The language of the mother–child relationship. In M. Woodhead, R. Carr and P. Light (eds) *Becoming a Person: Child Development in Social Context, Vol 1.* London: Routledge.

Stevens, E., 1977. Marianismo: La otra cara del machismo en Latino-América. In A. Pescatelo (ed.) *Hembra y macho en Latinoamérica: Ensayos.* México: Diana.

Suizzo, M.A., 2004. Mother–child relationship in France: balancing autonomy and affiliation in everyday interactions. *Ethos*, 32(3), pp. 293–323.

Taylor, J., 2008. *The Public Life of the Fetal Sonogram: Techology, Consumption and the Politics of Reproduction.* New Brunswick, NJ: Rutgers University Press.

Torche, F. and Wormald, G., 2004. *Estratificación y movilidad social en Chile: entre la adscripción y el logro.* Santiago: CEPAL.

Unicef, 2001. *Estado mundial de la infancia. Primera infancia.* New York: Unicef. PDF available online at: www.unicef.org/spanish/publications/files/pub_sowc01_sp.pdf [accessed 25 January 2012].

Valenzuela, E. and Cousiño, C., 2000. Sociabilidad y asociatividad. *Revista Centro de Estudios Públicos, 77.* Online, available at: www.cepchile.cl/dms/lang_1/ doc_1220.html [accessed 25 January 2012].

Valenzuela, J. and Duryea, S., 2011. Examinando la prominente posición de Chile a nivel mundial en cuanto a desigualdad de ingresos: comparaciones regionales. *Estudios de Economía,* 38(1), pp. 259–293.

Wall, G., 2010. Mothers' experiences with intensive parenting and brain development discourse. *Women's Studies International Forum*, 33(3), pp. 253–263.

Warner, M., 1985. *Alone of all her Sex: The Myth and the Cult of the Virgin Mary.* London: Picador.

Weisner, T., 1999. Values that matter. *Anthropology Newletter* 40(5), pp. 1–5.

Part IV
Parenting and/as identity

10 *"Spanish*[1] people don't know how to rear their children!"

Dominican women's resistance to intensive mothering in Madrid

Livia Jiménez Sedano

Introduction

> ALTAGRACIA[2] (27,[3] THREE CHILDREN) "There? I say to my neighbour, I say 'keep an eye on the child, I'll be back in a moment', maybe you go out in the morning, and you say 'keep an eye on him' and you come back at night (…) it's easy-going in Santo Domingo (…) here it's too much work, too much work."

Although the ideology of intensive parenting has been established in recent decades as the appropriate model for parenting by some scholars (Hays 1996) and has become the pattern of reference for social intervention professionals, this does not mean that it has been automatically accepted without challenges to its authority. This chapter shows an example of resistance: a group of mothers who emigrated from the Dominican Republic to Spain and now live in Madrid. Here I describe how they resist the ideology of intensive parenting when it is imposed by social workers and a certain sector of society. Instead of accepting it, these women transform the experts' picture of "good intensive parenting vs. bad neglectful parenting" into another picture based on ethnicity: "*Spanish* mothering vs. *Dominican* mothering." Through creating this ethnic scenario, they reverse their inferior position so that the ignorant, abusive, and neglectful "bad mothers" are the *Spanish* women who think that intensive parenting is the best way for rearing children; and the "good mothers," full of wisdom, skills, and proper maternal feelings, are themselves, the self-labeled *Dominicans*. Although they do not use the term "intensive parenting," the characteristics ascribed to *Spanish* mothering are very close to those that Hays uses to define the concept: child-centeredness, expensive in time, energy and money, and expert-guided (Hays 1996).

I must say here that I do not defend the idea that these models (*Spanish* parenting style and *Dominican* parenting style) exist as such, as there is a great variety of cultural parenting practices in both countries, and even among my informants. What I will do in this text is focus on the women who show open resistance to the intensive parenting ideology. I will reproduce and analyze the emic discourse of ethnic difference through which these informants make sense of their conflictive experience of mothering in a new context. From the theoretical point of view, ethnicity is understood here as a dynamic process of selfing and othering (Barth 1976) that is contextual (Okamura 1981; Eriksen 1991; Díaz de Rada 2007), created in concrete situations of practice (Bentley 1987; Díaz de Rada 2007), and multidimensional (Jenkins 1994; Díaz de Rada 2007).

The philosophy of intensive parenting has spread from the US and the UK, but it has been appropriated and adapted in different ways in each context (see Faircloth, introduction to this book). In order to understand the ethnographic context of this chapter, it is necessary to say a few words about kinship ideologies in Spain from a historical point of view. The Catholic Church has had a deep influence on the dominant model of "a good mother" and her duties (see Göknar's chapter to compare the role of religion in a Muslim context). A basic reference model for a mother in Catholic countries is the image of the Virgin Mary and the baby (see Murray in this volume for the case of Chile). Religious institutions were an important centre of production of legitimate ideas about mothering, linking it to sacrifice. But they were not the only ones. During the civil war and post-war period in Spain, under Franco's dictatorship, this set of ideas based on religion and women's self-sacrifice was codified and transmitted by the "Sección Femenina," an expert institution that became very important during Franco's dictatorship for producing and legitimizing gender roles. It defined womanhood and associated it with purity and a specific way of mothering (Roca 1996). Later on, when psychological theories about intensive parenting reached Spain in the 1970s, they fit well with these previous ideologies. The model of the Virgin Mary, the perfect self-sacrificing mother, and the picture of God as a baby that must be adored made child-centered theories easy to accept. It could be said[4] that this mix of religious and political elements shaped the base of "common sense" parenting that spread preferentially, although not exclusively, among the conservative high-middle class in Spain. Psychologists and social workers developed it further and claimed that this kind of parenting was scientifically legitimate. Probably the later spread of this intensive parenting ideology in the middle classes in Spain is related to economic growth (as in the case of Chile analyzed by Murray): it led to improvements in standards of living and the relatively fast process of enrichment produced changes in the reproductive model (fewer children and a bigger investment in each one).

In contrast, in the Dominican Republic, the economic situation is weaker and this intensive parenting ideology is not so popular in the broad working class sectors. Most migration projects from the Dominican Republic to Spain are headed by women (Gregorio 1998). The majority of my informants are working-class women who got their first job in Madrid as domestic workers. In the imaginary of these people, domestic workers are the extremely poor women from Haiti, who are labeled *Blacks*. In contrast, they label themselves as *Whites* or other mixed categories (*Rubio oscuro, Trigueño*, etc.) (see Gregorio 1998). In this way, becoming immigrants in Spain implies two processes of changing position in society: their class position gets lower and the racial category assigned shifts from *White* (or categories of mixes) to *Black*, in a context where most people have lighter skin than theirs. This situation, the legal barriers to getting a better job, and the feeling of rejection (perception of racism) by certain sectors of society, makes them feel distant from what they call *Spaniards*.

Moreover, they find it very hard to play their role as mothers in the new context: they see that most mothers in the city of Madrid rear their children on their own, instead of creating the care-giving networks they were used to in the Dominican Republic. In addition, their shared cultural ways of correcting and punishing children become labeled as mistreatment by social workers so that they are never free of suspicion (see the chapter by Berry for a discussion on how structural violence is obscured by blaming immigrant parents). All these factors mixed together constitute the context in which they produce the shared discourse about *Spanish* mothering and *Dominican* mothering analyzed in this text. The different processes of othering in the field of parenting in order to create social distinction ("we" parent/mother better than "they" do) are not always based on ethnic categories: examples for comparison can be found in the chapters authored by Jensen, Edwards and Gillies, Hoffman, Berry, and Hinton *et al.*

Methodology

The empirical materials provided are part of the ethnographic work carried out for my dissertation (Jiménez Sedano 2011). The research was based mainly on participant observation, interviews, life stories, discussion groups, analysis of documents, and statistical data. From 2002 to 2007, I conducted fieldwork in two ethnographic settings, one in Madrid and one in Andalusia. Here I focus on the case of Madrid, where many families with parents from the Dominican Republic live. I covered five neighborhoods in different parts of Madrid and I resided for some months in the homes of two of the families, joined them for family meetings, religious celebrations, and parties, and played with the children in the streets. I also went to cafes, bars, *Dominican* discos, *Dominican* beauty shops, and other places of socialization. I should say that I was labeled as a *White Spanish* woman, so they tried to explain their cultural patterns of child socialization to me by comparing them to what they thought was familiar to me: the *Spanish* way of socializing children in the family.

Child-centered *Spanish* mothering vs. adult-centered *Dominican* mothering

When I started doing fieldwork with my informants from the Dominican Republic, one of the things that surprised me the most was how unimportant children seemed to be in their everyday life. This perception was the product of my own socialization in a middle-class family in Spain, with a mother who is a specialist in child psychology, and of my own studies in educational psychology. As an anthropologist, I was ready to see cultural patterns of child-rearing that were different from my own experience, but I had a real culture shock that I did not expect. As an example, I will give part of the description of a *picapollo*[5] bar and the presence of children there:

The bar is well lit, small and with big windows (…). As we arrive (around 17:00 PM), people start asking for alcoholic drinks. (…) They all drink. The music is *bachata*[6] at a low volume. Some of them dance every once in a while. (…) Most of the children are playing outside the bar. We can see some of them through the window, but some keep out of sight. The small children are also roaming around, unwatched by their parents or by any adult. Some babies circulate from the arms of one to another. The barman serves hot feeding bottles. I see a baby who almost falls down the stairs to the toilet. Nobody was watching him. I see a woman sitting by the bar, drinking a beer with one hand, giving milk to her baby with the other, and flirting with a man beside her (…). As times goes on and it gets dark, the atmosphere changes. Some women enter the *picapollo* pushing baby carriages and they leave them at the entrance with the babies inside. Then they go to drink, dance, and flirt with the men. There is a baby sitting in his stroller crying but nobody cares. (…) I see small heads running through the knees of drunk men.

(Fieldwork diary)

I was shocked by the way these people were mixing things that, from my own experience of socialization, should be separated (see the seminal work by Mary Douglas on purity and the symbolic construction of space, 2007 [1927]). On one hand, the sphere of socialization at night in clubs and discos, with alcohol and sex-charged interactions; on the other, that of women playing their role of mothers, at home, keeping quiet to let the baby sleep, watching over the baby and attending to her or his needs, protecting him or her from any risk from the outside world (see Layne and Murray in this volume for contrasting ethnographic cases and analyses). That night I could not help thinking that if a social worker turned up, she would not know where to start. But the scene was not one of an isolated woman doing something at home that would be labeled neglectful by an expert (see Edwards and Gillies' chapter for a discussion about the changes in the concept of neglectful and over-protective mothering from a historical perspective for the case of UK). Instead, there was a whole social atmosphere where that was considered proper behaviour. Children were not the main focus of attention for their parents; they were simply there; where parents wanted to socialize with other adults, children had to adapt to the environment as secondary actors. For these women, their social life did not suffer dramatic changes after having children, unlike the cases of post-partum depression analyzed by O'Dougherty in this volume. It took me some time to break through the initial feeling of moral suspicion and an automatic tendency to protect the children that I regarded as unprotected, but I finally got used to it and considered it normal. There was a whole world to discover beyond the mentality of intensive parenting in which I lived.

Nevertheless, discourses and practices were not homogeneous among my informants. For example, that night at the *picapollo* I was sitting beside Gladis (28, three children). When the atmosphere started changing as described above, she said to me in a low voice: "Can you see this? This is what I don't like, now I don't think this is a proper place for children, with people drinking too much, and see all those baby carriages left by the door." A few minutes later she left the place with her children and went back home. Another example is Laura (29, three children), who lived in the same neighbourhood with her husband and children. She described herself as a Catholic woman who reared her children "from a Catholic point of view," and she rejected going to the *picapollos* or *Dominican discos* of the area. She thought that these were not good atmospheres for anyone based on moral religious arguments. It was quite clear that there was no one single way of *Dominican* mothering.

Another day, Gina (19, one child), one of my informants, had a baby and I went to visit her at the hospital with Ruby (35, one child), another friend of hers. Again, the situation was shocking for me: first, she had not received many visits, apart from her mother. Not even her sister had been there to see her and her new nephew. Having a baby was not such a big event. The situation had nothing to do with the picture I had seen so many times of all the family members around the mother and the child, adoring the baby in the hospital room. When we got there, Gina and Ruby spent most of the time talking about what had happened last night in the *Dominican Disco* they used to go to. Gina was upset because she had missed the party, as she was giving birth at that moment. They started talking about who was flirting with whom, who danced with whom, what they said, and which men were suspected of being unfaithful to their girlfriends and wives. The baby that was nursing at Gina's breast was not an important topic; they just exchanged a few words about how painful giving birth was and how difficult learning to breastfeed him was, before switching to a subject that was much more interesting for them: the events of the disco and the news about relations among the men and the women. A central issue in life for them was how to get a man and keep him by their side, and social information about new couples, break-ups, other women's strategies, and men's behavior was central to this. It was not only a matter of romanticism or gossip, but also a very important economic issue, as the economic support of a man (or some men) who was sexually interested in them was essential to supplement their poor and weak monthly income (see Jiménez Sedano 2011). Unlike the case described in Layne's chapter, this was a highly man-centered ideology: women invested a lot of time and energy in relations with men, they changed partners often, and children were used to it and learned how to stay in the background and not be bothersome. This phenomenon was interpreted as "non-structured families" by social workers, but actually it can be analyzed as a different way of structuring (Jiménez Sedano 2011).

The receiver *Spanish* child vs. the giver *Dominican* child

An important element to justify the idea of child-centeredness is that the child has a series of needs that have to be fulfilled in order to achieve a correct psychological development (Ochaita, 2004) (see also Murray and Faircloth in this volume for discussions of this idea). For this reason, all parenting practices are focused on these needs assigned to the child: her/his basic role as a child is that of receiving. The receiver child has no responsibility over others because s/he does not yet have the capacity to take care of him/herself, and adults must take care of the child until s/he has acquired these abilities. The child just has to "learn," which is understood as going to school and acquiring formal academic learning and obeying his/her parents. S/he is not supposed to satisfy the needs of adults or other members of the family.

In contrast, in some contexts children are considered to be able to do activities which are important for the social group: this is the giver child. From when they are very young, they have economic responsibilities. For example, all of my informants agreed that in the Dominican Republic girls from around six or seven years old were expected to start helping in reproductive tasks such as cooking, cleaning, and taking care of their younger siblings. These children are supposed to be able to think about others' needs. In the context of this ideology, if they are not pushed to do it, they will grow up selfish and they will be unable to socialize properly. They are responsible for others during childhood and for the future:

> CANDELA (42, THREE CHILDREN) "In my country children are ... for our parents we are like their investment; they have children so that we will take care of them when they grow older. That's it, children are an investment."

But children socialized in Madrid lacked the wider social context that legitimized the idea of the giver child. For example, Candela's children sometimes played the role of receiver children that they had seen at their friends' homes. Candela interpreted this as selfishness and it made her angry. She did not want to play the role of servant mother and feed this cultural model that was strange for her.

> After shopping in the supermarket with her two younger children, Raquel (eight) and Leo (ten), Candela puts everything in order in the kitchen. Leo says: "Mama, give me the orange juice cartons!" and then Raquel adds: "No, Mama, give them to me, I want orange juice too!" Candela gets angry: "You know these cartons of orange juice are the only thing I buy for myself and I take them for work! You know I buy nothing for me, everything is for you, but still you want them! You are worse than the children of the spider, who eat her after they are born."

> (Fieldwork diary)

Resource-consuming *Spanish* mothering vs. low-demand *Dominican* mothering

The conception of the receiver child needs the figure of a servant mother, dedicated full-time to satisfy his/her needs. In the ideology of intensive mothering this is not regarded as being a slave or a servant of the child, but a responsible and conscious woman who takes care of her child in the appropriate way. The self-sacrificing mother is the most highly valued figure in this cultural conception. It leads us to another feature that defines intensive parenting: it requires a high investment of time, energy, and money (Hays 1996). The mother (sometimes the father, also) is considered the only actor responsible for the child. She must work on the attachment link and become the main reference for her child by spending long hours beside her/him. She should not delegate too much to other people to do that work or the attachment link will become weaker and it could harm the child psychologically. For this reason, it is important for the mother to hold the predominant position over all the other actors who may collaborate in socialization practices. This assumption has the consequence of individualistic mothering practices, something rather difficult to accomplish for women working outside the home. It leads to practical problems of organization (and guilty feelings for the women who have interiorized this ideology). In the case of my informants, the main worry was the practical problems.

Selfish *Spanish* mothering vs. shared *Dominican* mothering

> ALTAGRACIA (27, THREE CHILDREN) "There you have four, five, you leave them at the neighbor's house, at the aunt's house, at anyone's house (…) Fuck, here nobody gives you a hand. It is rather difficult, nobody can, here everybody's time is limited."

In contrast to the individualistic intensive mothering model, my informants explained that, according to their experience, in the Dominican Republic there was a feeling that children belong collectively to the community. The ways people organize things to take care of them are shared strategies based on trust. But there is a big difference between the ideal version expressed in an interview situation and real daily life. The rules are not so clear and they have to be negotiated again and again. On some occasions the practice of leaving children at a friend's house is interpreted as an abuse, to the point that it can break up friendships and trust networks.

Nevertheless, the women I worked with idealized this model of collective socialization of children, and they called it the *Dominican* way, based on solidarity and trust.[7] In this ethnic scenario, they contrasted it with the *Spanish* individualistic model, in which they claimed that mothers do not trust their relatives and neighbours and want to do it all alone. It is not only that they do not want to help other women, but also that they do not want to receive any help. When someone tries to help them, they get angry instead of being grateful. I heard many stories like this:

> MARIBEL (39, THREE CHILDREN) "I would not dare to correct a *Spanish* girl (…) because her mother does not think the same way a *Dominican* mother does. I mean, her mother is going to say: 'you shouldn't mess with my girl, that is none of your business, mess with your own children.'"

These kinds of stories feed the idea of an opposition between the good collectivism and solidarity of *Dominican* culture and the bad individualism and lack of solidarity of *Spanish* culture. My informants blamed *Spanish* mothers: they believed their mothering style was like this because they want it to be like this, not because they do not have many options. Instead of believing that all women have similar structural problems and confront similar challenges for mothering, they build a scenario in which things are difficult because *Spanish* women are selfish and ignorant, and have made it this way. In contrast, *Spanish* fathers are pictured as responsible, loving, and tender to children, compared to *Dominican* fathers (see O'Dougherty in this volume about the link between involved fathering and modernity).

> ELEONOR (26, TWO CHILDREN) (talking with other women in the *Dominican* beauty shop). "Do you know the only nice thing that you have here? Here the man helps, collaborates (...) I see that men here collaborate a lot, and they help take care of their children, they don't mind staying with their children, taking them so that the mother doesn't have to go and things like that, this is the most beautiful thing that you have here. But the Dominican man loves his children and collaborates, but not to the same extent."

Through this discourse, an individualistic society is imagined to be the product of *Spanish* women's wishes. In such a scenario, where caring women are not present in the neighbourhood, they are afraid of losing control over their children; as they see it, nobody would care for them if they relaxed control just for a moment. Altagracia told us a story in the beauty shop, a story I heard in many different versions: the legend of the child lost in the middle of the city.

> ALTAGRACIA (27, THREE CHILDREN) "Look, I have a friend who has a son, Juanito, two-and-a-half years old, he crossed all this avenue, the main one, he crossed all that, all that and even beyond, until he arrived in Maribel's neighbourhood, more or less, there where she lived before, and once there he crossed four avenues, the people saw him so small walking alone and nobody said a word and nobody asked (...) he entered a neighbour's house, and they took him, they called the police, and everything, everything ... and nobody asked, a small three-year-old child..."

This legend of the lost child subsumes the main assumptions about the difference between two cultural models of parenting: in the Dominican Republic, everybody would know the child and the family he belongs to, someone would take him and look for his relatives, and even if they did not know him, they would be surprised by seeing a child alone and they would ask.

The experience of mothering as an individual task and being totally responsible for the child in Madrid is stressful and frustrating for these women. For this reason, they tried to build new collective mothering networks in Madrid (see the chapter by Jaysane-Darr for another ethnographic example of collective mothering practices), but it was a hard task. In some cases they used Dominican-ness and appealed to ethnic solidarity, but not always. Let us see two different examples: the case of Ruby and the case of Candela.

Ruby Torrente (35, one child) was born in Cibao, a rural region of the Dominican Republic. When she arrived in Madrid, she was single and had no children. She started living with an elderly woman who hired her as a domestic worker, and some years later she got pregnant by a boyfriend who simply disappeared. Afterwards she changed jobs and apartments every few months, trying to support herself and her daughter. She developed dense social networks among her friends from the Dominican Republic who were living in Madrid. By that time, she no longer had any relatives living there. She met most of the people she knew in *picapollos*; in these places many people who considered themselves *Dominicans* tended to gather. She met Lupita Santos (40, three children), one of her best friends, in a *picapollo*. Lupita helped Ruby when, for example, she could not pay the rent and was evicted from her home with her little child, Anai (four years old at that time). Lupita allowed mother and daughter to stay in the flat she had rented, where she lived with her three children. She did not ask for money until Ruby was able to find a new job and had an income again. Some months later, Ruby rented a room in another friend's flat. It was difficult to raise Anai and work away from home, but she met other women with similar problems and they organized a solid network through which children circulated. Each participant would take care of the others' children at some time.

This is an example of the reconstruction of a network of solidarity based on shared ethnicity. In contrast, we will now observe the case of another informant who managed to extend her networks without appealing to shared ethnic symbols.

Candela (42, three children) got married in Santo Domingo when she was 20 years old. She had her first baby, a girl named Ingrid. After a few years, she decided to get a divorce because her husband was running around with other women. Afterwards she met Darío Pérez and agreed to marry him. They had a boy, Leo. Things were getting worse in the country and they decided to go to Spain. Candela thought of leaving the two children with her mother but the elderly woman replied that it would be a horrible, unnatural act to force such a separation. Finally, the four of them took the plane together. The beginning was harder than they had expected. They arrived in a small village in southern Spain and, as Candela recalled, "there were no other *Dominican* people but us" in the area. She met nobody else and could not leave her children with someone as she was used to doing in Santo Domingo.

> CANDELA: "I had no option other than socializing with *Spaniards*. What did you want me to do, to lock myself in at home and say: 'I am a *Dominican*, I am going to put some meringue on?'"[8]

Darío spent the whole day working away from home and she had to work in a restaurant from morning to evening. Ingrid and Leo were home alone for long hours. Candela worried that something might happen to them. She was also afraid that a social worker might find out what was happening and take her children away from her. She started making friends with her next-door neighbour. She knew about the situation and came every once in a while to take a look and check that the children were all right. This is the way she started to build new solidarity networks, although they were much weaker and less dense than the ones she had had in Santo Domingo. Later on she found a new job as a domestic worker in the home of the Gómez family. By that time, Candela was pregnant again. Her new boss and her friends decided to help her and paid a private doctor and everything she needed as the months went by. They also looked after Ingrid and Leo, and finally the Gómez family became the main domestic solidarity network for the Garcías.

> CANDELA: "My children have enjoyed travelling and everything, and I didn't have to pay at all, you (*Spaniards*) have taken my children everywhere. 'Leave the girl with me, I am going to take her to the beach.'"

Some years later Candela and Darío went to Madrid with their three children, because Candela's brother had found a place for them there. But the Gómez family was integrated as part of Candela's kinship network; they would come to Madrid often to visit them and the children would go to spend months at the beach every summer.

Planned *Spanish* mothering vs. natural *Dominican* mothering

A consequence of this investment of time and resources in Madrid was that my informants felt unable to have as many children as they considered normal. They had to make plans about mothering: number of children, economic investment in each one of them, possibilities for organizing time, etc.; something they were not used to doing to that extent. Mothering had to be rationalized, analyzed and carefully planned in Spain.

> ALTAGRACIA (27, THREE CHILDREN) "(If my children had been born in the Dominican Republic), I am sure I would have had one more, it depends on the woman, on each one, but I would have more and all of them running around in the streets, like little cats and little dogs that people have there, heaps of children (...). There children are had just for having them, here people think more about it."

All of my informants coincided in perceiving and contrasting a high birth rate for the Dominican Republic with a low one for Spain. The metaphor most frequently used for speaking about this was that of cats and dogs: according to this metaphor, *Dominican* people have children without any previous plan, and the limits are left to nature, just as happens with animals. With regard to this planning, intensive *Spanish* mothering was considered a movement away from nature. This poses an interesting contrast with the association of intensive mothering and going back to nature explored in the chapters by Faircloth, Dow, and De Graeve and Longman. This idea of *Dominicans* being closer to nature than *Spaniards* was considered by some of my informants as a criterion of social prestige, but for others it was the opposite, something wrong but proper for an "underdeveloped culture." In the first group we find Candela and her daughter Ingrid (18), both of whom believe that *Spanish* people have become denaturalized. In this sense, Candela told me what her mother said the first time she went to Madrid to visit them: "What *Spaniards* get with their hands, they destroy with their feet." It means that the advantages she saw in terms of technology and economic development (in contrast to her context of origin) had not been directed toward improving the quality of life. On the contrary, this development had been carried out at the expense of what she considered basic social needs: a big family with a man working and a woman at home. Instead, women were working outside the home and they had dramatically reduced the number of children, which astonished her.

Expert-guided *Spanish* mothering vs. context-guided *Dominican* mothering

Another important characteristic of intensive parenting is the need for expert advice: parents are supposed to lack essential knowledge that cannot be transmitted through domestic socialization processes (for example, from mothers to daughters). In this way, experts make themselves indispensable. Common sense and also traditional and institutionalized cultural practices are now under suspicion of being mistaken and potentially damaging for the correct development of the child, and experts become the legitimate agents to pass judgment over them. But most of my informants still found the practices they had learnt at home more appropriate and better than those they could hear from social workers and psychologists. They just picked up some tips from the advice of experts that could fit in better with their previous conceptions. But there were important points of conflict: for example, instead of seeing the child as a vulnerable and limited being full of needs, they saw it as a flexible being whose limitations depended on how far the adults pushed them. Instead of seeing a weak child as the starting point to work on, they saw it as the product of a certain kind of socialization. And they preferred tough children who were competent and able to get along in difficult situations. From their point of view, avoiding hard work produced delicate children who would be incompetent for a hard life.

Delicate *Spanish* children vs. tough *Dominican* children

The day of Raquel's First Communion, Raquel's best friend came. He was a *Spanish* boy called Mario (nine). Candela had to take care of him. Once Mario's father had left the boy with Candela, she said: "now I have to take care of you the whole day as if you were a very soft and delicate thing, just like your father does … I don't even do that with my children! Otherwise your father will kill me…"

In this sense, Candela was worried because she believed that their children were becoming too soft and weak because of the cultural influence of their *Spanish* friends. One day, Raquel came back from school crying because she had hit her head against a wall. Her mother said: "Come on, that's nothing, stop crying because that will make your head harder. In my country children don't cry about everything…". These kinds of expressions were frequent and very efficient for making them change their attitude (see De Graeve and Longman's chapter for a contrast with a different way of working the ethnicity of children in the case of adoptive parents). Raquel and Leo did not want to be regarded as "unauthentic *Dominicans*" (Jiménez Sedano 2011).

For this reason, Candela wanted to make sure that Raquel and Leo would become tough and strong. Another day, on the way back from the supermarket, Candela gave them heavy bags to carry, and they protested. She was upset: "You are always protesting about everything! You don't look like Dominican children, in my country they carry much heavier things!" Raquel started crying. As I noticed that my bags were lighter than theirs, I offered myself to take some of the children's bags, but Candela refused: "It doesn't matter if you are older and bigger, because your mother didn't make you get used to carrying weight when you were younger and now your body is soft. But they are still very young and they can still get used to it and become strong."

Weak *Spanish* mothering vs. strong *Dominican* mothering

Another important issue of conflict with social workers was the physical punishment of children. Most of my informants found that hitting children in order to correct them was necessary. According to them, showing a strict pedagogical style was something positive, a performance of real preoccupation for children. Although not all of my informants agreed that it was the best way to punish a child, all of them coincided in that it was "the normal thing there." Nevertheless, they established a difference between the kind of physical punishment they had received as children and the kind they displayed now as parents. The first kind was seen as "excessive" and they preferred a "moderate" version of it. Anyway, this "moderate" punishment was interpreted as "excessive" by Spanish institutions and experts, so that it was not permitted at all and it was not considered "normal."

> ELEONOR (26, TWO CHILDREN) (TALKING WITH OTHER WOMEN IN THE DOMINI-
> CAN BEAUTY SHOP) "I agree that you don't have to mistreat and hit your
> child because that is not correct, but there is a day that the child makes
> you … he can make you really angry and you may hit him bad, right? (…)
> In my country they take children and they hit them hard, they kill them,
> that's not the way, you see? (…) but here even for a little punishment they
> call it mistreatment. If you call him: "Pay attention!!!" when he is going

to cross the road, that is mistreatment here, because he may be damaged psychologically (general laughter in the beauty shop). In my country you scream at a child when he is going to do something wrong, and the child limits himself (…) and you have the same problem on TV, more there [in the USA] than here, every two minutes you have the ad of calling social services if your father or your mother screams at you or hits you."

These women considered that not hitting or screaming at children in these situations was neglectful. If the child did not have the opportunity to learn the limits, s/he would be exposed to danger (see Berry's chapter for another ethnographic example of this kind of reasoning). But there was another consequence that was even more dangerous: children would not learn to respect the elders and that might result in social disorder.

ELEONOR (TALKING WITH OTHER WOMEN IN THE DOMINICAN BEAUTY SHOP)
"I have seen young children saying to their mothers, 'asshole, stupid' … I would kill him. If a child of mine disrespects me on the street I would kill him (…) here children are the ones who rule and give orders to parents!"

From their point of view, the biggest problem in Spain was that the power structure was reversed: in the first place, administrative institutions had the power to impose a certain parenting style on parents; in second place, children were empowered by the possibility they were given to report their parents. My informants were sure that children were accustomed to insulting their mothers in Spain and that it happened because these women were afraid of being reported if they answered back. For this reason, they were not strong enough: they were weak, and their children were out of control. In this *Spanish* parenting style, children ruled over parents.

Conclusions

This chapter shows how intensive parenting can be translated in ethnic terms when it is experienced as an imposition in a context of unbalanced interethnic relations as a result of immigration. In this situation, the authority of experts is not taken for granted by immigrant mothers under suspicion; instead, they delegitimize the experts' discourse by interpreting it as a cultural conception of an ethnically strange other. The power of claiming a scientific basis and objectivity for intensive parenting theories is thus neutralized. The symbolic efficacy of experts' status is weakened, and these mothers empower themselves. By constructing and sharing discourses of ethnic contrast, they stress their right to socialize their children according to their own cultural conceptions.

But there is another set of power relations at the base of this conflict: the one between parents and children. These mothers' resistance is about the fear of losing control over their own children. It was very important for them to keep that balance of power in order to maintain social stability: they express that fear in ethnic terms, saying that *Spanish* mothers let children rule, and so *Spanish* society is upside down. The main problem for my informants was not being threatened by social workers, but being threatened by their own children, who were empowered by Spanish institutions. The ethnic other is, thus, regarded as a new actor that provokes an illegitimate disruption in the relation between parents and children. Mothering is not a unidirectional process, but part of a complex set of relations where the agency of different actors comes into play (the chapter by Hinton, *et al.* shows this very well). It might be interesting to create a reciprocal concept such as "childing": the ways of performing the role of child in relation to ways of performing the role of parent. Both processes (parenting and childing) shape one another and are shaped by one another, although in a context of an imbalance of power. In this way, we may make these tensions and the agency of children in parenting studies more visible.

Notes

1 Ethnonyms appear in italics in this text because they are considered emic categories, and in this way they will be differentiated from etic categories (Jiménez Sedano 2011).
2 All the names of informants are pseudonyms in order to protect their anonymity.
3 For every informant cited in this text, I will indicate first the age and then the number of children. For children, only the age is indicated.
4 A deep study of this issue is lacking for the Spanish context; some of the hypotheses I depict here were suggested by Professor Jordi Roca in informal conversations.
5 *Picapollos* are bars where drinks and foods labeled as "typically Dominican" are served.
6 A musical style that is very popular in Santo Domingo.
7 This invention of a paradise lost in which ideal parenting/mothering can be displayed can be compared to other cases explored in this book. In Edwards and Gilles' chapter, the paradise lost is situated in the past, distant in time. We can see something similar in Dow's chapter, where it is imagined as going back to an original state of healthy relations with nature; here, it is situated distant in space, projected in the place of origin.
8 A musical style that is very popular in Santo Domingo.

References

Barth, F. (ed.) 1976. "Introducción," *Los grupos étnicos y sus fronteras*. México: FCE.
Bentley, G. 1987. "Ethnicity and practice." *Comparative Studies in Society and History*. 33: 1, 169–175.
Díaz de Rada, A. 2007. "¿Dónde está la frontera? Prejuicios de campo y problemas de escala en la estructuración étnica en Saapmi." Madrid: CSIC.
Douglas, M. 2007 [1927]. *Pureza y peligro: un análisis de los conceptos de contaminación y tabú*. Buenos Aires: Nueva Visión.
Eriksen, T.H. 1991. "The cultural context of ethnic differences," *Man (N.S.)*, 26: 1, 127–144.
Gregorio, C. 1998. *Migración femenina. Su impacto en las relaciones de género*. Madrid: Narcea.
Hays, S. 1996. *The Cultural Contradictions of Motherhood*. New Haven/London: Yale University Press.

Jenkins, R. 1994. "Rethinking ethnicity, categorization and power," *Ethnic and Racial Studies*, 17: 2, 197–223.

Jiménez Sedano, L. 2011. *Los niños y niñas como creadores de estilos locales de etnicidad. Una etnografía basada en la comparación de dos contextos* (unpublished dissertation).

Ochaita, E. 2004. *Hacia una teoría de las necesidades infantiles y adolescentes. Necesidades y derechos en el marco de la Convención de Naciones Unidas sobre los derechos del niño*. Madrid: McGraw-Hill.

Okamura, Y. 1981. "Situational ethnicity," *Ethnic and Racial Studies*, 4: 4, 454–465.

Roca, J. 1996. *De la pureza a la maternidad. La construcción del género femenino en la postguerra española*. Madrid: Ministerio de Educación y Cultura.

11 Becoming a mother through postpartum depression

Narratives from Brazil

Maureen O'Dougherty

Introduction

According to public health and psychological research, postpartum depression is an important problem and growing diagnosis for women globally. Public health data worldwide find a high prevalence; the more conservative estimates are one out of every eight mothers experiences depression during pregnancy or postpartum (O'Hara 2009; Bina 2008).[1] The mainstream position in Western biomedicine is to support the diagnosing and treatment of perinatal depression as a common mental health condition in motherhood with potentially serious consequences for the mother, child and family, if untreated. Some feminist and anthropological researchers question the pathologizing of postpartum depression. Critics question whether postpartum depression is an illness rather than an ordinary experience of the transition to motherhood (Ussher 2010; Lee 2003; Nicolson 1999).

I gathered narratives of pregnancy, childbirth and new motherhood from 68 women of diverse social classes in Rio de Janeiro between 2004 and 2009. Several accounts were marked by difficult experiences; these included eight stories of postpartum depression among women in a broadly defined lower-middle to upper-middle class. This chapter examines how these Brazilian women, who self-identify as having (had) "postpartum depression," represent experiences of early motherhood in their narratives.[2] My main focus is on several questions relating to challenges these women faced in the transition to motherhood. I ask: What does it mean for these Brazilian women to name postpartum depression as a significant part of their experience of new motherhood? What is the process by which their new identity of "mother" is coupled with "depression"? How do they narrate their personal transformation and characterize their accompanying emotions? Before and after addressing these questions, I consider the relevance of motherhood imperatives for contemporary middle-class Brazilian women. Doing so raises the idea of broadening the definition of "intensive mothering" (Hays 1996) to include the work of transforming one's life and identity in motherhood and in turn the possibility of postpartum depression in response.

Maternity as a totalizing experience

Middle-class motherhood has received little attention in the anthropology of Brazil. One relevant work for this discussion, however, is Tania Salem's "trajectory of the pregnant couple." This enlightening study from the 1980s followed pregnant couples in Rio de Janeiro who were determined to cast off childcare traditions dependent on heavy grandparent involvement and reliance on nursemaids. Once the baby was born, however, unforeseen circumstances presented themselves. As Salem explains:

> the intended plan that only the parents should take care of the baby, linked with the fact that the man continued his regular involvement in professional life, contributed to *the woman living maternity as an absolutely totalizing experience*, observing the inflation of one aspect of her personality, that of mother, in detriment of others.
>
> (1985: 51, emphasis added)

Salem suggests intensive concern with maternal care when noting the "absolute centrality conferred on the child, and the fear that any false step [by the mother] could compromise the baby's emotional equilibrium" (1985: 50).[3]

This work prefigures the concept developed by Sharon Hays (1996) of intensive mothering, that is, maternal practices entailing a great deal of time, energy and money focused on the child. Hays grapples particularly with the evident inconsistencies of this form of childcare at a time of high maternal employment. Intensive motherhood has been described in the context of women's paid employment outside the home, smaller family size and the nuclear rather than extended family. In this regard middle-class Brazilian women appear to share circumstances with counterparts in the Global North. Smaller-sized families in Brazil have occurred in all regions and social classes in an impressively short period of time, from six births per woman in 1965 to 1.9 in 2009 (Gorney 2011). Women's own professional pursuits, economic changes in the 1980s–1990s, ongoing costs of children's private schooling as the necessary means to higher education and a growing commitment to global consumption have provided an added push to paid employment and delayed childbearing among middle-class mothers.

Some notable differences between middle classes in Brazil and the Global North, however, raise the question of whether the concept of intensive mothering can be applied without distortion in this context. As Salem reports of her study participants, the modern parent–caregiver experiment did not take hold. Sooner or later in the postpartum period the extended family, formerly barred, was reinstated with grandmother(s) on site almost daily or in extended stays. Nursemaids, who, until recently received very low pay, were contracted. In the more prosperous households, housekeeping staff (one or more workers to cook/houseclean/do laundry) were already in service. Besides the difference in direct labor, there is the question of dedication to mothering practices. Comments of

Salem's study participants suggest a less than reverent view of motherhood as an intensive vocation. One woman said being restricted to the home and being a mother exclusively was bad for her. Another woman, who constantly talked to the first baby in the womb, said that with the second baby she "didn't have as much space for this kind of delirium ... it's a less totalizing maternity than the first" (Salem 1985: 57).

In the narratives I collected among women in Rio two decades later the same model of infant care among Brazilian middle classes remained in vigor, entailing active support from the new mother's mother and/or mother-in-law during the early postpartum and/or a nursemaid. A father's direct caregiving signaled a modern couple, but this was not common. Caregiving was thus intensive and gendered but aside from the important labor of breastfeeding,[4] it was usually dispersed across two or more women rather than concentrated on the mother. A kind of counter example from an upper-middle class participant proves the rule. Regina simultaneously chose the range of traditional methods and rejected them in favor of taking care of the baby herself during the first several weeks postpartum. As she reported with good humored self-irony, Regina rallied her mother, mother-in-law and domestic worker to her home then forbade them all from even holding her baby.

While extensive time, money and effort are bestowed on these Brazilian children, and while the women in the full sample generally voiced support for a more hands-on parenting approach than what they envisioned was done in the past, middle-class Brazilian mothers still delegated a (variable) portion of the direct labor. This is a salient difference from intensive mothering as understood to occur in the Global North. Precisely this difference offers an opportunity to consider intensive mothering beyond physical labor. While Hays takes due note of imperatives to be highly invested emotionally in the child (1996: 157), of less interest in her work are transformations to women's identity. Yet life crises events are dynamic moments entailing regulations of gender. For many women I met, a battle that emerged (either instantly in early motherhood or later on) was for a self independent of motherhood, an effort to pursue their lives without having motherhood be or remain a "totalizing experience." The challenge of reconciling motherhood and their broader lives (especially their professional lives) constituted a major drama (see Vaitsman 1994). For some women, as this chapter illustrates, this drama became a prolonged crisis.

This chapter is part of a larger study entailing semi-structured to open-ended interviews with Brazilian women aged 21–50 residing in Rio de Janeiro on experiences and decisions of fertility controls, pregnancy, childbirth and early motherhood. One third of the 31 interviews with low-income women were conducted with employees of a Flamengo neighborhood beauty salon. Another third took place in a shantytown above Santa Teresa and the remaining third at a maternity clinic in Laranjeiras among women waiting for an ob-gyn check-up. I met the middle- to upper-income women through two sources: friends and through announcements by a Flamengo fitness club instructor at her classes. These women resided in the Zona Sul, Zona Norte (Tijuca) and Niterói. I conducted follow-up interviews with about a dozen of the women, often over subsequent pregnancies and outcomes.

In the following sections, I use narrative analysis to explore explanatory models of postpartum depression from the stories and perspectives of the women themselves. Doing so affords the opportunity of assessing theoretical debates on postpartum depression as a psychiatric condition and as a response to the contemporary model of intensive motherhood. My approach draws mainly from sociolinguistic theories of narrative structure. Sociolinguist Labov (1997) identified key properties of personal narrative: complicating events (unexpected events that create challenge or adversity); resolution of plot complications; and evaluation (significance and meaning) of what occurred. From analysis of complicating events, we are able to derive a close understanding of the storyteller's beliefs of how (from what set of circumstances) and possibly why (from what cause[s]) she came to have perinatal distress. Capp and Ochs underscore in their work on agoraphobia that "all stories, whether historical, scientific, or personal, contain at least one theory about events" (1995: 16). Attention to resolution entails tracking what actions the women took in response to this personal crisis. These acts include developing a new critical perspective on motherhood as obtained through postpartum depression.

Complicating events

Carla's story: "You're the queen until he's born, then they take away your majesty"

Carla's story was the most elaborated of all in the sample: she had three children, and three experiences of postpartum depression; her recollection was of births that had occurred more than a decade earlier. Carla spent most of her time describing her second and worst experience of postpartum depression. As the passage below indicates, her story is filled with what might be called explanations of cause. I have put them in italics.

> You're extremely in love with your husband, and he's extremely in love with you and you have a baby coming, another! The pregnancy went smoothly [foi tranquila]. What surprised me was the depression. I had a very strong depression with him. *Perhaps because my twin sister had postpartum depression and today is schizophrenic....* And I lived through this pregnancy with this phantom, that I would have depression. And then, perhaps, I looked back at the sadness of my first pregnancy and said [to myself]: "that was depression and now I know the name!" The second was really hard; I can't talk about it without crying. I never thought I would suffer so much. Because it was like this: all the happiness that I imagined I would have I didn't. I suffered a lot with this child, I couldn't handle it. [...] It was really hard, because I was in love – I'm in love until today with my husband – and *I demanded of myself to be a perfect mother, and I couldn't identify that child as mine. Understand? Because I divided my husband with him.*

Carla's first potentially causal evaluation presents a genetic possibility. She then gives some description of her symptoms and a growing sense that she was depressed. The puzzling set of potentially causal statements that close this excerpt lead one to wonder why being in love with her husband made new motherhood hard. One might envision an ecstatic, newly forming nuclear family. But no, the presence of the second baby appears to have created a conflict of demands (of perfection as a mother in conflict with a lack of identification with the baby) and of passions (divided time between her husband and her baby). This pregnancy, Carla explained, came far sooner than expected in her second marriage to the love of her life. Consider what Carla told a pregnant friend earlier the day of our first meeting: "you're the queen until he's born, then they [*sic*] take away your majesty. But this will pass. The baby is going to be the center, and you are going to want this...."

Carla returned later to debate whether she herself overly expected to have postpartum depression but then reversed her line of thinking with: *"Because I didn't have any reason [motivo], but I never felt sadder. I never felt sadder in my life."* It is striking that Carla dismissed all the reasons she had put forward that might explain her having become depressed postpartum, in favor of saying there was no reason for it. Immediately after this denial, Carla spoke further of her twin. During her pregnancy, she was asked by her sister's doctors to recall her childhood, as her sister had lost her memory. This exercise was very painful for her.

Teresa's story: The anxiety came out of nowhere

> Physical. It's a physical pain. You wake up with it. It's horrible, you know, to wake up with it. [...] *I didn't have any reason* [motivo].... Work was great, my relationship with my husband was great, my relationship with the children, great. [...] *It was with the arrival of the second. It started the minute he came. I thought I wasn't going to be able to love him as much as [the first child].* [...] Time passed and I didn't feel anxious or depressed. It took a lot of energy (mothering the second child). *It was more or less one to two years after that the anxiety came from nothing [veio do nada].* [M.O'D.: Really?] *From nothing. From nothing. I really didn't have any reason.*

Teresa's account starts with a description of symptoms of overpowering, constant, unbearable pain (like a stab in the heart) as well as feeling unable to breathe throughout the entire day. Like Carla, Teresa maintained she lacked a motive for having postpartum depression; the constant pain of anxiety "came from nothing" (literal translation). The reason there was no reason for her anxiety and unhappiness was that "work was great, my relationship with my husband was great, my relationship with the children, great." Yet she, too, provided a counter explanation, potentially a causal one: she feared she wouldn't love this child as much as her first. Teresa also described many difficulties she had with this second child. Much later in the interview she reflected:

This is perhaps what happens to other women, too, when they have a child. Now you have to raise it! So how long will it be? I can't sleep anymore, I can't go out. I remember saying, "I want to go out! I don't want to come back!"

Carla and Teresa's accounts are marked by multiple statements that might be meant to indicate the "cause" of postpartum depression, but these are strikingly reversed. At a certain moment both declare a lack of motive. By doing so, they recast the potentially causal reasons as merely contextual ones. Carla wanted her second marriage but not for it to lead to a baby, at least not so soon, and not after what she had witnessed during her pregnancy: her twin sister diagnosed with a major mental illness evidently precipitated by postpartum depression. Carla's distress seems over-determined. Teresa, a person who generally exudes high spirits, presented her story most emphatically as under-determined – as coming out of nowhere given the all-around happiness. Yet Teresa too supplied a counter explanation: her sense of motherhood and family did not allow her to have just one child; she had to give her first child a sibling. Of Teresa and Carla, we might say that there was no motive, or rather, no motive for them to have another child: weren't things fine as they were?! Their happiness was cut short with motherhood.

Luciana's story: "It's one thing for you to have a moment of sadness; it's another to be permanently sad"

Luciana's experience of postpartum depression was not over at the time of first interview. In all, Luciana spent six years trying to get pregnant, had recourse to infertility treatments and suffered a miscarriage before finally carrying a pregnancy to term. After a detailed discussion of infertility treatment, Luciana then provided the immediate context for postpartum depression after childbirth. Finding she hadn't much breast milk, Luciana read on the internet about a pill for nausea (plasil) that increases the amount of milk and tried it. It did increase her milk, but, as she said:

> *It's just that it's a medication that makes you get depressed.* It makes you depressed, not immediately, the person is fooled and thinks it's okay.... As time went on taking this medication, I was also sensitive, you know, *I am a sensitive person, and all these things, having gone through this period* [...] I got neurotic about this breastfeeding story and I would cry and cry about it. *And the medication didn't cause it. For sure. But it made it worse. I am sure that the pill didn't cause the depression out of nothing. It's not that strong of a pill...*

In the passage above, Luciana replicates her own process of awareness first that the medication could but then could not cause depression "out of nothing." Like Carla and Teresa, Luciana's narrative also contains a reversal in the representation of the cause of depression, but hers is in the opposite direction. I asked Luciana when she became aware this was depression. She said:

> From the beginning I started to feel that this thing [negócio] wasn't real normal, because I would cry, be sad, all the time with the breastfeeding. I'd think, "gee, but what happened?" All those years that I tried to get pregnant. Of course I had times that were bothersome, times I was sad, but I wasn't sad the whole time. It's one thing for you to have a moment of sadness, and it's another to be permanently sad, permanently sad. After [baby's name] was born, I came to be always sad, permanently sad. [...] With postpartum depression, it was permanent sadness, 24 hours a day.

Luciana underscores that with postpartum depression her feelings of sadness were qualitatively different from prior sad or depressed feelings.

Luciana's experience appeared to be most directly, demonstrably contradictory. As she said herself before the baby came, she felt

> my only problem in life was that I didn't have a baby. On the day I had a baby, I discovered that no, I had other problems. I hadn't any money, I was in debt, the family was fighting about the debt, it was partly my fault ... and I started to see that I wasn't such a good mother as I had thought I would be. I used to think what could be difficult? It's enough for you to love the baby and everything will be fine. This didn't happen because the baby didn't respond. I'm affectionate, I'd come and take her, hug her and the baby didn't like this. She didn't like to be hugged, she didn't like affection. She had reflux, at 20 days she started to have reflux, so she started crying a lot and was nervous.

Luciana pointed out that the problems she was having at home, financial and familial ones, were difficult, but not the kind of problems to put her "in mourning," as she put it. The problems with breastfeeding and the baby vomiting from reflux weren't such terrible problems, Luciana noted, but she overly focused on them while suffering from postpartum depression. She also spoke of how she had felt the baby seemed to be more comforted and happy with others (and Carla said the same as well). She believed the baby sensed her anxious feelings.

For Luciana, there were the years of desperately trying to have a child and then the contrary experience of new motherhood – against which she immediately reacted in deep, unrelenting sadness, distaste and uneasiness with the difficulties with mothering, and in disappointment with her own inadequacies (lack of breast milk, lack of mothering skills, lack of ability to get the child to want to hug her). The success of finally becoming pregnant became a failure with the child's birth. Luciana suggests she was set up and/or set herself up for postpartum depression.

Plot resolutions

Carla's recovery at six months postpartum could be called the "working cure."
In a brief statement Carla indicated the resolution to her postpartum depression:
"going back to work is what saved me." Specifically, she was completing her
doctoral dissertation, which she felt she had to finish before dying, that the work
"stabilized" her, allowed her to "forget" her "guilt" and was "a moment that was
mine." She also said that she resolved her problem "intellectually" by reading
about postpartum depression, including a book on myths of motherhood (probably *Motherhood: Myth and Reality* by Élisabeth Badinter). Yet Carla declared
later on:

> breastfeeding saved me. I breastfed until the seventh month; it saved me
> from sadness because it gave me great pleasure to nurse my baby. I felt
> useful! It was the only moment I felt useful! All the rest of the time, I felt I
> could absolutely be thrown out.

At this point, Carla offered two divergent resolutions to her depression crisis:
her professional work as well as a key mothering practice, breastfeeding. At
the end of our first talk, Carla suddenly announced: "I think motherhood is
what saved me. Even though it was where I lived through the saddest experience, depression, I think it's what saves us. Because it gives meaning to our
life. I am very happy with the children I have." Carla said this after having told
me that she had wanted to end her life, but decided that she would force herself
to live until her children reached the age of 18 (so that they wouldn't lose a
parent before adulthood as she had lost her father), and then she would kill
herself.

Teresa had wanted to flee her home, but instead, her path to recovery entailed
first psychiatric medication and then psychotherapy. She quickly sought a doctor
(explaining she does not tolerate pain at all), was prescribed anxiety medication,
but this, she quickly noted, did not really help. Instead, her solution was talking
in therapy where she determined the reason for her trouble was motherhood.

> The medication didn't solve the problem. The medicine didn't solve it. So I
> looked for a psychologist, I went into therapy. I thought I had to speak about
> this pain. The more I spoke of the pain, the better I felt. In therapy, I talked,
> which made me cry; when you cry the pain lessens, you know. It seems that
> ... the pain comes and appears and it's all ... it's an unloading. It was a
> relief. The pain would come back later, but it was a big relief. [...] Now it
> was three years ago, and the pain doesn't come back. Therapy really worked
> and today I know that the pain was because of motherhood. [...] [M.O'D.
> And what made you get better?] Talking. Talking about the children, about
> motherhood, about motherhood, about motherhood. About things that hap-
> pened during the week, I would go through the whole week with her, every-
> thing I had done.

Teresa's was the classic talking cure where she identified her distress in therapy. She also developed a critical perspective on cultural scripts of motherhood. She emphasized what she called the "mandate" not just to be a mother, but the best mother. Teresa repeated on several occasions quite simply, flatly, as if it were a prison sentence, that she had to be good, a good mother. As her statements below indicate, Teresa was awed by the great responsibility and power she had over her child as well as by how difficult it was for her to be confronted by a toddler defying her power. She also returned to her initial dilemma: not believing she could love another child as much as the first, yet following through on a sense of obligation to have two children.

> What left me anxious was the responsibility. I felt responsible for every-thing that happened to them. If I didn't do this they'd get sick, if I didn't do that they wouldn't do well in school, if I didn't – I had to be … perfect. Because if I wasn't they would be deeply unhappy, bad, sick, you know? So it was an enormous weight on top of me! […] The responsibility. I had to be good, I had to be a good mother. You can't have just one child. In my head. Ridiculous.

I imagined Teresa was worried about her abilities to perform as a mother and suggested she may have had such doubts. Teresa responded: "No, I didn't have doubts about being a mother. I always thought I was a great mom. It was the weight. I understood that it was a lot of responsibility that I was shouldering. This gave me pain." In therapy Teresa reconsidered that she really "didn't have all this power to control everyone and everything." Finally, work also helped, Teresa said, because it allowed her to get out of the house. Teresa was thriving in her profession.

Luciana did not take medication, as she feared what it might do to her and her baby, and she didn't have help or ask for it, including not from her mother, who lived on the floor below but didn't have a way with babies, and she couldn't afford a therapist, as she had lost her job during the process of getting infertility treat-ment. In several snapshots, Luciana presented how she moved toward recovery:

> After six weeks or so, I'd take her out to go the little square nearby where no one went. A very small square. I became friends with a flower salesman at the square; we'd chat. He was the only person who'd listen to me, he and the internet – people my age, all these people that had had a baby. I always did this ever since I had infertility treatment, I'd get into the chat rooms.

Luciana eventually found a babysitter and started to attend church every day. She started feeling better, not only by praying, but also by comparatively reflect-ing on her youth vis-à-vis older women who were

> happy with life, active, visiting people, they have a perspective on life. And me. I have years in front of me, more time to live than them, why am I

crying? So, I kept going to church, and I started feeling better, better and better. [...] Little by little, I felt more adapted to motherhood. As she started to crawl – she took a long time to crawl – and move about by herself, she didn't need me so much to carry her up and down [...]. At about nine months I started to have fun with her. I started to adapt. But I'm still not 100 percent.

Perinatal distress in theoretical perspectives

Given the multiplicity of emergent theories without direct statements of cause, we find ourselves at an impasse. But wait: we have framed the issue as why the postpartum depression when the complicating event was, of course, the baby. In the bare sequence of events, the multitude of potential causes becomes context, and the cause unitary: the baby arrived, then the problematic feelings these women came to call postpartum depression started. Carla lost her majesty with the baby's arrival; Teresa identified motherhood as the trouble; problems started right away with the baby, for Luciana. Notably, Luciana's symptoms of permanent sadness were symmetrical with the permanent change in life. While space limitations prevent discussing all eight stories, it is important to note that their stories followed the same structure as those discussed in detail here. What medical anthropologist Gay Becker (1997) calls "embodied distress," distress occasioned by critical disruptions to people's lives, is relevant. The women seemed to be trapped into a context where the baby's birth meant the end of the mother's happiness. Their language is of a dire, mortal, chronic hell. Unlike people in Becker's study, who faced socially recognized misfortunes, here it is the socially recognized good fortune that disrupts.

Interpretive lenses abound to reflect on the theories emergent in the narratives. Numerous feminist works have exposed saccharine idealizations surrounding motherhood. Poet Adrienne Rich is unique in directly naming children as the cause of pain. Her classic work, *Of Woman Born*, opens with this statement: "My children cause me the most exquisite suffering of which I have any experience. It is the suffering of ambivalence: the murderous alternation between bitter resentment and raw-edged nerves, and blissful gratification and tenderness" (1976: 21). Psychoanalytical approaches view motherhood as a crisis of selfhood.[5] Oberman and Josselson believe "at no time ... is the clash between a woman's struggle against an apparent loss of one's self and adjustment to the acquisition of another so painfully raw as during the first few months of motherhood" (1996: 345). Similarly, social scientist Tina Miller emphasizes the magnitude of the existential crisis – so huge as to potentially threaten "ontological security," that is a sense of order and continuity to one's life and one's self (2005). One new mother in Miller's study felt her life had so utterly changed that there was nothing left from before. Another went through the motions of mothering.

To my knowledge, one theorist links perinatal distress to the current model of intensive motherhood. Social policy analyst Ellie Lee (2003) asserts that the current rise in postpartum depression may stem from the new child-centered ideology of intensive motherhood, as well as from a contemporary rendering of motherhood as the most meaningful vocation. The influence of an intensive motherhood model is suggested in the women's narratives. Teresa's sense of having to be perfect indicates she had been burdened by an ideology of intensive mothering. Other stories point to conflicts with the vocation. Luciana finds that the difficult but mundane infant care was not truly the cause of her trouble, but rather, she had become totally invested in the promise of motherhood as her reason-for-being only to find herself limited by motherhood. Another woman protested her dismay at this reduction, shouting angrily to her husband and mother: "have I become only two breasts?!"

Anthropologist Edward Hagen (2002) argues from an evolutionary perspective that becoming depressed postpartum is akin to going on strike; women "bargain" for support in contexts where relinquishing maternal care is not an option. Hagen and Barrett (2008) suggest from empirical research among the Shuar of the Ecuadorian Amazon that perinatal sadness or depression ("psychic pain") is a response to opportunity costs: that is, to invest in the newborn would require undesirably reducing investment in other siblings and/or in activities beneficial to (even vital to) the mother herself. Somewhat surprisingly, this bottom line interpretation is not inconsistent with philosopher Judith Butler's theory of performativity (1990; see also Schwartz 1994). Applied to perinatal distress, the theory would suggest the women suffering from postpartum depression fail to perform normative motherhood, which requires not solely childcare practices, but, in this context, corresponding feelings and an acceptance of sacrifice of the self as mothers. With postpartum depression, the failure among these Brazilian middle-class women to emotionally perform as mothers might be said to constitute unvoiced objection or resistance partially to intensive mothering and more broadly and directly to the imperative of motherhood.

How the Brazilian women discussed here find a way out of their crises is also in keeping with the theoretical perspectives. In all narratives wanting to get out of the house was an early response to a sense of entrapment (Mallinson et al. 1996). Another vantage point for viewing this response can be drawn from Petra Büskens' case study of a woman who left her family and later held joint custody. In "When Eve left the garden," Buskens affirms that "mothers who leave are forging an historically unique pathway out of the current impasse between mandatory selflessness and/or cultural contradiction" (2005: 276). Buskens concludes "the mother who leaves is a creation myth of sorts for she promulgates the possibility of a mother in possession of her own desire: a desire to be a free individual and a mother" (2005: 279). The women discussed here did not leave their marriages or households. Instead, for all, reclaiming their own work, rather than what seemed like unending self-abandonment, was a viable solution (see also Miller 2005). Carla and Teresa returned to their work in academia. Luciana declared:

> What I want to do now is go back to work. I wanted to be this housewife taking care of a baby, but when I stayed with her, I discovered that to only stay at home, for me, is not something that gives me much fulfillment [realização].

Carla's account differs from Luciana's and Teresa's in one important way. She not only emerges victorious over serious depression, she also comes to find her selfhood no longer diminished but rather enhanced through motherhood (see also Rich 1976: 348).

Evaluations of events and one's own and other people's acts is an integral part of narrative structure. Labov has noted that without narrator evaluation, the sense and meaning of the story may be lost. Besides the women's sense of the experience in their lives, what Somers (1994) calls the ontological narrative, the accounts speak to cultural scripts of motherhood most explicitly through such evaluations. In the next, and final section, the women's evaluations place perinatal distress in context.

Evaluating postpartum depression/evaluating the woman

Near the end of the interviews, the women presented critiques of normative views of motherhood, as well as on the social censure of and disrespect for postpartum depression. Luciana said her sadness was obvious, but as to the naming, "no one is going to give it the least bit of importance just because I changed the name [from sadness to postpartum depression]." She pointed out that the term postpartum depression does come up on occasion in the media,[6] but that she herself

> always thought it was something that happened to silly people, you know, that it was silly, something that neurotic people had. So obviously it's a bit difficult to admit that you have something that you always said ... not to mention that I always said that if I managed to have a baby all my problems would end.

Luciana braved harsh critique over her postpartum depression. When she told people she had "stopped everything to be a mother" only to find she "didn't have a good way with the baby," people derided her, saying " 'you took years to have a baby and now you give yourself the luxury of complaining?!' " One of the other women with postpartum depression and anxiety said that at first she didn't tell anyone about her severe distress "because people don't understand and think it's foolishness [bobeira], that it's a joke [palhaçada – literally clowning], that it's silly [frescura]." This woman received these comments from family members.

Carla, who bore her distress silently and without recourse to therapy or medication, closed a painful experience of revisiting her depression with the following statements emphasizing that postpartum depression develops in relation to multiple factors, including social constraints on speech.

> I think postpartum depression has a hormonal component, but it also has to do with space for you to dialogue, right? [...] I think it's hard to separate postpartum depression from a number of things. I don't think any postpartum depression manifests in isolation. It comes in a time and context.

For her part, Teresa criticized Brazilian society's upholding of motherhood as "sublime" and for considering childless women abnormal. Without over-generalizing, one might infer that one perspective in Brazil represents postpartum depression as a frivolous, illegitimate "sick role" (Parsons 1951). Another highlights the imperative of motherhood as the ultimate fulfillment for women. These statements all point to a context in popular culture censoring negative emotional responses to motherhood.

In narrative codas (bringing the story back to the present), the women underscore that developing a discourse on postpartum depression and/or on motherhood is itself a way to confront a context that is unaccepting of negative responses to motherhood. Luciana communicates widely about her experience on the web. Carla speaks to pregnant women she knows about the possibility of postpartum depression and presents herself as someone they can turn to for help. Teresa is critical of Brazilian ideologies of motherhood. Through such discursive interventions the women present counter-narratives (Riessman 1993) to a unitary motherhood script.

This chapter opened with the question of whether diagnostic labels like "postpartum depression" problematically medicalize and pathologize a normal life crisis transition. Ussher argues that the diagnostic label "decontextualizes social problems" (2010: 15) and leads to medicating women. Hagen and Barrett warn that medication in particular could "inhibit a mother's motivation to act in her own interests, and in the interest of her older children, and could interfere with her ability to learn from experience" (2008: 36–37). Lee criticizes a "quite powerful tendency in British and American cultures to represent motherhood as an ordeal and, in particular, as an experience that is linked to the development of mental illness" (2003: 225). She maintains that while contemporary mandates for intensive motherhood could account for negative responses, it is a "big jump" – a mistaken one – to label these experiences as psychiatric conditions (2003: 245).[7] The result of this medicalization, Lee believes, is to make women more passive and disempowered. Her recommendation is social network support rather than biomedical intervention. Regarding social networks, sociologist Verta Taylor's study of the grassroots development of self-help postpartum depression support groups in the U.S. begins with a skeptical prediction that the diagnostic label could denigrate women's experience and "ironically reaffirm the model of self-sacrificing and blissful mother by insinuating that therapy and medication are the keys to normal motherhood" (1996: 165). Her research leads her to conclude that these networks do not disempower or re-essentialize motherhood, but rather, encourage a critical stance that "maternal sacrifice undermines women's identities and well-being" (1996: 179).

While I generally agree with the tenor of the critical approaches presented above, I also have some practical and theoretical reservations. I have concerns first and foremost because of the undue burden placed on the individual women to champion their cause especially in the absence of broader societal support. What is needed is a larger effort to confront the socially reproduced gender norms that make objections to the normative motherhood script – which, in the current iteration, is ideologically and morally intensive – appear pathological. Second, I would caution that the transition to motherhood these women undergo should not be characterized lightly as merely a challenging role change when what is entailed is a powerful process of gender regulation. It is worth recalling that Nicolson (1999), who was the first to argue that the transition to motherhood should not be pathologized, nonetheless represented it as a life crisis event in which the old self, now lost, is mourned. This idea makes sense; remember Luciana herself used the word mourning, albeit ironically. In a way, my concern is that both medicalization and its absence could dismiss rather than acknowledge and validate women's experiences.

Third, I would emphasize that our theories need to include an expectation of women's agency as active, discerning and critical, and our approaches need to be attentive to how they represent and evaluate their experiences. In the eight stories I gathered in Brazil on postpartum depression, medicalization was not a large part of the experience. Medication was only relevant for two and in a limited way. While my sources are few, they do not lead to a straightforward conclusion about the implications of taking on the diagnostic label of postpartum depression. The diagnostic label, mainly self-assigned, seemed to provide a means for the women to process and acknowledge their own negative experiences of motherhood.

Let's return, finally, to the idea raised in the introduction of broadening the definition of intensive mothering to include the work of transforming one's life and identity in motherhood. What I found from the women's narratives is that the "new" model of intensive motherhood reiterates an old one: to embrace a consistent, coherent identity of the (literally) self-sacrificing mother. The women's narratives attest to the ongoing strength of that imperative, once a duty, now called a choice. Their stories lead me to conclude that for now, the earnest theoretical attempts to decouple psychiatric pathology from the experience of motherhood appear to be at cross-purposes with these women, who come to accept and incorporate the social and psychiatric classifications of their motherhood. By taking on the name "postpartum depression," these Brazilian women countered the silencing they faced. By accepting this label and diagnosis even without social approval, they moved toward reclaiming their voices and reconstructing their lives.

Notes

1 In biomedicine, postpartum depression is said to come in three forms: baby blues, postpartum depression and psychosis. The literature is most concerned with the middle range, longer lasting postpartum depression. The limited research in Brazil, mainly among low income women, reports high estimates of 19 percent (Moraes *et al.* 2006).

2 Perhaps I should make it clear from the outset that I'm not concerned here with the genealogy of how postpartum depression came into social existence, nor as Jerome Bruner puts it in his work *Acts of Meaning*, "ontologically obscure issues as whether the account is 'self-deceptive' or 'true' [but] only in what the person thought he did, what he thought he was doing it for, what kind of plights he thought he was in, and so on" (Bruner 1990: 119–120).

3 It is important to note that a call to more intensive mothering is not unique to the late twentieth century. Historian Susan Besse (1996) discusses a parallel shift at a time of lower fertility rates among wealthier households in early twentieth century Brazil.
4 Breastfeeding took center stage in early motherhood narratives, emerging as a classic plot complication with challenges and adversities, but where the mother eventually triumphs.
5 Another second-wave feminist, psychiatrist Ann Dally (1982), believes that maternal depression develops in lieu of a solution to the impossibility of escape and/or the feeling of having lost something vital.
6 In recent years, the mainstream media has occasionally reported on global public health research emphasizing postpartum depression as serious and warranting medication and therapy.
7 Nancy Chodorow argues that in the contemporary context women "mask conflicts and ambivalence about motherhood, by turning those conflicts into ones between motherhood and career" (2005: 137–138).

References

Becker, G. (1997) *Disrupted Lives: How People Create Meaning in a Chaotic World*, Berkeley, CA: University of California Press.

Besse, S.K. (1996) *Restructuring Patriarchy: The Modernization of Gender Inequality in Brazil, 1914–1940*, Chapel Hill, NC: University of North Carolina Press.

Bina, R. (2008) "The impact of cultural factors upon postpartum depression: a literature review," *Health Care for Women International*, vol. 29, no. 6, pp. 568–592.

Bruner, J. (1990) *Acts of Meaning*, Cambridge, MA: Harvard University Press.

Büskens, P. (2005) "When Eve left the garden: a modern tale about mothers who leave their families," in M. Porter, P. Short and A. O'Reilly (eds.) *Motherhood: Power and Oppression*, Toronto: Women's Press, pp. 265–284.

Butler, J. (1990) *Gender Trouble: Feminism and the Subversion of Identity*, New York: Routledge.

Capps, L. and Ochs, E. (1995) *Constructing Panic: The Discourse of Agoraphobia*. Cambridge, MA: Harvard University Press.

Chodorow, N. (2005) "Ambivalence about motherhood, choice, and time," in S.F. Brown (ed.) *What Do Mothers Want?* Hillsdale, NJ: Analytic Press, pp. 131–149.

Dally, A. (1982) *Inventing Motherhood: The Consequences of an Ideal*, New York: Schocken Books.

Gorney, C. (2011) "Brazil's girl power," *National Geographic*, September, vol. 220, no. 3, pp. 96–119.

Hagen, E.H. (2002) "Depression as bargaining: the case of postpartum," *Evolution and Human Behavior*, vol. 23, no. 5, pp. 323–336.

Hagen, E.H. and Barrett, H.C. (2007) "Perinatal sadness among Shuar women: support for an evolutionary theory of psychic pain," *Medical Anthropology Quarterly*, vol. 21, no. 1, pp. 22–40.

Hays, S. (1996) *The Cultural Contradictions of Motherhood*, New Haven, CT: Yale University Press.

Labov, W. (1997) "Some further steps in narrative analysis," *Journal of Narrative and Life History*, vol. 7, no. 1/4, pp. 395–415.

Lee, E. (2003) *Abortion, Motherhood, and Mental Health: Medicalizing Reproduction in the United States and Great Britain*, New York: Aldine de Gruyter.

Mallinson, T., Kielkhofner, G. and Mattingly, C. (1996) "Metaphor and meaning in a clinical interview," *American Journal of Occupational Therapy*, vol. 50, no. 5, pp. 338–346.

Miller, T. (2005) *Making Sense of Motherhood: A Narrative Approach*, Cambridge/New York: Cambridge University Press.

Moraes, I.G., Pinheiro, R.T., Silva, R.A., Horta, B.L., Sousa, P.L. and Faria, A.D. (2006) "Prevalence of postpartum depression and associated factors," *Revista de Saúde Pública*, vol. 40, no. 1, pp. 65–70.

Nicolson, P. (1999) "Loss, happiness and postpartum depression: the ultimate paradox," *Canadian Psychology/Psychologie Canadienne*, vol. 40, no. 2, pp. 162–178.

Oberman, Y. and Josselson, R. (1996) "Matrix of tensions: a model of mothering," *Psychology of Women Quarterly*, vol. 20, no. 3, pp. 341–359.

O'Hara, M.W. (2009) "Postpartum depression: what we know," *Journal of Clinical Psychology*, vol. 65, no. 12, pp. 1258–1269.

Parsons, T. (1951) *The Social System*, Glencoe, IL: The Free Press.

Rich, A. (1976) *Of Woman Born: Motherhood as Experience and Institution*, New York: Bantan Books.

Riessman, C.K. (1993) *Narrative Analysis*, Newbury Park, CA: Sage Publications.

Salem, T. (1985) "A trajetória do 'casal gravido:' de sua constituição à revisão do projeto," in *Cultura da Psicanálise*, S.A. Figueira (ed.) São Paulo: Brasiliense, pp. 35–61.

Schwartz, A. (1994) "Taking the nature out of mother," in D. Bassin, M. Honey and M. Mahrer (eds.) *Representations of Motherhood*, New Haven, CT: Yale University Press, pp. 240–255.

Somers, M.R. (1994) "The narrative constitution of identity: a relational and network approach," *Theory and Society*, vol. 23, no. 5, pp. 605–649.

Taylor, V. (1996) *Rock-a-by Baby: Feminism, Self Help, and Postpartum Depression*, New York: Routledge.

Ussher, J.M. (2010) "Are we medicalizing women's misery? a critical review of women's higher rates of reported depression," *Feminism and Psychology*, vol. 20, no. 1, pp. 9–35.

Vaitsman, J. (1994) *Flexíveis e plurais: identidade, casamento e família em circunstâncias pós-modernas*. Rio de Janeiro: Editora Rocco.

12 Sacrificial mothering of IVF-pursuing mothers in Turkey

A. Merve Göknar

MERVE: Can you tell me why you want a child?

EDA:[1] When we get older, we need someone to take care of us. You know, one injection is 130 TL (about 80 US$). I don't have the money for any more injections (her eyes welled up). If we had a house or a car, I would definitely sell them. I feel cursed. When I see a baby, I don't look directly into his eyes, I am afraid of cursing him with the evil eye. I adore them. I put all other dreams on hold: I never purchased a house or a car, not even a new dress, and I never travelled anywhere. I visited doctors; that's all I have done with my life. I have sacrificed my life and anything I had in order to have a child. If I have money again, I will spend it on fertility treatments. I have tried artificial insemination (by husband) four times. I attempted IVF (in vitro fertilization) once. I am already deep in debt.

The vignette above is from my field notes, which I took while I was conducting research about the demand for IVF and the experience of childlessness in Turkey. I met Eda, a 36-year-old woman married for 17 years, in a private IVF clinic in the European part of Istanbul. She was in the waiting room, along with 20 other women (all in various stages of IVF treatment) and their husbands or friends. Eda was there to meet the doctor for a second cycle of IVF. She hoped the doctor would perhaps find free medications for her. Eda is one of many women I encountered, who were ready to sacrifice anything in their lives in order to have a child. Selling a car, quitting work, and not spending any money for personal leisure are among many things women readily do in their quest for motherhood.[2] Not enjoying life is another type of sacrifice. The underlying belief is that parents sacrifice much from their lives while raising their kids; so why shouldn't parents-to-be, or expecting parents-to-be do the same?

This chapter explores the concept of intensive mothering as it pertains to Turkish women pursuing IVF. Intensive mothering actualizes these women's adult gender identities. In their efforts to conceive a child via IVF, women usually exhibit a certain notion of parenting: intensive parenting, as it is increasingly referred to in anthropological literature. To date, studies on intensive parenting have focused on parents, as described in the introduction of this book. Studies on IVF have focused on the efforts by childless people to conceive a child, before they become parents. Different from those two approaches, this chapter argues that childless women engage in intensive parenting before they give birth or even before conceiving a child. "Perfect mothering," an ideal shared by parents, can start from the day a woman decides to conceive a child.

The word "intensive" in this paper describes the zeal and meticulous care women exhibit in performing perfect parenting. Their readiness to make sacrifices ranges from quality of life (often beginning before conception), to the variety and abundance of activities they engage in to birth and raise their child, and to their efforts to prove to themselves as well as others that they are good at parenting. The intensity and type of the effort varies according to contemporary parenting ideologies (for example see Faircloth, this volume for attachment parenting). Intensive (*yoğun*) is not commonly used to describe parenting practices in Turkey. I use it in order to enable a theoretical comparison across different studies.

Sacrifice, a stereotypical concept for mothers in Turkey, can also shape childless women's efforts to conceive. This chapter scrutinizes how the concept of intensive mothering fits into the concept of sacrificial mothering, an ideal shared by Turkish mothers. It not only examines the politics of sacrifice, but also questions what "parenting" represents in "intensive parenting": it explores how women negotiate their adult gender identities through the act of intensive mothering before the birth of their children.

The chapter also includes a section on pregnant women's intensive parenting practices. I reflect on my experiences as a pregnant woman in order to understand the intensive parenting efforts of women who pursue IVF. I discuss the ways in which my experience as a pregnant Turkish woman in Los Angeles, California is informed by sacrificial motherhood. My own experience of pregnancy, my upbringing in Turkey being immersed in certain motherhood ideologies, my feminist academic position, and current life in Los Angeles have informed my interpretation of intensive parenting (before birth). I follow Mauthner and Doucet (2003, p. 419), who in their critique of reflexive methodologies used with qualitative data, note that too much attention has been paid on reflexivity regarding the data collection phase. They suggest that "the interplay between our multiple social locations and how these intersect with the particularities of our personal biographies needs to be considered, as far as possible, *at the time* of analysing data" (emphasis original).

This chapter is based on research conducted in northwestern Turkey in 2006–2007. The research project consisted of two distinct environments related to each other by the theme of childlessness; one was in two IVF clinics and the other was in two villages. The "North" IVF clinic was in Istanbul and the "South" IVF clinic was in the outskirts of Istanbul. I conducted 137 interviews with women who underwent IVF treatment at these two clinics. The interviews ranged from a few minutes to a couple of hours. My questions explored women's reasons for wanting a child as well as for pursuing IVF. The clinics attracted couples from all over Turkey (as well as some from abroad such as Turkish immigrants from Germany). The second research environment took place in two neighbouring villages in the northwest part of Turkey. In the villages, I explored the consequences of being childless in daily life.

IVF arrived in Turkey in 1987 and the number of IVF centres in Turkey significantly increased in one decade, from 22 in 1998 to 121 in 2010. The Turkish Ministry of Health does not disclose any statistics regarding IVF with the public (except the names of active IVF clinics). According to a newspaper article (Çelebi 2011), it is estimated that over 50,000 IVF babies have been born in Turkey, and Turkey is the seventh country in terms of the number of IVF treatments after Israel, France, Spain, the United Kingdom, the United States and Germany. The total number of IVF cycles per year is over 40,000. However, the article mentions that according to Bahçeci, a well-known IVF specialist in Turkey, there are 500,000 people who are in need of IVF, a statistic that indicates that state financial support for IVF is insufficient.

IVF is available only to heterosexual married couples in Turkey (third-party-assisted reproduction treatment is illegal). Unlike the Shia Muslims in Iran and Lebanon (Clarke 2006a, 2006b, 2007a–2007d, 2008, 2009; Inhorn 2004, 2006; Tremayne 2006), gamete (sperm or ova) donation and surrogacy are not possible in most of the Sunni Muslim world. The Turkish Republic of Northern Cyprus is a notable exception and is preferred by Turkish couples who seek IVF via donated ova, sperm, embryo or who want to try surrogacy. However, with the latest legislation (March, 2010), it is illegal for Turkish citizens to have a third-party IVF even outside Turkey.[3] Those who have donor IVF treatment abroad are persecuted along with the doctors who conducted the procedure. The ideology behind this legislation is to protect the sanctity of the institution of family, which upholds a heterosexual family model. The mother in this ideal family picture is a sacrificial mother (*fedakar anne*), which is discussed below.

In Turkey, where everyone is expected to get married and eventually have a child, the rhetoric of sacrifice (*fedakarlık*) is inherent in the ideals of parenting. Parents are expected to "sacrifice their lives" for their children. This is expressed in the discourse of *hayatını çocuklara vermek* (giving one's life to one's children). During my research, I met childless women who were doing well financially, and who kept secret their efforts to conceive a child. They frequently heard the question "what are you going to do with that money, you do not have a child." These women (and their husbands) were scorned for "working in vain." In fact, some of them had internalized this perception of working. They were sad about working and earning money in vain. They wanted to spend their money on their children, not on themselves. They would feel better if they sacrificed their dinners out, avoided travel in summer and so forth for their children's education or other expenses. The more they sacrificed, the better they felt.

Sacrifice is a common script with which parents, especially mothers, reproduce their adult identities. Popular culture enhances these hegemonic femininities to the extent that motherhood is reified via the ability to sacrifice. In one of the popular Turkish television series, broadcasted in 2006–2009, a woman called

Şehrazat (Scheherazade) slept with her boss for money in order to fund her son's bone marrow transplant. Şehrazat's behavior created a public conversation about the extent to which mothers can sacrifice for their children. The commentaries about Şehrazat's act in popular media highlighted people's approval of her behavior as an example of being a sacrificial mother. Views of celebrities who defended the woman's act established mothering as a sacred role that embraced sacrifice.

The reification of sacrifice as a marker of mothering makes it something only mothers are perfect at. It is a stage of adulthood that only mothers can attain. Childless women in this respect remain at the periphery of adulthood, as beings not capable of even understanding what constitutes sacrifice. Their womanhood lacks a major skill that only women with children possess. Hegemonic femininity as such puts considerable pressure on childless women. I have encountered women protesting this fact during my interviews in IVF clinics and also during my stay in the villages. In one case, a childless woman I met in one of the villages, told me: "I have done so much for my niece. She even thinks I have done for her more than her mother. But neighbours think that I cannot understand what it takes to act like a mother. I can."

Despite their complaints, childless women adopt the script of the sacrificial mother who engages in intensive parenting. Intensive mothering and the sacrifices it entails begin even before conception in those cases. They start early on while trying to conceive and continue during pregnancy (see Murray, this volume for an example of sacrificial motherhood during pregnancy in Chile). Below, I classify childless women's engagement in intensive mothering into five categories to elucidate the variety of sacrifices they are ready to make.

Material sacrifices

As mentioned above, parents earn money to raise their children, and they also make plenty of material sacrifices while raising a child. Material sacrifices begin even before they become parents. I met women in IVF clinics who were ready to do anything to find money for the IVF treatment. Some began knitting children's clothing and selling those to friends and acquaintances. For most of them, since the treatments were time consuming, starting a daily job was not an option. Many of them started by selling the gold bracelets and gold coins they received as wedding gifts. I consider these sacrificial objects since they have symbolic as well as material significance. They represent the high stakes women must pay in order to conceive a child. Engaging in such sacrifices, women themselves are transformed into sacrificial objects. Since it was primarily women who pursued an IVF treatment, they were also the ones burdened with finding funding. They asked kinsfolk and friends (to whom they could disclose the treatment) for money, avoided the purchase of any "non-essential" items for the house, avoided travel expenses and when these were not sufficient, they sold what they could in order to pay for the IVF treatment. In addition to the women, husbands engaged in material sacrifices to fund treatments. Cars, houses, electronic appliances from their homes and fruit trees from their gardens were among the items sold to raise money. I even met a couple that sold the property that was their sole source of household income.

Career sacrifices

I maintain that intensive parenting is characterized by a willingness to sacrifice everything for the family and the generation that follows. Giving up a career after marriage appeared as a common script of femininity during my research, especially among working-class people. These women explained that they wanted to give their full attention to taking care of their families and homes. Sometimes, it was so because they (or their husbands) saw no reason for them to earn money (the husbands felt they earned enough to provide for the whole family). Additionally, sacrifice as an ideal informed their decisions. Sacrificing career for the family was not limited to working-class families. One woman undergoing an IVF treatment was a university graduate with a remarkable career in business. She gave up her career the moment she decided to have a child. She conceptualized mothering as another type of career. She told me: "If I cannot embark on the career of mothering (if the IVF treatment fails), I will start a new career." Her ideal for mothering involved the constant presence of the mother in taking care of her children. Like many others she believed that children needed their mothers constantly with them during the first for few years of their lives, and she felt ready to sacrifice her career in business for her new career in mothering.[4]

Relationship sacrifices

Managing relationships with kinsfolk and friends remained a critical element of IVF treatment. Most of them preferred not to disclose the treatment to anyone. They wanted to avoid the stigma attached to infertility. Within the social circles of some women whom I met in the IVF clinics, infertility was commonly associated with sexual impotency for the man. A man proved his "maleness" by impregnating a woman. IVF made it explicit to everyone that the couple struggled with conceiving a child and raised doubts about the man's virility. Remaining discreet about treatment proved a challenging task for those women who were under constant scrutiny by intriguing neighbours and affines. Some women lived close to their affines (in the same apartment building for example) if not in the same house. For them, creating excuses for their visits to the IVF clinic was daunting. One woman complained to me that her mother-in-law was so suspicious of her frequently leaving the house without explanation that she accused her of having an extramarital affair. When the woman admitted to her mother-in-law that she was visiting her gynaecologist, she was accused of having an affair with her doctor. The woman was nearly in tears while narrating this story as it represented a substantial hurdle for her to manage. She continued the IVF treatment despite the strained relationship with her mother-in-law.

There were others who did not disclose the treatment because they did not want to make their parents nervous about the process or the results. The constant questioning from their parents about the progress of the treatment was a bother. Moreover, they avoided frustrating their parents in case of a negative result from the treatment. These people usually had close relationships with their parents. Not only it was hard to conceal the treatment but also it was hard for them to lie to their parents.

Most women had a hard time convincing their husbands to go for an IVF. However, the hardest moments were when they wanted to continue with another cycle of IVF after a failed cycle. In those cases, husbands sometimes blamed their wives for wasting time and money, and they did their best to stop them from undergoing any further cycles of IVF. The constant struggle between women and their husbands upended matrimonial harmony.

Sacrifices in lifestyle

Some of the women in the IVF clinics were housewives who were not accustomed to physical exercise. Some of them smoked. Some did not have the best nutritional knowledge or habits. The director of the North IVF clinic would always suggest lifestyle changes to each couple in his first meeting with them. Below is an example:

> You need to work out. You cannot sit down all day and expect your body to function optimally. Your bodies need activity, so start moving. Walk a couple of kilometres everyday. You cannot smoke and wait to be a parent. Smoking is poison, it is unhealthy for both of you, and it kills sperm. Do not poison yourself. Additionally, it is bad for the child; so stop smoking now. Do you eat pastries all day? Avoid that and eat nutritious food. You need to take care of your bodies. Your bodies will produce this child. You are going to be parents; so be responsible.

"Be responsible" highlights this physician's perception of parenting which starts even before conception. Responsibility, which one would expect from a parent, is also expected by parents-to-be. I observed that women were usually willing to behave like parents, and make all the necessary lifestyle changes that were asked of them.

It is important to note that the couple's adoption of a parenting mindset was fueled by the woman's efforts. This finding supports the theoretical concept of sacrificial motherhood. Although men begrudgingly joined the cause (they became involved in the IVF treatment, quit smoking, etc.), women were more unanimously willing to start parenting than their husbands, who were reluctant to attempt treatment. These women's narratives expressed the pride they felt for making radical changes in their lives.

Sacrifice as proud suffering

Some women considered IVF a battle to be won, and welcomed the hardships related to treatment. I was surprised to witness a sense of comfort from those hardships. Suffering such as health complications, funding problems, or failed cycles bolstered their self-esteem. Suffering emerged as an essential component of parenting and the onset of suffering signalled the onset of parenting. Many of them considered completing a cycle of IVF as a great accomplishment on the path to having a child. The more suffering they endured, the greater their sense of pride for having accomplished a daunting project ("project" being my idiom). In the example below, a woman from the North IVF clinic undergoing IVF for the first time explained her willingness to struggle in order to conceive a child. The more she must endure, the more satisfying her success will be:

> There are people who struggle to conceive a child for years, my uncle and his wife for example. I want to struggle for this as well. I know I will love the child more if it is my achievement. I will say: "I did this. I fought for it, and I made it come true." The child will be the fruit of my battle. It will be my child.
>
> (23-year-old woman married for three years. She had been a textile worker when she was single, now she is a housewife)

The sacrifices made for treatment become a rhetorical tool women use to identify with parenthood. They can downplay such hardships in the greater context of parenthood, accepting that sacrifice is precisely what parents do. This approach naturalized the sacrifices made for the IVF treatment and even prepared the women for the permanent mindset of parenthood.

Paxson's (2004, pp. 98–99) research on ethics and family planning in Athens and her reference to Dubish (1995, pp. 212–217) about Greek motherhood, describe a rhetoric of self-sacrifice by which women demonstrate the difficulties in performing their social roles. Middle-class women reify sacrifice to the extent that chores such as housekeeping become a fetish among them. The women in Paxson's research assess being good mothers by the extent of their giving. The reification of giving as a marker of good mothering corroborates my research findings about the ideals of mothering. Self-sacrifice as a rhetoric of mothering also appears in the narratives of women whom I met in IVF clinics. However, unlike the women in Athens, these women hardly emphasize any difficulties, which is consistent with the rhetoric. Rather than complaining about self-sacrifice, they emphasize their *efforts* and *accomplishments* such as finding money for the treatment or managing relationships with their affines.

The phases of conception and pregnancy are transformational for a woman. The transformation may be challenging when a woman needs to make major life decisions at the same time. Choosing between career and full-time mothering is a common conundrum. During this phase of transformation, it is easier to choose from available identities. Sacrificial motherhood is one of these. For others, sacrificial motherhood may not be a choice: they may be reproducing a hegemonic form of femininity whereby sacrificial mothering is the only way to become adult women. Nowadays, sacrificial mothering has increasingly become intensive mothering, when a woman engages in mothering "activities" and behaviors to the fullest.

Intensive mothering during pregnancy

At the time of interpreting my research data for the purpose of writing this chapter, I am expecting a baby. My personal experience as a pregnant Turkish woman who lives in Los Angeles, California has informed my interpretations. Therefore, below I reflect on my pregnancy experience.

I had not been aware of how I might have appropriated the ideals of intensive parenting until one day during a conversation with a friend. When my friend learnt that I wanted to have a natural birth, she exclaimed: "Are you crazy? Why is that? Do you know that down there it will always be too large for good sex? Have a c-section, you will be thankful … unless of course you want to act like a perfect mother."

I still want to have a natural birth, but this conversation awakened me to the fact that I might also be reproducing the hegemony of perfect mothering. I chose not to have a home-birth with a midwife as opposed to the growing trend in Los Angeles among many of my friends. I wanted to consider every major decision concerning the baby's safety as opposed to those moms-to-be who in my view acted based on their birth fantasies. Now, I look at myself, and consider that may be I have been acting like a perfect mother, and they are just taking it easy.

I realize I am not taking it very easy. I searched for the best birth class, but now I am dissatisfied because I feel another class may have been better, but I failed to find it. I have also taken breast-feeding and baby-care classes in order to learn the best methods of nursing and baby-care. I do prenatal yoga, walk daily for an hour and work out. I do squats everyday in order to strengthen my legs, because the doulas in Los Angeles describe it as the ideal pose for birthing. I have tortured myself with hours of squats, and I am not even in labor yet. Each day I read about pregnancy, childcare, lactation, vaccinations, coping with a crying baby, and ways to put the child to sleep. Spare time at my computer is spent selecting nursery items, or perusing pregnancy and parenting websites. I consult the "my pregnancy" application on my smart phone every day. I am working on our "birth plan." It is a letter to the hospital outlining the procedures and overall experience that I prefer for childbirth. It also includes my preferences regarding the environment (dim lights during labor and birth, for example), and procedures immediately following the birth (skin to skin contact with the baby for an hour before he is washed, no use of pitocin (synthetic oxytocin) for postpartum contractions, and so forth). I just downloaded dolphin sounds onto my iPod for the baby to listen to. Before going to bed I write in a journal about that day, so our son will have an idea of our experience while expecting him.

Among all these parenting activities, I try to fit in writing an academic journal article, completing job applications, or launching my website. At the end of the day, when these projects are incomplete, I feel guilty that I have not done enough. Thank goodness for the discourse of sacrifice, with which I am justified in shifting priorities towards motherhood. I am practising perfect parenting by these intensive parenting activities. This necessitates sacrifice and my incomplete projects confirm this. As a mom-to-be, I am sacrificing my career and my achievements for my son-to-be while I prioritize mothering activities. I am already intensive parenting.

My husband has also shown signs of prenatal intensive parenting. One morning, after reading a section from his book *The Expectant Father* (Ash and Brott 2001), he started poking my belly. After one poke, he says "one." After two pokes, he says "two." To my surprise, he explained that learning starts in the womb. Teaching the fetus how to count certainly seemed to raise the bar on intensive parenting! As I was telling him I don't want us to be overzealous parents, who read Shakespeare to their babies in utero, he told me about the benefits of the poking exercise for brain development and mentioned a product called "prenatal university." I discovered that Rene Van de Carr,[5] who is considered a pioneer in prenatal learning, suggests that learning for a baby starts as early as five months into pregnancy. Babies who receive prenatal stimulation he admits, have better skills for coping with the outside world. In my view, prenatal teaching efforts by couples make an exemplar of intensive parenting before birth.

The idea that parenting begins with conception is not uncommon. Our prenatal education instructor stated, "parenting starts before birth." Among the documents she has given us to read, one of them states:

> An additional reason for parents to begin active parenting at conception is the discovery that babies in the womb are also developing more rapidly than previously thought possible. From the second month of pregnancy, experiments and observations reveal an active prenate with a rapidly developing sensory system permitting exquisite sensitivity and responsiveness.
>
> They seem especially interested in the larger environment provided by mother and father, and react to individual voices, stories, music and even simple interaction games with parents. The quality of the uterine environment is determined principally by parents (...). Now there is mounting evidence for memory and learning in utero and for precocious communication before the stage of language. These abilities of unborn babies underlie the successes reported in a series of scientific experiments with prenatal stimulation and bonding.

This approach of "active parenting" turns the womb into a classroom where the parents are teachers and the fetus is a student.[6] The teachers (the parents) need to be persistent, giving the same instructions every day at the same time. Their persistence and high involvement in teaching enhances the "quality of the uterine environment" aka the prenatal classroom. The student is expected to cooperate. She is expected to give responses to visual, audio or tactile stimuli from her parents. She is also expected to show the positive outcomes of her training in the prenatal university: To be a calm, peaceful postpartum baby and to show early and easy learning skills. Nonetheless, the document where the above quote comes from does not speak of the ways in which children are affected by the high expectations set by their parents for learning even before they are born.[7]

Intensive parenting appears differently in Los Angeles than in Istanbul. Had I been in Istanbul during my pregnancy, a great deal of the preparation, training and support for childbirth would not have taken place simply because those concerns are not prevalent there yet. Activities and concerns such as prenatal yoga, birth or breast-feeding classes, swaddling techniques, midwives, doulas and birth plans are the results of a society steeped in the information age and a constant striving for a "best practice." In Istanbul, the doulas would have been replaced by family members and friends keen to share their expertise in baby-care. The tension between a male-centered medical birthing world and a female-centered natural birthing world is not yet apparent as the patriarchal tendencies in Turkey are still firmly set in place. In Istanbul the intensive parenting would appear in the form of excessive concern for the well-being of the child, and in the sacrifice of self for the needs of the child. In Los Angeles, one can be more pro-natural in terms of the activities one does or products one purchases.

Despite the parenting differences between Istanbul and Los Angeles, there remains a distinct similarity. Having been immersed in an ideology of sacrificial motherhood in Istanbul, I have felt at home here with the intensive, child-centered prenatal practices. My practices and purchases may be different but the pressure to be a responsible and perfect mother even before birth is the same. I naturally adhere to such intensive parenting practices now due to an internalized sacrificial motherhood script from my formative years. I am able to claim certain positive credentials (such as sacrifice) related to being a good mother before I give birth to my son.

Conclusion

As a mother-to-be who is already engaged in intensive parenting, I have insight into the experience of IVF-pursuing women and their intensive parenting. My enthusiasm for mothering is directly related to my intensive parenting activities. The ideals of parenting to which I subscribe are shaped within a habitus composed of my social life in Los Angeles among artists, my feminist academic career, and my upbringing in Turkey where sacrificial motherhood is hegemonic. I am also shaped by my reaction to certain aspects of these hegemonies (such as deciding against home-birth with a midwife which opposes feminist ideals and the popular trends of my social circles in Los Angeles). As a "responsible parent" (as the director of the North IVF clinic described) I am prepared to alter my lifestyle and be intensively involved in parenting for the "best interests" of the child. These best interests are informed by the contemporary ideals and trends of raising a child. By exhibiting this involvement in parenting even before giving birth, I reproduce the ideals of sacrificial mothering.

The women in my research who undergo IVF are also excited about the prospect of being a mother. During the IVF treatment, after a woman's ova is extracted and fertilized with sperm from her husband, the embryo is transferred to the uterus of the woman.[8] After the transfer, there is a waiting period of about two to three weeks before the pregnancy test. During this time, many of the women are hopeful, and consider themselves pregnant with the baby–embryo in their womb. Despite anxiety about the result, many of them start seeing themselves as moms-to-be and act as such. For their babies, there is nothing they would not do. They start sacrificial activities sometimes from the onset of the treatment. They spend time visiting fertility websites, sharing their experiences, fears and hopes. On cocukistiyorum.com (which means: I want a child.com), I have read about women praying (citing a sura from the Koran) for each other many times a day. The women discuss what is good to eat and drink and to do during the waiting period. They are already intensely engaged in mothering before being mothers – just as I am.

Enthusiasm for parenting is not the whole picture for IVF-pursuing women. Since IVF is usually a last resort to conceive a child, the extent to which women can engage in parenting or sacrificing can be high. Some of these women have tried to conceive a child for years. They have had to encounter stigma attached to childlessness in Turkey. The types of stigma they had to abide with include the perception of infertility as sexual impotency for men, making their maleness (*erkeklik*) ambiguous. Another kind of stigma is related to women's adult identities. For many women, motherhood is essential to achieving complete adulthood or womanhood. Some women start IVF treatment because they need a son to negotiate their adult gender identities. Negotiating gender identities is a process, whereby women want to have children (or sons), and then eventually they expect their children to get married so that they become powerful mothers-in-law one day. Once she has a grandchild (or a grandson), a woman's womanhood and power within the female members of her extended family are firmly established. For these women, having a child is the initial step in this long path to womanhood. Not all women in Turkey need grandchildren or daughters-in-law to negotiate their gender identities. However, most of the women in my research needed a child to complete their adult gender identities.

Complete adulthood or womanhood entails mothering and all of its implications. Being capable of sacrifice, and doing whatever is required to care for a child are the ideal markers of mothering. Childless women are left at the periphery of womanhood when they are viewed as lacking the capacity to understand mothering or making sacrifices for a child. For some childless women, this is a motivation to engage in intensive parenting and sacrifices even before they conceive. It is their method of re-establishing their contested adult gender identities. They reproduce themselves as mothers and complete women while they reproduce with IVF. Intensive parenting is a Western concept but it easily fits into mothering discourses and practices in Turkey under the rubric of being a perfect mother, aka a sacrificial mother. This article argued that, IVF-pursuing women reproduce a hegemonic femininity of intensive mothering even before they become mothers as a means to negotiate their adult gender identities.

Notes

1 The names of the research participants and IVF clinics are pseudonyms.
2 According to Inhorn (1994, 1996), urban poor women in Egypt also go to great lengths in their "quest for conception" (Inhorn 1994).
3 For a discussion regarding the latest legislation in Turkey, please see Gürtin-Broadbent (2010) and Gürtin (2011).
4 According to Dally (1982, pp. 97–103), the discourse that the child needs her mother's constant presence started with a report written by Bowlby in 1951 regarding a study for the United Nations about the needs of homeless children. The UK government generalized the findings of the research to all children, and started promoting the idea that mother–infant love is essential to the mental health of children. The idealization of motherhood with such propaganda became widely prevalent both in the UK and USA. Dally notes that such idealization of motherhood appeared at a time when women started to have careers and more power. Keeping the women at home with their children also was useful for politicians who did not have to worry about creating solutions for the care of children of working mothers.
5 Available at www.brillbaby.com/early-learning/experts/rene-van-de-carr-1.php.
6 It should be noted that, as I choose to use the word "fetus" in order to emphasize my view that pregnancy is too early for starting any education, the people who support prenatal learning prefer the words "prenate" or "unborn child," and totally avoid the use of "fetus," so that parents can be conceived to the logic of prenatal education.
7 Elkind (2001) argues that the pressure for early intellectual attainment, rather than having any advantages on learning, is a major source of stress for children.
8 At the time of my research, up to three (in certain cases up to four) embryos could be transferred in one cycle of IVF in Turkey. As of March 6, 2010, the latest legislation on IVF permits only SET (single embryo transfer). In certain cases such as women over age 34, transfer of two embryos is allowed.

References

Ash, J. and Brott, A. 2001. *The Expectant Father.* New York: Abbeville Press.
Clarke, M. 2009. *Islam and the New Kinship: Reproductive technology and the shariah in Lebanon.* New York/Oxford: Berghahn Books.
Clarke, M. 2008. New kinship, Islam and the liberal tradition: sexual morality and new reproductive technology in Lebanon. *Journal of the Royal Anthropological Institute,* 14(1), pp. 153–169.
Clarke, M. 2007a. The modernity of milk kinship. *Social Anthropology,* 15(3), pp. 1–18.
Clarke, M. 2007b. Closeness in the age of mechanical reproduction: debating kinship and biomedicine in Lebanon and the Middle East. *Anthropological Quarterly,* 80(2), pp. 379–402.
Clarke, M. 2007c. Children of the revolution: 'Ali Khamene'i's "Liberal" views on *in vitro* fertilisation. *British Journal of Middle Eastern Studies,* 34(3), pp. 287–303.
Clarke, M. 2007d. Kinship, propriety and assisted reproduction in the Middle East. *Anthropology of the Middle East,* 2(1), pp. 71–91.
Clarke, M. 2006a. Shiite perspectives on kinship and new reproductive technologies. *ISIM Review,* 17(1), pp. 26–27.
Clarke, M. 2006b. Islam, kinship and new reproductive technology. *Anthropology Today,* 22(5), pp. 17–20.
Çelebi, E. 2011. SGK kesenin ağzını açtı, Türkiye tüp bebekte dünya yedincisi oldu [SGK (Social Security Association) started spending more, Turkey became the seventh in

global ranking. *Hürriyet*, [online] 13 February 2011. Available at www.hurriyet.com. tr/yazarlar/17008882_p.asp [accessed on 2 May 2011].

Dally, A. 1982. *Inventing Motherhood: The consequences of an ideal.* New York: Schocken Books.

Dubish, J. 1995. *In a Different Place: Pilgrimage, gender and politics at a Greek island shrine.* Princeton, NJ: Princeton University Press.

Elkind, D. 2001. *The Hurried Child: Growing up too fast too soon.* Cambridge, MA: Perseus.

Gürtin, Z.B. 2011. Banning reproductive travel? Turkey's ART legislation and third-party assisted reproduction. *Reproductive Biomedicine Online*, 23(5), pp. 555–564, online, available at: www.rbmojournal.com/article/S1472-6483%2811%2900470-6/fulltext.

Gürtin-Broadbent, Z. 2010. Problems with legislating against "reproductive 'tourism." *Commentary for BioNews*, pp. 550, online, available at: www.bionews.org.uk/page_56954.asp.

Inhorn, M.C. 2006. Making Muslim babies, IVF and gamete donation in Sunni versus Shi'a Islam. *Culture, Medicine and Psychiatry*, 30(4), pp. 427–450.

Inhorn, M.C. 2004. Middle Eastern masculinities in the age of new reproductive technologies: male infertility and stigma in Egypt and Lebanon. *Medical Anthropological Quarterly*, 18(2), pp. 162–182.

Inhorn, M. C. 1996. *Infertility and Patriarchy: The cultural politics of gender and family life in Egypt.* Philadelphia, PA: University of Pennsylvania Press.

Inhorn, M.C. 1994. *Quest for Conception: Gender, infertility and Egyptian medical traditions.* Philadelphia, PA: University of Pennsylvania Press.

Mauthner, N.S. and Doucet, A. 2003. Reflexive accounts and accounts of reflexivity in qualitative data analysis. *Sociology*, 37(3), pp. 413–431.

Paxson, H. 2004. *Making Modern Mothers: Ethics and family planning in urban Greece.* Berkeley, CA: University of California Press.

Tremayne, S. 2006. Not all Muslims are luddites. *Anthropology Today*, 22(3), pp. 1–2.

13 Intensive parenting alone

Negotiating the cultural contradictions of motherhood as a single mother by choice

Linda L. Layne

Introduction

Single mothers by choice (SMCs) have been increasing in numbers and visibility in the US since the 1980s. Such women not only buck the nuclear norm, they do so in an era of 'intensive mothering' (Hays 1996; Furedi 2001; Douglas and Michaels 2004; Warner 2006; Katz 2008, 2012), an approach to parenting which places enormous responsibility on mothers to assure that their children have every possible advantage, and judges them by how well their children turn out. Despite empirical data to the contrary (Golombok *et al.* 1997; Golombok and Badger 2010), these maverick mothers are frequently accused of jeopardizing the well-being of their children by not providing a father. In this chapter, I use an in-depth case study to describe how one American single mother by choice (SMC) practically and discursively manages the demands of intensive parenting.

In *The Cultural Contradictions of Motherhood* (1998) sociologist Sharon Hays argues that working mothers in the United States are faced with a cultural contradiction: the challenge of being nurturing and unselfish while engaged in child rearing at home, while competitive and ambitious at work. This case study shows how one mother combines two of the current ideologies of intensive mothering – 'Attachment' and 'Tiger Mothering' – despite the fact that proponents define these approaches as antithetical. These approaches each address one side of the cultural contradiction Hays identifies between the ideologies of private and public spheres. Combining them is one practical way of negotiating competing demands and bridging the spheres. This case shows that it is possible for an SMC to meet the demanding standards of 'intensive mothering,' and suggests that, in several important ways, SMCs may actually be more able to do so than heterosexually-partnered parents. Whether or not this is a good thing is debatable.

'Carmen'[1] is typical of American SMCs in that she is heterosexual, highly-educated, financially stable, and was over 35 when she joined the organization Single Mothers by Choice to explore the possibility of having children on her own. She differs from most SMCs in that she is an ethnic minority. Born of an Asian immigrant mother and an Eastern European-American father, she identifies herself as Asian-American.

In 2005, at the age of 40, Carmen gave up a tenure-track teaching position at a prestigious university to move back to the Northeast in order to be closer to her aging mother and her brothers and their families. She used her savings to make a down payment on a triplex. She occupies the ground floor which includes a back yard and garage. Rent from the two upper units covers her mortgage, property tax and insurance. During the study period she was fixing up the house she had inherited from her father in order to rent it. In supplementing her wage income this way, Carmen resembles many other American SMCs (Hertz 2006: 226).

At age 42, after a period of internet dating, Carmen bought five vials of 'open identity sperm' from California Cryo Bank and was inseminated in her fertility doctor's office, in what is ironically termed 'spontaneous IUI.' She did not get pregnant and the next cycle used 'stimulated IUI' which entailed self-administration of daily shots to encourage multiple eggs to develop. That insemination resulted in the birth of Maria in June 2007.

Her fertility specialist emphasized that if she wanted to have another child, she should not delay. There were no more 'specimens' from the donor she'd used, so the sperm bank contacted him and he agreed to donate more. When Maria was 15 months old, Carmen used the same method that had worked before and was successful on her first try, becoming pregnant at age 44, three months after having being hired as the manager of a division of an engineering firm. To her utter surprise, an early sonogram revealed twins. Maternity leave allowed her to stop going to office two weeks before Nel and Toby were born.

Methods

As is typical for case studies (Reinharz 1992; Stake 2000; Yin 1993), multiple methods were used. I interviewed Carmen two evenings in July 2011, after her children were asleep, about whether she considered her parenting to conform to Hay's (1996: 8) definition of 'intensive parenting,' i.e. 'child-centered, expert-guided, emotionally absorbing, labor intensive, and financially expensive.' Following our interviews Carmen shared further thoughts she'd had, completed Hay's questionnaire and interview questions (which are included as appendices in her book), and answered additional questions via email. This process continued over subsequent months with over 100 exchanges relating to this study taking place between July 2011 and February 2012.

Another source of data was participant observation. I have known Carmen since 2005 when she rented a room in my house. It was during that year that Carmen became what in SMC parlance is 'a thinker,' someone considering undertaking parenthood in this way. We developed a close friendship, and when she became pregnant, I was happy to accompany her to childbirth classes. My partner and I are her children's godparents and our families regularly celebrate birthdays and holidays together. During the designated research week, I made a point of spending extra time with them. We had four get-togethers that week including a Godfather's Day barbecue. Because of our close family ties, I have an extensive cache of photos of her family which provided additional documentary evidence. Carmen, in turn, mined her own photo archive, discovering photos that document aspects of her early mothering practices she had overlooked.

Because of our close personal relationship, the advantages and limitations of such a study are similar to those of doing autoethnography. I have explored these methodological issues in the piece I wrote about having a critically-ill newborn in an intensive care unit (Layne 1996). Does my personal involvement make the work un-objective, flaky, and soft and/or does it mean that I have a breadth and depth of knowledge about this family that permits a richer, thicker, more complete, more accurate, more nuanced account? Our relationship can be seen as similar to that of many anthropologists with their 'key informants'[2] – individuals with whom the researcher develops a close, long-term, multifaceted relationship. Given our similar social statuses, my approach is perhaps most akin to collaborative ethnographic projects like Whitaker's (2007) intellectual biography of his friend, a revolutionary Tamil journalist. Whatever its anthropological heritage, such a case study complements the more common methods (clinic ethnographies, semi-structured interviews, questionnaires, textual analysis) used by sociologists and anthropologists studying new reproductive technologies and the family forms they help to create.

'Child-centered': child-led v. parent-led interpretations

Hay's first characteristic of 'intensive mothering' is 'child-centered.' When I asked Carmen whether she considered her parenting to be 'child-centered,' she pointed to the double parlor in which we sat (see Figure 13.1).

> All of this space is dominated by their stuff, clothes, toys, books, and, you know, bills and logistical paperwork for their life. The front parlor is their play area; this half is the living room, but it's really a laundry area, and an overflow play area.

She explained that the filing cabinets by the computer were now filled with files relating to the children:

> That used to be where I kept my graduate research work but now that has all been supplanted with logistical paperwork for their lives – bills, college savings, medical reports, information on our medical and dental insurance, and articles about parenting and budgeting and vacations.

Carmen addressed the term, 'child-centered,' explaining that when she'd seen it on the interview questions I'd provided in advance, she hadn't been 'sure if it meant that children are the highest priority in this parent's life, or if it meant the child supplants everything else, what were formerly single-person-centered projects and interests.' I asked how those two meanings differed and she explained,

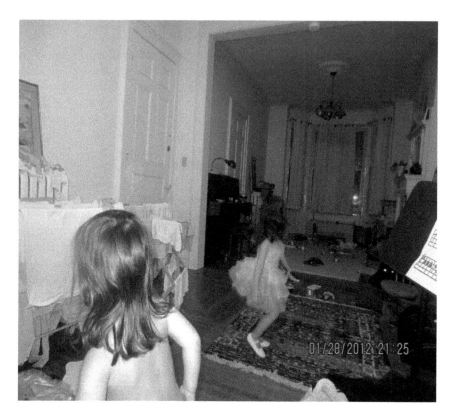

Figure 13.1 Maria and Nel dancing in the parlors, January 2012 (source: photo by
       Carmen).

I think someone could lead a balanced adult life and still keep your child's
interests the highest priority, but I've never seen a single mother by choice
keep that clear, straight, or balanced. What I've seen is the child's (or in my
case children's) priorities overtake, eclipse everything else.[3] You could call
that 'child-centered' or 'child-dominant' or 'child-...', I don't know, some
word like 'overrun' or 'eclipsed,' but those sound pejorative. If I wanted to
force fit my parenting into a compartment of my life I could, but at their det-
riment, and it would be a compromise of how I want to parent and how I
was parented.

For Hay's (1996: 57), 'child-centered' means the mother 'will 'follow the baby's
lead' allowing the child 'to guide the process of child rearing' because they
know who they are and what they need. Carmen understands the term in a completely different way, one that 'rings true' to her 'Asian background.' She
elaborated,

Growing up I often heard, 'Those parents don't care enough about their kids to do X. . . .' like make them wear a helmet when they ride a bike, or make them exercise manners, or make them wait, to enforce structure in their lives, or to make sure they do their best at school, lessons, sports, you name it. You know, all the hard stuff. The reason given to me as I was growing up was that such parents don't care enough to do that work for their kids. They are not 'child-centered', would be one way to put it.

Carmen then brought up *Battle Hymn of The Tiger Mother*, the controversial book published in 2011 by Amy Chua, a professor at Yale's law school and mother of two daughters. Carmen had emailed me the article by Chua (2011), 'Why Chinese Mothers Are Superior,' the day it was published in *The Wall Street Journal*. She bought and read the book, followed the animated public response to it, and discussed it with her mother. Her mother was critical of 'the extremity of Chua's approach and her single focus on achievement (Carnegie Hall, Harvard, etc.)' deeming it 'very old-fashioned and psychologically damaging.' But Carmen says she and her cousin (the daughter of her mother's sister) agree that the mothering described by Chua felt very familiar to what they had experienced – 'There were very hard consequences to disappointing their expectations, especially for their daughters.' But Carmen also noted that because her mom was a single mom (Carmen's parents separated when she was in eighth grade), she couldn't 'enforce those expectations or structure our lives to the same degree' that Chua did.

Carmen feels her upbringing and the approach she is adopting in raising her children differs significantly from that of the other members of the neighborhood kids group she helped found. This contrast informed a recent conversation Carmen had had with the director of Maria's school during which she shared something she says,

> I'm not allowed to say in the downtown community of moms[4] – that I desire a structured environment for my children. A lot of the other moms are at least ten years younger, and they are all for 'the joy of learning, child-guided learning', and it is like, 'What would you like to learn today child?' That's not me. I'm all for structure, nurturing structure. . . . There needs to be an agenda.

The parenting philosophy Carmen attributes to the other moms in her group is often labeled, at least by critics, 'the permissive approach' and is the approach advocated by those enormously popular child-rearing experts, Spock, Brazelton, and Leach, upon whom Hays focuses (1996: 51). When it comes to discipline, these experts 'recommend the careful molding of the child's self-discipline as opposed to demands for compliance to an absolute set of rules' (Hays 1996: 60).

Carmen's approach to discipline is more in line with Tiger Mothering. Carmen said, 'I am so glad that I read [*Tiger Mother*], because it gives me permission to be a hard ass, because that is so out of fashion.' Later in the interview she returned to this issue.

I don't think I'm a child abuser but I can be real rough with them, not physically, although I will plunk them down in a chair pretty quickly or the new timeout is with the bathroom door shut for as many minutes as how old they are (2 or 4) and I feel guilty about it but I think it is good for them because they are not saying 'stupid' anymore, biting is down, pinching is down, and only because I am being a real hard ass and I hate doing that.

Carmen receives support for this approach from her mother and one of her brothers. She explained why she sets store in their views, reminding me that her mother has a Master's in social work, and that her brother took courses in early childhood development for his PhD. 'They say, "Children feel secure with limits … If you don't provide them, you are doing them a disservice. They need them, so you better step up to the plate and provide them."'

'Expert-guided'

When we turned to the second characteristic, 'expert guided,' Carmen asked whether that term 'implied that the mother is the expert or that she seeks expert advice?' I indicated the latter whereupon she suggested we 'count all the parenting books in this house.' Members of the 'middle and professional classes' have been found to be particularly active consumers of the multi-billion dollar child-care advice literature industry (Hoffman 2009: 16–17).[5] In this regard, as in so many others, Carmen is at the 'intense' end of the continuum (cf. Geyboy 1981, Han n.d). That evening she showed me 33 books and two magazines she considers sources of expert guidance for parenting. Of these, 14 books and one magazine were explicitly on parenting including many best sellers such as *Dr. Spock's Baby and Child Care* [1946] which her mother had given her, Faber and Mazlish's *How to Talk so Kids Will Listen and Listen so Kids Will Talk* (1982), and *Parenting Magazine*. Four books were about things to do with children; six books and one magazine were publications not generally considered as parenting resources but which she found useful in her role as a parent, e.g. *The New Yorker*, a book on investments, and the just-issued biography of Obama's mother. She also had eight scholarly books on reproduction which had either been written by or recommended by me. In addition to these printed sources of expertise, Carmen also mentioned documentaries, web-based resources, and a host of people she consults, including friends, family, and professionals.

In a follow-up email she added, 'It occurs to me that expert guidance may mean tons of lessons in the context of intensive parenting' and she listed the lessons Maria has taken (ballet, gymnastics, swimming, Spanish, and violin) and her plans for the twins. This is another way she diverges from the approach to intensive parenting Hays focuses on. One of the authors Hays uses as an exemplar, Leach, is against pushing 'a child to do things early or to be the best at gymnastics or dancing class' because it conveys the message that the parent's love is conditional on achievement and 'that is very damaging' (Lawson 1991).

After our interview, I realized I had not seen the book on 'attachment parenting' (AP) she had discussed with me during her first pregnancy. 'Attachment parenting' is an approach to parenting pioneered by pediatrician William Sears, building on British psychoanalyst John Bowlby's attachment theory, distilled into seven attachment tools, or 'Baby B's,' designed to 'bring out the best' in the baby and the parents (www.askdrsears.com).

'Attachment parenting' falls within the same 'permissive' approach' advocated by Spock [1946], Leach [1977] and Brazelton, all of whom are against 'detached handling, strict scheduling,' and corporal punishment. (Indeed, it is curious that Hays does not address 'attachment parenting', since its principles seem to epitomize what she calls intensive parenting.) Carmen had come across the term on the SMC list serve and searched for books on that topic on Amazon. The one she bought was *Attachment Parenting: Instinctive Care for Your Baby and Young Child* by Katie Allison Granju. Carmen recalls that she was already familiar with the benefits of birth bonding and nursing, but that the book introduced her to the other AP tenets, most importantly, baby wearing and co-sleeping. 'I was convinced that was the way to go, especially for me a single mom. I knew I'd have to work and be away from my child, so wanted to optimize her "positive attachment" to me.' The local SMC contact person with whom she'd developed a friendship advocated AP saying 'it's certainly the more exhausting parenting route, but much more rewarding and healthy for all.'

Box 13.1 Carmen's adoption of Dr. Sear's 7 Baby B's

YES	Birth bonding
YES	Breastfeeding
YES	Bed sharing
NOT APPLICABLE	Belief in baby's cry
SOMEWHAT	Baby wearing
NO	Avoid experts who advocate schedules
NO	Balance – don't neglect your own needs
NOT APPLICABLE	Balance – don't neglect your marriage

Carmen breast fed the twins until 30 months in order 'to try to make up for having held them less, to maximize bonding.' The result, though, was that she now 'felt guilty for not nursing Maria longer' whom she had weaned at 14 months, when she started working again and was ready to try for 'baby #2.' With the twins, she 'pumped at work and came home with plenty of supply for the nanny.' She mixed nursing with bottle feeding of breast milk (sometimes mixed with formula) so that Maria and others could help and to give her nipples a rest. Because she nursed her children for significantly longer than average in the US, her mother and aunt kept asking when she was going to stop breastfeeding. She told them she planned to stop when they turned two but didn't do so because 'all of us seemed to love the nursing so much' (Figure 13.2).

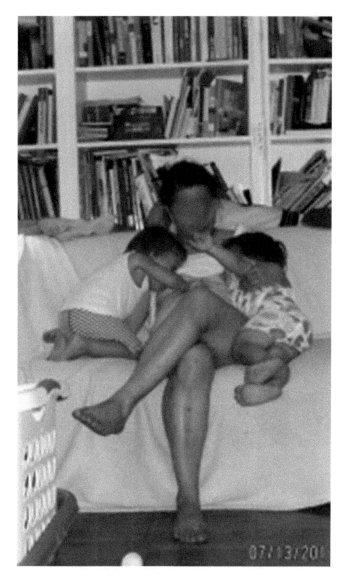

Figure 13.2 Double nursing in parlor, July 2011 (source: photo by Jess Bouchard, reproduced with permission).

Baby wearing proved to be the most challenging for Carmen. 'I needed my hands free to do housework, etc. but didn't find a sling that worked for me.' 'As for wearing the twins, forget it, didn't even try. Still feel guilty about that because they were held much less as infants than Maria was.'

Co-sleeping was easier. Carmen started sleeping with the twins while in the hospital and once home, 'was so grateful that I did not have to get up at all hours to fix formula for them, but could roll to this side or that to feed while remaining half asleep.' During the initial weeks she used 'arms-reach' sleeping, placing the twins on an adjoining mattress or in their car seats, for safety reasons. Carmen explained that one of the reasons co-sleeping worked so well for her is that she doesn't have a sexual partner trying to share the bed. She recalls the book talking about how 'to resolve the competing demands of a sex life in a marital bed with co-sleeping. I remember feeling like the co-sleeping decision is such an obvious 'yes' without that competing and incompatible factor for a single mom.'

Although Carmen has moved the children to their own cribs or beds, she still ends up bed sharing for part of the night. She usually falls asleep with Maria in Maria's bed then gets up and works for two to three hours (from eleven to one or two) 'or until they start migrating to my bed. Maria's usually first, and sometimes I continue working with her beside me in bed[6].... To make up on sleep, about once a week, I just sleep right thru in Maria's bed.'

Carmen diverges from the principles of attachment parenting when it comes to scheduling. Dr. Sear's sixth 'B' is 'Beware' of parenting experts who advocate 'rigid and extreme parenting styles that teach you to watch a clock or a schedule instead of your baby.' In contrast, Carmen imposes a daily routine, remarking that '*If I didn't have a schedule I'd be dead!*' Their 'fixed' daily activities include 'wake up time; breakfast; school drop off; lunch; nap; wake up time; school pick up; afternoon activities/lessons/playdates; dinner; music/practice time, pajamas; teeth; story; bed.'

In addition to her emphasis on bonding, breastfeeding, baby wearing, and co-sleeping, her choice to keep the children home with one primary care-giver (the 'nanny'), rather than sending them to a day-care center, is in keeping with Attachment Parenting advice, whereas Carmen's approach to education, discipline, and daily schedules is more in line with 'Tiger Mothering.'

'Financially expensive'

Carmen and I agreed that the characteristics 'emotionally absorbing' and 'labor intensive' had already been amply demonstrated in her responses to my questions, so we turned to the final defining characteristic of 'intensive parenting' – 'financially expensive.' She addressed this saying,

> I grew up impoverished, I mean really poor and I always worked. I was never a waster of money. I have a respect for it. But since having the children, I've never written so many big checks in rapid succession in my life. Oh, a $1,000 check for school this month, oh, a lesson here, a lesson there, violin, everything is like, 'Okay, here is a few hundred dollars,' every single time. I'm always drained. I would never do it differently. In fact, I love doing it. I love getting the best violin teacher. I love thinking I have the best school placement for her. I love that she is speaking Spanish and I love that

if she wants pink nail polish then I'll buy it for her. I like that. I don't want
her to be a spoiled brat, and there might be some things I need to address
there. I know there are, but I like being able to be her sole provider for
everything, even 'the nice-to-have things.' That is very, very fulfilling for
me, because I don't have to be married to some jerk for that or to have to
negotiate over what is important.

Carmen speculates that she spends a greater part of her household income on her
children than do her married counterparts.

She then told me about a conversation she'd had with another mother at gymnastics. Carmen asked her if her daughter took dance lessons too. The woman
explained she wanted to send her to a well-regarded studio in a nearby city but
her husband thought it was too far away and too expensive and wanted her to go
to the shop down the block. Because they couldn't agree, she wasn't taking
lessons. Carmen's reaction – 'Get a divorce! Of course I wasn't serious, but
what a pain in the butt. I would hate that. So the finances are definitely key.'

Are SMCs better able to be intensive parents; and if so at what cost?

Carmen's case demonstrates that it is possible to carry out the demands of intensive parenting without a second parent helping with bread winning and/or child
care and housework. If Carmen is any indication, the women who choose to
undertake SMCing may be particularly energetic, able, smart, innovative adults;
in other words, those best equipped to engage in this type of parenting.

Furthermore, 'attachment parenting' is premised on the theory that infants
are hard wired to bond with *one* primary caregiver – the mother, who is in turn
literally attached to the baby for as many hours of every day as possible – by
breastfeeding on demand, bed-sharing, and wearing the baby throughout the
day. It is hard to imagine how one could do this and tend to the needs of one's
marriage.

The last of Dr. Sear's '7 B's' is 'Strive for Balance in Your Personal and
Family Life, ensuring that everyone's needs – not just the child's – are recognized, validated, and met to the greatest extent possible.' One of their tips for
maintaining family balance is to 'Be creative in finding ways to spend couple
time.' The picture that illustrates this is of a man and woman dancing, but not as
a couple, but rather as a three-some; the baby is attached to the mother in a front
carrier and thus positioned between them.

Indeed, in some of the attachment families Faircloth studied, the husband had
moved to another room in order to get enough sleep to go to work. One of her
participants, Lauren, a 42-year-old mother of a two-and-a-half-year-old daughter
she was still breastfeeding reported the disastrous effects of these mothering
practices on her marriage. 'I have a strong relationship with my daughter, we are
very close, physically. But with my husband, it is a catastrophe.' Other women
also described the negative effects attachment parenting had on their physical

relationship with their partner. They 'would frequently talk about being "touched-out"' by 'breastfeeding their children, and disinclined to be in physical contact with their partners.' Several felt their husbands were jealous of the breastfeeding. One woman suggested that mothers should 'compensate' for the fact that their partner is 'left out' of attachment parenting by having sex with him even if they don't feel like doing so (Faircloth 2013, Chapter 6).

Furthermore, numerous studies show that the number of hours that American women devote to house work increases significantly when they marry. For example, a 2005 study (Swanbrow 2008) based on time-diary data of a nationally representative sample of US families found that 'having a husband creates an extra seven hours a week of housework for women.' Because of cultural norms about wifely roles and gendered standards of cleanliness, having a man in the house does not decrease the amount of work to be done because it is shared; on the contrary, it significantly increases, the amount of housework women feel obliged to do.[7]

In SMC families, it may be that women are devoting less time to housekeeping and meal preparation than in coupled families. In contrast to the way her own mother managed her household, Carmen explained, 'I always choose to engage my kids emotionally or their interests or lessons or homework over doing housework.'[8] The result is that her house could be described as in a state of 'severe untidiness,' much like that of a British SMC, Julie Wise, who explains that as she raises her adopted son there is no one to help with 'cooking, washing up, cleaning, tidying, gardening...' and that she is often torn between doing chores and playing more with her son. By the time he is asleep she is usually 'too wacked to catch up on chores that I've missed. It can pile up' (Wise 2007: 9, 83–84). Carmen remembers wistfully one nanny she fired because she was not good with the children but who was great at straightening up. 'I would come home and say, "Oh my God I can just boil an egg. I don't have to wash the pot first."'

If the critics of the ideology of intensive parenting (Hays 1996; Douglas and Michaels 2004; Warner 2006; Katz 2008, 2012) are right and this type of mothering hurts women, are SMCs particularly vulnerable to this harm? By her own report, Carmen's self-care is poor.

> It is really taking a toll on my health and on my fuse. More self-care needs to be happening here but I am not quite sure how to achieve that. One concrete way is to purchase a bigger home, because I need an office. I need space. I can't do anything here, not even pay my bills in peace. The bills get scattered all around and my files are on top of toys. I think it is emotionally unhealthy for me, because I have always had only my space. Then suddenly I have none. Even my bed, my breast, it is all available to them. I don't think a boyfriend is going to balance that. I should go to a gym or run. Before having the children, I always ran or did something aerobic. I have gained weight. I just look awful. They even thought I had an enlarged thyroid because I had gained this weight.

Furthermore, in terms of work, she is definitely on 'the mommy track.' One month after the designated research week she lost her job; her company down-sized and the unit she managed was eliminated. In some ways Carmen is relieved. The strain had been enormous.[9] She doesn't foresee returning to a 9–5 job as she found it very difficult to be 'fully there' at work and noted she could no longer put in the hours as she had done before children.

Conclusions

The cultural contradictions that concern Hays stem from the opposing 'logics' of private and public spheres that working mothers must negotiate. A mother's 'primary responsibility is to maintain the logic that dominates family and inti-mate life, a logic requiring a moral commitment to unremunerated relation-ships grounded in affection and mutual obligations' (Hays 1996: 152). At the same time, 'as a paid working woman,' she must operate according to the logic of the public sphere, 'a logic emphasizing the individualist, calculating, com-petitive pursuit of personal gain' (1996: 152). This late twentieth/early twenty-first century concern is a variation of one that arose in the US during the first half of the nineteenth century. Meyer observes, 'With fathers steadily more intent upon the marketplace, obviously mothers would be spending more time with the children.' Given 'the ... maternal pedagogy stressing love as the proper means of a mother's suasions,' how were mothers supposed to 'prepare' their sons 'for the challenges of the competitive democratic marketplace?' (1987: 272). Whereas in the early nineteenth century, the contradiction between the logics of home and marketplace was problematical only for sons, today children of both sexes are expected to enter the world of work. The opposing approaches to parenting whether labeled 'romantic' v. 'rational-efficiency' (Buskens 2001: 75), 'unstructured' v 'structured' (Faircloth 2013), or 'Attachment' v. 'Tiger', can be understood as aligned with the opposing logics of the private and public spheres. 'Attachment Parenting' is patently about forming loving, close, relations within the home; the essence of Tiger Mothering is to prepare children for a lifetime of stellar achievements out in the world (Chua 2012: 49).

As we saw, Carmen combined these two purportedly contradictory approaches – 'Attachment Parenting' to 'maximize bonding' and 'Tiger Mother-ing' to prepare her children to succeed. 'Attachment parenting' was popular among her local parenting community, but alien to her family of origin; Tiger Mothering was familiar to her family of origin, but rejected by her local parent-ing community. Carmen used books by proponents of both approaches to justify her choices.

Watching Carmen deploy these philosophies makes plain that despite their marked differences, both are forms of 'intensive parenting', i.e. they are 'child-centered, expert-guided, emotionally absorbing, labor intensive, and financially expensive' though, as we saw, what is meant by 'child-centered' and 'expert guided' are quite different. As for 'labor intensive,' advocates of each approach each approach claim that theirs is 'the hardest', and therefore, the most praise-worthy, and that the outcomes are worth it (Chua 2012: 53, 148; Hays 1996: 120).

A case like this, that shows how one actual mother puts multiple philosophies of parenting into practice, illustrates some of the challenges that face middle-class American parents today, as well as some of the unique challenges of being an SMC. Hays asks, why do career women engage in intensive mothering practices that 'drain away her time, interfere with her pursuit of financial rewards, diminish her status, and leave her feeling exhausted and inadequate by the end of her daily double shift?' (1996: 152). Carmen would answer: because there is nothing she would rather be doing, nothing she'd rather be spending her money on, and though she is often exhausted, she is also exhilarated by the challenge. This is how Carmen feels on her way to work:

> I am very happy after I leave home and the twins are set up for breakfast with the nanny, and I take Maria to school and we have our hugs goodbye. She is all set with her lunch and her bathing suit and her sunscreen and everything, and I'm on my way to work, *and I'm on time*. I was just screaming to myself in the car, *'I am by far happier than any other time in my life, by far. Hands down, no comparison to any other time.'*

But are the critics right in claiming that intensive mothering is an ideological trap which serves the interests of those in power, 'men, whites, the upper classes, capitalists and state leaders' (Hays 1996: 153)? Let's concede that 'intensive mothering' serves the interests of those in power. That does not mean that it does not also serve the interests of those women privileged enough to engage in it. American middle-class women who are SMCs like Carmen belong to a category of persons who enjoy power, enjoying an unprecedented level of freedom.

Acknowledgments

Obviously, this paper could not have been written without Carmen's generosity and cooperation. I would not have ventured into this study were it not for Carmen's encouragement and Charlotte Faircloth's pioneering work on intensive parenting. I am grateful to Rensselaer for the sabbatical leave which enabled me to write this while a visiting Fellow at Cambridge's Centre for Family Research, which, thanks to the direction of Susan Golombok, was the perfect environment for such a project. I benefited from regular conversations with Martin Richards, and with Barbara Bodenhorn, whose appreciation of my methodological innovations emboldened me. As ever, G.J. (Ben) Barker-Benfield, remains, my cherished, invariably positive intellectual companion.

Notes

1 At my invitation, she selected the pseudonyms for herself and her children.
2 'Key informants' are defined as 'individuals selected on the basis of criteria such as knowledge, compatibility, age, experience, or reputation who provide information about their culture' http://oregonstate.edu/instruct/anth370/gloss.html
3 Similarly, Julia Wise, a British single woman who adopted her son reports in her memoir, *Flying Solo* (2007: 79), 'my entire life became "Alan-centric" and "I" started to disappear along with my personal aspirations.' Wise contrasts her situation with single mothers 'who are divorced where child goes to other parent for a weekend or even week and allows mum to establish a separate life' (2007: 81).
4 This group of mothers operates as a negative reference group for Carmen, much as the Spanish mothers do for the Dominican mothers described by Jiménez Sedano (this volume), and the parents who appear on *Supernanny* (as well as the show's presumed viewers) do for the parents described by Jensen (this volume).
5 Hoffman (2009: 17) notes that 'while parenting advice is saturated with expert opinion, "expert" is a rather ambiguous term' and the 'advice given by well-known parenting experts' is often different from 'best practice standards supported by academic research.'
6 Forgoing sleep is a very common strategy used by working mothers, even those who are married. Hochschild (2012) notes how frequent the subject of sleep was brought up by the married working mothers in two-income families (and how infrequent it was mentioned by the husbands).
7 See Hays (1996: 99–100) for data on this among her sample.
8 A related finding is that single mothers may feel less 'time strain' (i.e., the feeling that they aren't spending as much time with their children as they would like) than married mothers 'because they are generally able to spend … more one-on-one time' with their children (Milkie *et al.* 2004: 758). Married women report feeling less time strain if their husbands work long hours, i.e. if they are parenting in an environment more like that of a single mother (Milkie *et al.* 2004: 758).
9 See Layne (2012) for a discussion of the anxieties that stem from intensive mothering alone.

References

Buskens, P. (2001) 'The Impossibility of "Natural Parenting" for Modern Mothers: On Social Structure and the Formation of Habit' *Journal of the Association for Research on Mothering* 3(1): 75–86.
Chua, A. (2011) 'Why Chinese Mothers Are Superior' *The Wall Street Journal* January 8.
Chua, A. (2012) [2011] *Battle Hymn of The Tiger Mother*. London: Bloomsbury.
Douglas, S.J. and Michaels, M.W. (2004) *The Mommy Myth: The Idealization of Mother-hood and How it has Undermined All Women*. New York: Free Press.
Faircloth, C. (2013) *'Militant Lactivism'? Infant Care and Maternal Identity Work in the UK and France*. Oxford/New York: Berghahn Books.
Furedi, Frank (2001) *Paranoid Parenting: Abandon Your Anxieties and Be a Good Parent*, London: Penguin.
Geboy, M.J. (1981) 'Who is Listening to the "Experts": The Use of Child Care Materials by Parents' *Family Relations* 30(2): 205–210.
Golombok, S. and Badger, S. (2010) 'Children Raised in Fatherless Families from Infancy: A Follow-up of Children of Lesbian and Single Heterosexual Mothers in Early Adulthood' *Human Reproduction* 25 (1): 150–157.
Golombok, S., Tasker, F., and Murray, C. (1997) 'Children Raised in Fatherless Families from Infancy: Family Relationships and the Socioemotional Development of Children

of Lesbian and Single Heterosexual Mothers' *Journal of Child Psychology and Psychiatry* 38(7): 783–792.

Han, S. (n.d.) *Making Babies in America: An Ethnography of Ordinary Pregnancy.* Unpublished book manuscript.

Hays, S. (1996) *The Cultural Contradictions of Motherhood.* New Haven: Yale University Press.

Hertz, R. (2006) *Single by Chance, Mothers by Choice: How Women are Choosing Parenthood without Marriage and Creating the New American Family.* Oxford: Oxford University Press.

Hochschild, A. with Machung, A. (2012) *The Second Shift: Working Families and the Revolution at Home.* New York: Penguin.

Hoffman, D.M. (2009) 'How (Not) to Feel: Culture and the Politics of Emotion in the American Parenting Advice Literature' *Discourse: Studies in the Cultural Politics of Education* 30(1): 15–31.

Katz, C. (2008) 'Childhood as Spectacle: Relays of Anxiety and the Reconfiguration of the Child' *Cultural Geographies* 15(1): 5–17.

Katz, C. (2012) 'Just Managing: American Middle-Class Parenthood in Insecure Times' in *The Global Middle Classes: Theorizing Through Ethnography.* Edited by Rachel Heiman, Carla Freeman, and Mark Liechty. Sante Fe, NM: School of Advanced Research Press, pp. 169–187

Lawson, C. (1991) 'Growing up with Help from Penelope Leach: Advice from a Doctor and Mother' *New York Times* June 13, C1.

Layne, L.L. (1996) '"How's the Baby Doing?": Struggling with Narratives of Progress in a Neonatal Intensive Care Unit' *Medical Anthropology Quarterly* special issue, 'Biomedical Technologies: Reconfiguring Nature and Culture' ed. Barbara Koenig, 10(4): 624–656.

Layne, L.L. (2010) 'Donors and Daddies, Fathers and Lovers: The Presence of (Mostly) Absent Men in Narratives of Single Mothers by Choice' Special issue on Men and Motherhood, ed. Sallie Han. *Phoebe: Gender and Cultural Critiques* 21(2): 1–20.

Layne, L.L. (2012) '"I have a fear of really screwing it up": The Fears, Doubts, Anxieties, and Judgments in the Experience of One American Single Mother by Choice' presented at the workshop 'Parenting: kinship, expertise and anxiety' European Association of Social Anthropologists, Nanterre University, France, July, under review, *Journal of Family Issues.*

Meyer, Donald (1987) *Sex and Power: The Rise of Women in America, Russia, Sweden, and Italy.* Middletown, CT: Wesleyan University Press.

Milke, M.A., Mattingly, M.J., Nomaguchi, K.M., Bianchi, S.B., and Robinson, J.P. (2004) 'The Time Squeeze: Parental Statuses and Feelings about Time With Children' *Journal of Marriage and Family* 66(3): 739–761.

Reinharz, S. (1992) 'Feminist Case Studies' *Feminist Methods in Social Research.* Oxford: Oxford University Press, pp. 164–174.

Stake, R.E. (2000) 'Case Studies' in *Handbook of Qualitative Research.* 2nd edn. Edited by N.K. Denzin and Y.S. Lincoln. Thousand Oaks: Sage, pp. 435–454.

Swanbrow, D. (2008) Exactly how much housework does a husband create? *Michigan Today,* April 3, online, available at: http://ns.umich.edu/new/releases/6452 [accessed January 4, 2012].

Warner, Judith (2006) *Perfect Madness: Motherhood in the Age of Anxiety.* New York. Riverhead Books.

Whitaker, Mark (2007) *Learning Politics from Sivaram: The Life and Death of a Revolutionary Tamil Journalist in Sri Lanka.* London: Pluto Press.

Wise, Julia (2007) *Flying Solo: A Single Parent's Adoption Story*. London: British Association for Adoption and Fostering.

Yin, Robert K. (1993) *Applications of Case Study Research*. Newbury Park: Sage.

Websites

'Definitions of Anthropological Terms' http://oregonstate.edu/instruct/anth370/ gloss. html [accessed January 4, 2012].

Attachment Parenting International: www.attachmentparenting.org.

14 Power struggles

The paradoxes of emotion and control among child-centered mothers in privileged America

Diane M. Hoffman[1]

Over the last fifty years a powerful global convergence of ideas and practices regarding childrearing and parenting has emerged. This consensus, supported by a vast array of childrearing media and informed by expert advice, highlights the desirability of child-centered forms of parenting, in which parents focus on the developmental needs of the child, respect the child as an individual, and provide children with ample opportunities to exercise choice in order to develop a sense of individual agency (Bloch *et al.* 2003; Popkewitz 2000, 2003; Rose 1989; Canella 1997). In the United States, especially, such child-centered ideals and practices are widely valued, and have effectively come to constitute a key trend in the ways American parents raise their children (Penn with Zalesne 2007).

At the same time, however, definitions, perceptions, and potential outcomes of "child-centeredness" are topics of intense debate across the popular landscape of American parenting. What can be asserted, at the minimum, is that there are important social class-based differences in the extent to which parents adopt a child-centered approach (Kusserow 2004; Lareau 2003; Tobin 1995). As these authors illustrate, different perspectives on adult–child relationships are tied into diverging notions of individualism as well as cultural capital and social stratification. Adults of different social classes relate to their children with expectations shaped both by present circumstances and by future, envisioned adult roles in society. In this process, both children and adults are shaped by larger cultural and class-based goals for personhood and identity.

In this article, I deepen this argument by probing the ways in which privileged mothers confront issues surrounding parent–child relationships by focusing on a key notion in the landscape of contemporary American parenting: the parent–child power struggle. I explore how mothers' articulation of the "power struggle" encodes important insights concerning culturally situated notions of power, selfhood, and emotional control. Though they consciously reject what they identify as "mainstream" parenting ideas and practices, the mothers I interviewed hold cultural models concerning the relationship of emotion, power, and the development of self that are in fact widely shared in the mainstream parenting advice discourse. Further, as mothers articulate their views, it becomes clear that the power struggle is not just about the formation of child selves, but also about the identities of mothers themselves within contested fields of mothering.

Parental ethno-theory in communities of practice

Anthropologists have a well-developed literature on parental ethno-theories of childrearing and child development (Goodnow and Collins 1990; Harkness and Super 1996; LeVine *et al.* 1994). These ethno-theories are characterized by commonly held and largely implicit beliefs, values, and practices, influenced by local socio-moral ecologies and resources that parents use to raise their children. Yet some of these discourses are broadly distributed across communities of practice, often extending beyond those groups in which parents situate themselves. For Americans in particular, as Quinn notes, despite an emphasis on diversity in specific choices and strategies of childrearing, "the most fundamental tenets of the shared cultural model for raising a child to be a valued adult" are widely shared and often unquestioned. (2005: 488)

For the present study, I interviewed ten mothers, all of whom were residing in an upper-middle class mid-Atlantic community in close proximity to a major university. Semi-structured interviews took approximately one and a half hours, and were conducted in participants' homes (often with children playing nearby), or in public locations such as coffee shops. The participants were recruited using an online notice on a local parenting network about a study on mothers' views regarding child behavior and discipline.

All were white, currently married, and had least one child ranging in age from one to seven years old. All had college degrees and seven had professional work experience, either being currently employed in a professional capacity (one was a lawyer and another was a professor), or in the past (three had been private school teachers [including one former Montessori school teacher]; two others had worked in the business field). They thus represented an economically and educationally privileged group.

When asked during the interview about whether they had heard the term power struggle, all the mothers readily admitted familiarity with it and could provide examples from their own experience.

> INTERVIEWER: Would you say that you have power struggles with your child?

> Yes, for example we have a lot of power struggles over clothes. He [son] refuses to wear a collared shirt on Sundays. So if a conflict arises, I get him to tell me how he feels about it. And I can give him some choices.
> (GC, November 10, 2007)

> Yes, a lot of the tantrums are about power struggles. She might have a tantrum over eating a bowl of cereal, or when I try to put bib on her. When I put her diapers on she takes them off. Just about everything can be a power struggle.... She just wants to make choices.... But then I sometimes ask, who's making the choices here, me or her? Sometimes I have to bribe her...
> (CS, December 14, 2007)

Power struggles? Oh yes, definitely. She wants to exert her independence and control. She knows it is something we want and she knows she can control the situation. ... The more I push [potty training] the more she resists. I think of them like who has control in a situation.

(JC, December 8, 2007)

One mother who said her child could not "sit still long enough to eat a meal" and had trouble getting dressed in the morning offered her reasoning for this behavior: "Kids [his age] just want to control the environment" (GK, November 8, 2007). Another said, in reference to her son's food aversions, "It's totally a power thing" (BG, December 13, 2007). Mothers considered the power struggle as a natural event in parenting, taking it as evidence of the child's developing need to assert independence or control over the situation or environment.

The power struggle in the mainstream: parenting advice literature

In this sense, they participated in a discourse on selves and power influenced by the dominant frames of child development research and psychology in the U.S. – a discourse that has greatly shaped the contours of parenting advice in contemporary America (Apple 2006; Grant 1998; Hulbert 2003; Hardyment 1995). In this discourse the power struggle is understood as a common (though emotionally trying) event for American parents that is linked to developmental needs of the child's emerging sense of self. Power struggles happen whenever a child resists, over a (variable) period of time, a parent's efforts to get the child to comply with a rule, request or desire.

This need to exert control or experience one's personal power is naturalized as a developmental imperative linked to the emergence of an autonomous, independent self:

The power struggle is an inherent part of growing up. ... This is because as kids go through their developmental stages, they need to challenge their parents appropriately in order to get more autonomy.

(Lehman, 2011)

A preschooler's desire to dictate his outfits isn't only about creating a certain look. He's beginning to want more control over his environment.

(Skolnick 2005: 183)

Resisting a parent is a toddler's way of establishing autonomy. For the first time in his short life, he's his own little person. He's carving out an identity for himself.

(Banin 2005: 93)

Moreover, in the U.S. ethno-discourse, power and control are constructs of choice for explaining children's behavior across a wide range of situations, not only those characterized as power struggles. For example, the popular parenting magazine *Parents* brings in the idea of the child's need for control in a variety of situations:

> Q: I just got remarried, and my 5 year old is suddenly really possessive of all of his toys. What can I do?
> A: Find little ways to give him control, like letting him decide on snacks or a family activity.
>
> (Lee 2006: 38)

> Kids love to play make-believe because they're in control.
>
> (Garisto 2006: 192)

> Why do loveys have such magical powers? Quite simply, they help children control their emotions.
>
> (Miller 2006: 234)

The child's assumed need to assert control is a dominant explanatory framework for children's behavior in a wide variety of situations. Yet this privileging of control and power obscures the possibility of other equally plausible interpretations. For example, why can't playing make-believe be an occasion for genuine flights of imagination, rather than a chance to "be in control"? Why can't "the magical power of loveys" be about desires to be cared for and to show caring, rather than simply about control over emotions? Why is possessiveness in the case of divorce just about control, rather than genuine fear of loss? The emphasis on the theme of control precludes alternative explanations that might capture, for example, the richness of children's aesthetic sensibilities, imaginations, or the full range of their emotional engagement with the world. In this sense, adult narratives over power and control, though ostensibly "child-centered," may be anything but, as they obscure the richness and authenticity of children's own subjectivities and desires.

The power struggle as cultural trope: comparative perspectives

There is something in the transformation of the ordinary events of parent–child interaction into occasions for struggle and contest over power that is culturally very interesting. Why are these events glossed as "power struggles" but not "attention struggles" or "dependency struggles"? Indeed, why should parents "struggle" with their children in the first place? In comparing contemporary Chinese parenting discourses with American ones (Hoffman and Zhao 2008), we found that the overwhelming emphasis in the U.S. discourse on issues of power and control was absent in the Chinese case, where there was much more emphasis on mothers being "in harmony" with the child. Similar observations have been made in other comparative studies of Chinese and American parenting (e.g. Chao 1994, 1995) where researchers have found Chinese approaches to childrearing stress not power or control but strategies of training or "guidance" based on emotional warmth and close parent–child self-identification.

More evidence for the cultural particularity of the power struggle comes from exploration of Japanese childrearing. Hess and Azuma (1991) and Machida (1996) consider that the very concept of "parental control strategies" is based on Western assumptions: "As a construct, parental control strategies fit well within a unidirectional model of parenting wherein, as scholars have presumed until recently, mothers control children" (Machida 1996: 250). As Chen (1996: 125) notes, a mainstream Japanese approach emphasizes the quality of inter-subjective feelings of the mother–child dyad by creating an atmosphere in which the child will feel little psychological discrepancy or discontinuity. There is little discussion of power or control, but much emphasis on fostering a sense of empathic identification.

Moreover, even when there is an emphasis on growth of autonomy and/or independence, there is little in the cross-cultural literature to suggest that power or the adult–child power struggle is universally a dominant feature of a developing a socially competent self. Some cultures that are the most ostensibly "collective" or anti-individualist in orientation and where the maintenance of high levels of social conformity and cooperation are important also socialize for extremely high levels of individual autonomy, as can be seen in descriptions of child socialization among certain Native and South American groups (Chisolm 1996; Lee 1987[1959]; Rival 1996). In the case of the Navaho, Chisolm writes,

> Signs of this huge and abiding respect for individual autonomy are everywhere.... Navahos abhor the idea or practice of controlling other beings in the course of everyday life. ... This enormous respect for individual autonomy is expressed nonverbally as well as verbally.
>
> (1996: 178–179)

These cross-cultural examples suggest that it is important to consider the principles that underlie cultural discourses about power and control, and to investigate how these governing ideas are related to cultural formations of the individual in relation to others.

Mothers in and against the mainstream

Mothers in this study claimed they made an effort to distance themselves from practices and philosophies that they considered "mainstream." Three defined themselves as part of the local "holistic" mothers network and half had children enrolled in Montessori schools or otherwise claimed to be influenced by Montessori philosophy. Others said they had no specific identity but that they were not "mainstream."

In an effort to probe what they considered to be "mainstream," I asked what sources of information they used in parenting their children. All except one denied that they regularly read "mainstream" parenting magazines (except perhaps while in the doctor's office). Two mothers, however, said they did read a magazine called *Brain, Child* (which bills itself as the "magazine for thinking mothers"), and most said they did read some parenting books. The most important source of information by far, though, was the internet. They all said they consulted parenting sites on the internet (including mom blogs and sites devoted to Montessori and Holistic mothering, and a variety of *Yahoo* groups ["if there's any niche in parenting there's a group on *Yahoo*," according to one*)*, as well as getting parenting information from friends and from the schools their children attended, either through newsletters, individual consultations with teachers, or through parent education seminars.

What emerged from my interviews was a very critical perspective on what mothers considered to be "mainstream" parenting. When pushed to define "mainstream" further, one mom said, "A mainstream mom ... has a crib. She has babysitters more. We don't go out a lot or if we do we take her [two-year-old daughter] with us" [JC, November 10, 2007]. When asked what was a mainstream mom, another mother said: "Mainstream moms are commercial ... and they are more harsh than I'd like to be. It's top-down, less respectful of the child. There's a lot of 'nos' without explaining why" [GK, November 8, 2007]. For another mom, "Mainstream is what the doctors recommend" [LD, November 20, 2007]. Other moms identified the discipline technique of giving children "time outs" for misbehavior as mainstream:

> We don't call it "time outs." We give warnings, with consequences. Time outs are so trendy. Everybody uses time-outs except some of the people I hang with.
>
> (SB, October 29, 2007)

> [Parenting magazines] are very focused on mainstream things. I only read them in the doctor's office, but [generally] I don't subscribe to that philosophy. I like a little less of a mainstream, more alternative style. Like time-outs.... I don't want to use time-outs. It's more like a punishment to me, like I wouldn't be teaching anything.... I prefer the Montessori philosophy because it's more child-based ... kids are given a choice to be independent. ... Mainstream ignores the emotions....
>
> (CS, December 14, 2007)

The common thread in their views of "mainstream" parenting, beyond the presence or lack of certain discipline strategies such as time-outs, however, was that it reflected what mothers felt was a lack of attention to the individual child and his or her needs and emotions. For these mothers, in sum, it appeared to be insufficiently child-centered.

Handling power struggles I: controlling emotions

While denying that they were mainstream, however, mothers participated in a very prominent discourse, widely available through parenting advice sources in print and online, about power struggles and especially about the link between power struggles and the emotions. In the popular parenting literature, the power struggle is metaphorically an "emotional battle" where "no one wins and no one surrenders" (Osherson 2007). In the advice literature on power struggles, parents are often explicitly encouraged to "teach kids how to handle their emotions" by labeling emotions for their kids or using words to describe their children's feelings. Parents are told, "Your child can't really understand her feelings of anger or frustration at this age. But it's still a good idea to label these emotions for her. Try saying, "You must be so mad that Sam took that yellow bus," or, "I'll bet you're angry that Mommy won't let you climb onto the coffee table" (Schipani 2006: 194).

Mothers in this study also believed they should help their children verbalize emotions, because children don't yet have the ability to do so. These ideas are captured in the ways mothers responded to questions regarding the handing of emotions in relations with their children:

INTERVIEWER: How do you deal with your child's strong emotions?

Part of [the way I handle my daughter's emotions] comes from my Montessori training. In my approach we spend a lot of time on giving kids words to talk about emotions. In Montessori they have the Peace Table. If you have a conflict you go to the Peace Table.... [Daughter, age two] doesn't really have the knowledge or vocabulary to explain what she's feeling, so ... I talk with her. I acknowledge her feelings, give her the words, try to get her to express her emotions.

(CS, December 14, 2007)

They did this thing on emotion at school. You should try to talk about [emotions with your child]. If they are sad, for example. They had pictures up at school. We've just started to do this [at home] too. We got the idea from the school. [Before then] we hadn't really thought about it very much.

(BG, December 13, 2007)

Something I picked up from Montessori was helping kids with emotions ... instead of saying 'quit hitting your sister' you should say "hitting your sister might make her feel bad."

(GK, November 8, 2007)

One mother, ES, explained how she had created a "peace wand" based on the Montessori School's "Peace Rose." As I was interviewing her in her living room, her son was playing nearby with two other neighbor children. At one point he got into a scuffle with one of the other children. ES said, "You need to use your words. Do you want to try the peace wand?" The boy defiantly said, "No!" ES said, to me, "He doesn't know how to use the peace wand...." For about twenty minutes following, while the interview was ongoing, the mom continuously interrupted our conversation to try to get the children to use the "peace wand" but to no avail. Ironically, the mother interpreted her son's behavior as a case of *not knowing how to use the peace wand* rather than as a refusal – an act of resistance or power on the part of the child.

In the end interviews revealed that mothers adopted the same strategies to respond to their children's emotions that are advocated in the mainstream advice literature that the moms claim they rejected (see Hoffman 2009). This literature, predicated on a deficiency view of the child's emotional capacities, requires parents to need to step in and verbalize for the child what he or she cannot express. It was common for a mother to say, as CS does, "She really doesn't have the knowledge or vocabulary yet to explain what she's feeling" (December 14, 2007). Verbalization, combined with other "calming" strategies, narrates the child's emotions in ways that effectively channel and constrain along adult-sanctioned lines.

Frank Furedi (2008) makes a similar point, observing that the contemporary "therapeutic culture" of parenting is deeply ambivalent about emotions, for as it extols the value of emotional expression, it demands that emotions be kept under strict control. Similarly, Tobin (1995) also writes about the extent to which contemporary middle-class approaches to early education promote a kind of psychologized narrativity that stresses the substitution of techniques of verbal expression for other expressions of child-centered emotionality.

Handling power struggles II: choices

Another prominent strategy mothers recommended to defuse power struggles was to use "choices." As one said, "We use language with them that will give choices" (SB, October 29, 2007). Another said, "You just give the child a choice: Do you want to go upstairs by yourself or do you want me to bring you upstairs?" (CL, October 18, 2007).

Another mom, whose son was now out of toddlerhood, said that now she has fewer power struggles because "I got creative at offering alternatives and choices" (GC, November 10, 2007).

Using "choice" strategies to defuse a power struggle is also a prominent theme in the mainstream parenting advice literature. For example:

> For example, instead of a back and forth battle to get your child to go to bed, the situation may be defused before it starts by offering choices to the child: "Would you like to walk to bed or be carried?" ... Offering realistic, positive, and broad choices ... demonstrates to your child that they do have power in the world.
>
> (Landes 2007)

Give your child choices. ... Let them make as many choices as they can that will give them control over what happens to them. For instance, "Do you want to take your bath before I read you a story or after?"

(Kvols 2006)

Though Montessori education represents for these mothers an alternative to the mainstream, the Montessori approach too emphasizes a similar psychology of individualized choice and the need to grant children ways to feel powerful:

Give your child choices. We all like to feel powerful and influential and our children are no different. Let them make as many choices as they can that will give them control over what happens to them.

(Lighthouse Academy 2009)

While giving children choices seems to be aligned with the goal of allowing the child to exert power over the environment, effectively, there really is no choice for the child who doesn't want to go to bed at all – it's either walk or be carried. In the power struggle discourse, the adult represents the situation *as if* it were a real choice to the child, and in so doing grants the child "power," but only deceptively, since the choices presented to children are predetermined by the adult and non-consequential for the adult's ultimate goals in the situation. In no case is a child offered a truly consequential choice that would compromise parental aims. The child is thus manipulated into fulfilling adult desires, while being granted the illusion of autonomy.

Power struggles in the community: mothers, difference, and identity

Though mothers in my study defined themselves in opposition to the mainstream, analysis of their discourse on power struggles revealed that they shared many of the ideas related to power and emotion that are characteristic of the mainstream advice literature. They shared the notion that it is important to get children to label and talk about their emotions, and that giving children "power" to make choices is one way to manage adult–child conflicts.

This still leaves open the question to what extent mothers' views are shaped by their particular class position. As Kusserow (2004) shows, the construct of individualism has different versions that vary by class. In the "soft individualism" of the upper-middle class, while parents and teachers ostensibly value the child's feelings, they carefully manage and intervene in children's emotional expression, even to the extent of denying what the child is attempting to express:

Great importance is placed on letting the child express her true and natural feelings, and yet only certain feelings are allowed to be expressed. ... Sometimes a child was not allowed to say, "I wanted to hurt Jimmy," without the teacher saying, "No, let's think about this. That's not really what you meant. What do you feel? Do you feel *sad* that Jimmy took your blocks?"

(2004: 165, emphasis in original)

In this process, emotions are paradoxically more governed than they appear to be, as parents and teachers decide for the child what they are feeling and co-narrate the "right" feelings.

It may be that what mothers are identifying with in my study is very much a class-based, privileged self of the upper-middle class. This is the self that implicitly informs the ostensibly scientific expertise of the child development establishment, itself already intrinsically linked to and defined by education and social privilege. When mothers talk about managing power struggles by narrating emotions and proving opportunities for children to "feel powerful" via choice, they not only identify with an expert-guided "child-centered" view of parenting, but with a model of self defined through the lenses of control and power. The irony is that this "child-centered" self is always narrated and constructed by adults, and thus always exists in tension with, and potentially undermines, what may be children's own visions and experiences of the world.

When we came to the end of our interviews, and I asked about how mothers saw their community, a profound discomfort and critique inevitably emerged that centered on the competitive atmosphere of mothering:

INTERVIEWER: What do you feel are the significant issues in your community with regard to childrearing that you personally are concerned with?

There is a whole lot of judging going on. Other mothers are the most judgmental. There is a lot of pressure to do it right. You think you're right but then people will criticize you for anything.... There's an element of extreme mothering now.

(ES, November 8, 2007)

There are lots of ego moms. They take it to the CEO level, over the top, doing all this research. Very little laissez-faire parenting.... It's like cults, sometimes you run into these types.... I just can't deal...

(GK, November 8, 2007)

You need to find your tribe. I was part of a mom group in every city I've lived. Every city or place is different. In Missouri the mom groups tend to be religious. In Portland, it was like Holistic moms on crack: Oh my gosh! You eat meat!!!???

(BR, December 5, 2007)

I never realized how competitive it is ... you just get these looks from some moms. It's kind of surprising how competitive it is.

(CS, December 14, 2007)

It's really hard to be a mom nowadays. There's a hierarchy of moms here – a tyranny ... I've heard moms say they won't send their kids to a daycare because it has plastic toys. ... No mom wants to admit their kid watches TV. I sometimes feel it's a little bit like junior high school all over again...

(BG, December 13, 2007)

These accounts point to a deep tension that is centered on mothers' identities as parents. Here are moms who struggle to enact their vision of what is best for children, yet who find themselves in a pitched battle with other mothers over the best way to parent. What is so ironic is that in the end the "power struggles" are not just between adults and kids, but between parents themselves, as they struggle to carve out identities in a contested field of parenting. While the children are certainly the ostensible focus of their efforts, the mothers are waging their own battles over who they are, identities that are defined by the choices they make in the ways they raise their kids. Moms who don't send their kids to daycares with plastic toys are making as much a statement about themselves and how they want to be perceived as what they feel is best for their children. Parenting is, in this sense, a very public activity, with public consequences, in ways that mothers found surprising and disconcerting.

This suggests that the avoidance of identification with the "mainstream" can be read in two slightly different ways. In one sense it can be seen as an identity-choice that mothers make to define themselves as more educated, more aware, more sensitive to the needs of the child – somehow "better than" moms who have cribs and get babysitters. In this way, it represents a form of self-affirmation as "child-centered" that draws upon class-based ideals of privilege.

In a second sense, it reflects a need to define the self as individual, as unlike all other selves. This rationale is linked to an ideology of individual differences that exerts a powerful influence in America over the ways individuals see themselves in relation to others. Although none of the mothers used the word "unique" to describe themselves or their philosophy, some did convey a similar idea by talking about difference: how they (and their children) could not fit into a single type or a one-size-fits-all approach.

One mother who said she often goes online for parenting advice (and who identifies as a Montessori mother), also said that her "philosophy is different from my friends', it doesn't really mesh with theirs" (CS, December 14, 2007). Another said that while her approach was informed by Montessori, and that she has a few close friends who generally share her views, all the same she is "probably different from others" (SB, October 29, 2007). Her children, too, were seen as "different" from each other: "every kid is so different" (SB). As another said, "Different parenting books work with different children. Kids are just too different" (GK, November 8 2007). Believing that one and one's children are "different," perhaps, is a way both to distinguish oneself from the mainstream and to assert one's sensitivity to the unique needs and qualities of the individual child – in other words, to be "child centered."

But in this emphasis on their difference, as a number of studies have shown, these mothers are again quite mainstream. American parents on the whole tend to misperceive themselves, considering themselves more different from others than they actually are (Penn and Zalesne 2007; Quinn 2005; Weisner 1999). In fact, belief in one's difference enables a certain kind of blindness, allowing mothers not to recognize how similar they really are to the mainstream that they so vehemently criticize. Difference thus becomes a way to position oneself, but not to see oneself.

An emphasis on differences can also be seen a way to rationalize the difficulties that mothers perceived with putting the "child-centered" ideal into practice with their own children. In fact, enacting emotional control strategies and giving choices – considered 'the best' ways to deal with power struggles – did not always work smoothly in practice. Mothers themselves readily admitted frustrations and difficulties. Even as they described how they used choices or emotional talk, mothers said that it doesn't always work; e.g., "B[son] challenges all the things I thought were the right way to teach ... We are supposed to give choices, but, with him he has to have more routine, more structure. ... He needs more traditional techniques" (GK, November 8, 2007).

I also witnessed these difficulties, during the event with the peace wand, as well as on other occasions during our interviews, as mothers would sometimes stop our discussions in order to engage in lengthy negotiations with their children over behavior. For example, on one occasion while I interviewed two mothers together while their children played, each stepped away from our conversation for almost twenty minutes to engage in a serious negotiation with her child over behavior. Certainly, for these mothers, it was not easy to be "child-centered." The irony is that the methods that supposedly empowered children and validated them – talking about emotions, giving a child a choice – were still methods of control, and children seemed to know this. They could – and did – resist them, to parents' great discomfort. So in the end, the only the power that was fully legitimated was the power adults chose to "give" to children through emotional narration and choice, while children's authentic forms of power/resistance remained invalidated.

Conclusion: paradoxes of power and emotion in raising selves for society

The ubiquity of the power struggle as trope of choice for framing parent–child relations in contemporary America allows or even encourages a masking of the questions of autonomy, relatedness, and belonging that lie at the heart of producing selves in society. In the sense that it deflects attention to the questions of management, rationality, and the techniques of control, it permits disengagement with the ways in which emotion and power remain embodied, subjective, lived, and unavoidably present in everyday lives, both in families and in the wider society. It is a discourse about power, but it is a reductive and deceptive one: reductive, in that power constrains the view of the child's self, limiting it and providing an all-inclusive explanation for the child's being; and deceptive, in that the kind of power that ultimately is practiced is not that of genuine autonomy but the false exercise of manipulated choice. That such a conflict leads to practices that could be called emotionally deceptive – and that the greater lessons of emotional control may be those of emotional manipulation and deception – are surely not the ideals that the culture itself desires to teach.

From my vantage point, the discourse on power struggles in parenting, far from providing a solution to the problems of parent–child relations, re-inscribes mothers and children in unresolved cultural tensions over the power of the emotions to undermine relationships, and uncertainty over how to harness them for social good. As Jules Henry pointed out in his critique of American education many years ago, much of the incompetence in education is often due to fear and a sense of persistent vulnerability (1966). For the mothers in my study, who felt vulnerable to the criticisms of others in their efforts to carve identities for themselves as "good" mothers, struggles were not only with their children, but with the larger community, and even, one might speculate, with the larger culture and its pressures to get the job of childrearing "right."

Ultimately, though subscribing to the ideals of child-centrism, mothers chose the mainstream strategies of parenting that risked undermining its achievement. They did so because these strategies are deeply tied into unspoken and unexamined assumptions about the kinds of selves society ought to produce. In so doing they reproduced their own and their children's vulnerability, since they can never quite attain the ideals they set for themselves and for their children. For privileged mothers at least – those whom one would least expect to have problems with power – anxieties and fears about how to deal with emotions in the contested spaces of ordinary family life pose enduring difficulties to the fundamental tasks of raising selves for "success" in contemporary times.

Note

1 This article is developed from a prior publication in *Ethos, The Journal of the Society of Psychological Anthropology*, 41(1): 75–97.

References

Apple, R. D. (2006) *Perfect Motherhood: Science and Childrearing in America*, New Brunswick, NJ: Rutgers University Press.

Banin, J. S. (2005) What Makes a Toddler Tick, *Parenting*, June: 92–96.

Bloch, M., Holmlund, K., Moquist, I. and Popkewitz, T. (eds) (2003) *Governing Children, Families, and Education: Restructuring the Welfare State*, New York: Palgrave Macmillan.

Canella, G. (1997) *Deconstructing Early Childhood Education: Social Justice and Revolution*, New York: Peter Lang.

Chao, R. K. (1994) Beyond Parental Control and Authoritarian Parenting Style: Understanding Chinese Parenting Through the Cultural Notion of Training, *Child Development*, 65(4): 1111–1119.

Chao, R. K. (1995) Chinese and European–American Cultural Models of the Self Reflected in Mothers' Child-Rearing Beliefs, *Ethos*, 23(3): 328–354.

Chen, S. J. (1996) Positive Childishness: Images of childhood in Japan, in C. P. Hwang, M. E. Lamb, and I. E. Sigel (eds.) *Images of Childhood*, Mahwah, NJ: Lawrence Erlbaum.

Chisolm, J. S. (1996) Learning Respect for Everything: Navaho Images of Development, in C. P. Hwang, M. E. Lamb, and I. E. Sigel (eds.) *Images of Childhood*, Mahwah, NJ: Lawrence Erlbaum.

Family IQ (2007) Defusing Power Struggles with Children, online, available at: http://ebookbrowse.com/defusing-power-struggles-with-children-pdf-d351302175 [accessed November 26, 2012].

Furedi, F. (2008) *Paranoid Parenting: Why Ignoring the Experts may be Best for your Child*, Chicago, IL: Chicago Review Press.

Garisto, L. P. (2006) Imagine That! Let your Child Get Lost in Play, *Parents*, September: 192.

Goodnow, J. J. and Collins, W. A. (1994) *Development According to Parents: The Nature, Sources, and Consequences of Parent's Ideas*. Mahwah, NJ: Lawrence Erlbaum.

Grant, J. (1998) *Raising Baby by the Book: The Education of American Mothers*, New Haven, CT: Yale University Press.

Hardyment, C. (1995) *Perfect Parents: Baby-care Advice, Past and Present*, Oxford: Oxford University Press.

Harkness, S. and Super, C. (1996) *Parents' Cultural Belief Systems: Their Origins, Expressions, and Consequences*, New York: Guilford Press.

Hess, R, and Azuma, H. (1991) Cultural Support for Schooling: Contrasts Between Japan and the US, *Educational Researcher*, 20(9): 2–8.

Henry, J. (1966) Vulnerability in education, *Jules Henry on Education*, New York: Random House.

Hoffman, D. M. (2009) How (Not) to Feel: Culture and the Politics of Emotion in the American Parenting Advice Literature, *Discourse: Studies in the Cultural Politics of Education*, 30(1): 15–31.

Hoffman, D. M. and Zhao, G. (2008) Global Convergence and Divergence in Childhood Ideologies and the Marginalization of Children, in J. Zajda, K. Biraimah, and W. Gaudelli (eds.). *Education and Social Inequality in the Global Culture*, Dordrecht: Springer, pp. 1–16.

Hulbert, A. (2003) *Raising America: Experts, Parents, and a Century of Advice about Children*, New York: A. A. Knopf.

Kusserow, A. (2004) *American Individualisms: Child rearing and Social Class in Three Neighborhoods*, New York: Palgrave Macmillan.

Kvols, K. (2006) Avoiding Power Struggles with Children, online, available at: www.montessori.org/index.php?option=com_content&view=article&id=270:avoiding-power-struggles-with-children&catid=27:articles-on-parenting-the-montessori-way&Itemid=42 [accessed March 7, 2012].

Lareau, A. (2003) *Unequal Childhoods: Class, Race, and Family Life*. Berkeley, CA: University of California Press.

Lee, D. (1987[1959]) *Individual Autonomy and Social Structure: Freedom and Culture*. Long Grove, IL: Waveland.

Lee, S. (2006) Behavior Q & A, *Parents*, October: 38.

Lehman, J. (2011) Power Struggles Part I: Are You at war with a Defiant Child? Online, available at: www.empoweringparents.com/Power-Struggles-with-a-Defiant-Child.php# [accessed February 28, 2011].

LeVine, R., Dixson, S., LeVine, S., Richman, A., Liederman, P. H., and Keefer, C. H.

(1994) *Child Care and Culture: Lessons from Africa.* Cambridge: Cambridge University Press.

Lighthouse Academy (2009) Avoiding Power Struggles With Children, online, available at: www.kidslaf.com/2009/11/avoiding-power [accessed February 29, 2012].

Machida, S. (1996) Maternal and Cultural Socialization for Schooling: Lessons Learned and Prospects Ahead, in D. W. Shwalb and B. J. Shwalb (eds.) *Japanese Childrearing: Two Generations of Scholarship*, New York: The Guilford Press.

Miller, C. S. (2006) Life with Lovey, *Parents*, online, available at: www.parents.com/toddlers-preschoolers/development/behavioral/lovey [accessed June 15, 2012].

Osherson, S. (2007) Dissolving Power Struggles. online, available at: www.innerself.com/Parenting/dissolving_power.htm [accessed June 12, 2012].

Penn, M. J. with Zalesne, E. K. (2007) *Microtrends: The Small Forces Behind Tomorrow's Big Changes*, New York: Twelve Publishing.

Popkewitz, T. S. (2000) Globalization/Regionalization, Knowledge, and Educational Practices: Some Notes on Comparative Strategies for Educational Research, in Thomas Popkewitz (ed.) *Educational Knowledge: Changing Relationships Between the State, Civil Society, and the Educational Community*, Albany, NY: State University of New York Press.

Popkewitz, T. S. (2003) Governing the Child and Pedagogicalization of the Parent, in M. N. Bloch, K. Holmlund, I. Moqvist, and T. S. Popkewitz (eds.) *Governing Children, Families, End education: Restructuring the Welfare State*, New York: Palgrave Macmillan.

Quinn, N. (2005) Universals of Childrearing, *Anthropological Theory*, 5(4): 477–516.

Rival, L. (1996) Formal Schooling and the Production of Modern Citizens in the Ecuadorian Amazon, in B. A. Levinson, D. E. Foley, and D. C. Holland (eds.) *The Cultural Production of the Educated Person: Critical Ethnographies of Schooling and Local Practice.* Albany: State University of New York Press.

Rose, N. (1989) *Governing the Soul: The Shaping of the Private Self*, New York: Free Association Books.

Schipani, D. (2006) Attack of the Toddler, *Parents*, October: 193–194.

Skolnick, D. (2005) Fashion Frenzy, *Parents*, July: 183–184.

Tobin, J. (1995) The irony of self-expression, *American Journal of Education*, 103(3): 233–258.

Weisner, T. (1999) Values that Matter, *Anthropology Newsletter*, 40(5): 1–4.

Afterword

Ellie Lee

Having attended a workshop to discuss draft chapters for this volume held in April 2012 at the University of Kent, it came as no surprise to find that the final versions comprise a fascinating collection. They demonstrate the benefits of interdisciplinary engagement, and of seeking to make insightful cross-cultural comparisons. These are both projects that are frequently upheld as aims of excellent scholarship, but are difficult to genuinely achieve in practice. This book has managed to do these things admirably.

Perhaps one reason why it has been possible to do this so well arises from the contributors taking the concept 'parenting culture' as their collective starting point. All of the contributing authors have taken the meaning of 'parenting' to be not self-evident. They have rather begun their investigations from the premise that 'parenting', as the editors put it, 'might be seen as a particular historically and socially situated form of childrearing', that is 'understood as both the source of, and solution to, a whole host of social problems'. This fresh way of thinking through the everyday experiences of family life, and the connections of this experience to the wider socio-cultural landscape, manifestly employs the sociological imagination; a way of thinking that works to uncover the relation between personal experience ('troubles') and the wider context ('issues') (Mills 1959: 8). But approaches and ideas from a variety of disciplines have been used to great effect to bring to life the overall insight that 'parenting' is not just another word for bringing up children.

In addition to the creative engagement with a common theme across disciplines they offer, the chapters here are also notable for the insights they give about parenting culture in different societies. In regards to the development of the study of parenting culture, this is perhaps the most notable achievement of this book. It has, for the first time to my knowledge, brought together in one place a comparative set of enquiries and this feature of this book means it makes a vital addition to a growing body of work that has up to know been more restricted in its scope. Through the work included here, we come to know far more about the evolution of trends most studied hitherto in North America, Australia and the United Kingdom.

Looking to future, it is what emerges from this cross-cultural look at parenting culture that perhaps poses the most questions for further research. Probably the most striking finding to come out of this collection is the commonalities in the construction of the 'problem of parenting' in different cultures. Other research has demonstrated some commonalities across the industrialised world. For example, research on infant feeding has drawn attention to the moralisation of breastfeeding in the US, Canada, UK, Australia and New Zealand (Liamputtong 2011). Studies have also alluded to the way rules about parenthood transfer, or diffuse, between these societies, for example, messages projected at pregnant women about eating, drinking and other aspects of lifestyle (Bell *et al.* 2009; Leppo 2012; Lowe and Lee 2010). Efforts have begun to emerge to encourage comparative analysis with European culture.[1]

Highlighted here, however, is the global spread of themes and preoccupations presumed to be characteristic of and originating in parenting culture in the Anglo-American context. This is most notable when it comes to 'infant determinism', that is the notion that what happens in the early years of life determines all later development (Bruer 1999; Kagan 1998). In particular, the articulation of infant determinism through claims about early brain development far outstripped what certainly I was expecting, in its global spread. Investigating and documenting how this claim (and others) has spread in this way constitutes and important future project for parenting culture studies. It is one that might make good use of the existing tradition of social constructionist sociology centring on analysis of the cross-cultural diffusion of social problems (Best 2001; McAdam and Rucht 1993).

The spread of infant determinism brings with it the globalisation of what has been termed 'parent causality'; the idea that there is a direct and inexorable relation between 'parenting' and 'outcomes' measured by how successful in various ways a child might be. This cultural construct of the parent has, as the editors indicate, been developed and discussed extensively by Hays (1996) and Furedi (2008) the latter of whom in particular also points to a central contradiction of this construct. The parent in contemporary culture is, explains Furedi, not simply represented as 'God-like' in their influence over the child, but as also simultaneously incompetent, given the intimate and inextricable linking of parent-causality with the idea that parents need to be trained and given expert advice in how to raise children. The associated subject position of the parent – as God-like but incompetent – lies at the heart of what Furedi terms an experience of 'paranoia'. Others detect this in the ubiquity of anxiety among parents, who feel like they are never 'good enough', and in what is now frequently pathologised as 'depression' among both mother and fathers (Lee 2010).

In engaging with this, this volume considers the question of resistance, seeking to explore the ways in which parents may respond to and perhaps react against what is clearly an unliveable demand (how can anyone sustain a coherent identity over decades as a god and a fool? Clearly, something has to give). In doing so, interesting observations are made, again, about how resistance works itself out in different cultures, but perhaps a key insight to emerge is the way responses to the demands of parenting culture remain confined to and work within its premises. An interesting feature of our times is, indeed, the multiplication of apparently 'resistant' forms of parenting; the 'slacker mum', 'serenity parenting', 'benign neglect', or most recently the 'sh*tty mum'. Yet the question this poses is how far do efforts to develop these alternative forms of parenting style comprise more an alternative version of intensive parenting rather than an overthrowing of it, demanding in their own way that parents perform identity work, maybe of an especially self-conscious kind? This too is a important area for the future of parenting culture studies, opening up new possibilities for innovative research.

The importance of this volume and the research questions it engages with and develops is, finally, not simply intellectual. As this collection quite clearly shows, parenting culture in its current form generates significant personal troubles and anxieties that diminish the most human of human experiences – namely raising the next generation. Those who have written for this book for this reason have made an important contribution to scholarship, but also play a role, that hopefully will continue, in encouraging public debate about how we might better proceed in making a link with tomorrow.

Note

1 For example, the conference 'Science, evidence, experts and the new parenting culture' held at the University of Kent in September 2011 included papers from scholars looking at Norway, Spain, Denmark, Belgium, Italy, as well as the US, Canada and the UK. See: http://blogs.kent.ac.uk/parentingculturestudies/pcs-events/previous-events/parenting-science/.

References

Best, J. (ed.) 2001. *How Claims Spread, The Cross-National Diffusion of Social Problems*. New York: Aldine de Gruyter.

Bell, K., McNaughton, D. and Salmon, A. 2009. 'Medicine, morality and mothering: public health discourses on foetal alcohol exposure, smoking around children and childhood overnutrition'. *Critical Public Health* (special issue) 19(2): 155–170.

Bruer, J. 1999. *Myth of the First Three Years: A New Understanding of Early Brain Development and Lifelong Learning*. New York: The Free Press.

Furedi, F. 2008. *Paranoid Parenting*. London: Continuum.

Hays, S. 1996. *The Cultural Contradictions of Motherhood*. New Haven, CT/London: Yale University Press.

Kagan, J. 1998. *Three Seductive Ideas*. Cambridge, MA: Harvard University Press.

Lee, E. 2010. 'Pathologising fatherhood: the case of male Post Natal Depression in Britain'. In S. Robertson and B. Gough (eds) *Men, Masculinities and Health: Critical Perspectives*. Basingstoke: Palgrave.

Leppo, A. 2012. 'The emergence of the foetus: discourses on foetal alcohol syndrome prevention and compulsory treatment in Finland'. *Critical Public Health*, 22(2): 179–191.

Liamputtong, P. (ed.) 2011. *Infant Feeding Practices: A Cross-Cultural Perspective*. New York: Springer.

Lowe, P. and Lee. E. 2010. 'Under the influence? The construction of foetal alcohol syndrome in UK newspapers'. *Sociological Research Online*, 15(4)2, online, available at: www.socresonline.org.uk/15/4/2.html.

McAdam, D. and Rucht, D. 1993. 'The cross-national diffusion of movement ideas'. *Annals of the American Academy of Political and Social Science*, 528(1): 56–74.

Mills, C.W. 1959. *The Sociological Imagination*. London: Oxford University Press.

Index

Page numbers in *italics* denote tables. Please note that page numbers relating to notes will be denoted by the letter 'n' and note number following the note.

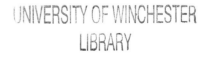